Clinical Management of Patients with Heart Failure

Clinical Management of Patients with Heart Failure

Guest Editors
Cristina Tudoran
Larisa Anghel

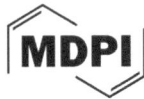

Basel • Beijing • Wuhan • Barcelona • Belgrade • Novi Sad • Cluj • Manchester

Guest Editors

Cristina Tudoran
Department VII. Internal
Medicine II. Discipline
of Cardiology
University of Medicine and
Pharmacy "Victor Babes"
Timisoara
Romania

Larisa Anghel
Internal Medicine
Department
University of Medicine
and Pharmacy
Iași
Romania

Editorial Office
MDPI AG
Grosspeteranlage 5
4052 Basel, Switzerland

This is a reprint of the Special Issue, published open access by the journal *Journal of Clinical Medicine* (ISSN 2077-0383), freely accessible at: https://www.mdpi.com/journal/jcm/special_issues/91TCP5E3S2.

For citation purposes, cite each article independently as indicated on the article page online and as indicated below:

Lastname, A.A.; Lastname, B.B. Article Title. *Journal Name* **Year**, *Volume Number*, Page Range.

ISBN 978-3-7258-3301-6 (Hbk)
ISBN 978-3-7258-3302-3 (PDF)
https://doi.org/10.3390/books978-3-7258-3302-3

© 2025 by the authors. Articles in this book are Open Access and distributed under the Creative Commons Attribution (CC BY) license. The book as a whole is distributed by MDPI under the terms and conditions of the Creative Commons Attribution-NonCommercial-NoDerivs (CC BY-NC-ND) license (https://creativecommons.org/licenses/by-nc-nd/4.0/).

Contents

About the Editors vii

Preface ix

Ana-Maria Vrabie, Stefan Totolici, Caterina Delcea and Elisabeta Badila
Biomarkers in Heart Failure with Preserved Ejection Fraction: A Perpetually Evolving Frontier
Reprinted from: *J. Clin. Med.* **2024**, *13*, 4627, https://doi.org/10.3390/jcm13164627 1

**Andrea D'Amato, Paolo Severino, Silvia Prosperi, Marco Valerio Mariani,
Rosanna Germanò, Andrea De Prisco, et al.**
The Role of High-Sensitivity Troponin T Regarding Prognosis and Cardiovascular Outcome
across Heart Failure Spectrum
Reprinted from: *J. Clin. Med.* **2024**, *13*, 3533, https://doi.org/10.3390/jcm13123533 27

**Emilia-Violeta Goanta, Cristina Vacarescu, Georgica Tartea, Adrian Ungureanu, Sebastian
Militaru, Alexandra Muraretu, et al.**
Unexpected Genetic Twists in Patients with Cardiac Devices
Reprinted from: *J. Clin. Med.* **2024**, *13*, 3801, https://doi.org/10.3390/jcm13133801 42

**Alexandra-Iulia Lazăr-Höcher, Dragoș Cozma, Liviu Cirin, Andreea Cozgarea,
Adelina-Andreea Faur-Grigori, Rafael Catană, et al.**
A Comparative Analysis of Apical Rocking and Septal Flash: Two Views of the Same Systole?
Reprinted from: *J. Clin. Med.* **2024**, *13*, 3109, https://doi.org/10.3390/jcm13113109 60

**Liviu Cirin, Simina Crișan, Constantin-Tudor Luca, Roxana Buzaș, Daniel Florin Lighezan,
Cristina Văcărescu, et al.**
Mitral Annular Plane Systolic Excursion (MAPSE): A Review of a Simple and Forgotten
Parameter for Assessing Left Ventricle Function
Reprinted from: *J. Clin. Med.* **2024**, *13*, 5265, https://doi.org/10.3390/jcm13175265 78

**Andreea Cozgarea, Dragoș Cozma, Minodora Teodoru, Alexandra-Iulia Lazăr-Höcher, Liviu
Cirin, Adelina-Andreea Faur-Grigori, et al.**
Heart Rate Recovery: Up to Date in Heart Failure—A Literature Review
Reprinted from: *J. Clin. Med.* **2024**, *13*, 3328, https://doi.org/10.3390/jcm13113328 89

**Larisa Anghel, Cristian Stătescu, Radu Andy Sascău, Bogdan-Sorin Tudurachi, Andreea
Tudurachi, Laura-Cătălina Benchea, et al.**
Impact of Newly Diagnosed Left Bundle Branch Block on Long-Term Outcomes in Patients with
STEMI
Reprinted from: *J. Clin. Med.* **2024**, *13*, 5479, https://doi.org/10.3390/jcm13185479 104

**Alina-Ramona Cozlac, Caius Glad Streian, Marciana Ionela Boca, Simina Crisan,
Mihai-Andrei Lazar, Mirela-Daniela Virtosu, et al.**
A Dual Challenge: *Coxiella burnetii* Endocarditis in a Patient with Familial Thoracic Aortic
Aneurysm—Case Report and Literature Review
Reprinted from: *J. Clin. Med.* **2024**, *13*, 7155, https://doi.org/10.3390/jcm13237155 119

Dragoș Lupu, Laurențiu Nedelcu and Diana Țînț
The Interplay between Severe Cirrhosis and Heart: A Focus on Diastolic Dysfunction
Reprinted from: *J. Clin. Med.* **2024**, *13*, 5442, https://doi.org/10.3390/jcm13185442 131

Jasmine K. Dugal, Arpinder S. Malhi, Noyan Ramazani, Brianna Yee, Michael V. DiCaro and KaChon Lei
Non-Pharmacological Therapy in Heart Failure and Management of Heart Failure in Special Populations—A Review
Reprinted from: *J. Clin. Med.* **2024**, *13*, 6993, https://doi.org/10.3390/jcm13226993 . . . . **144**

Catarina Silva Araújo, Irene Marco, María Alejandra Restrepo-Córdoba, Isidre Vila Costa, Julián Pérez-Villacastín and Josebe Goirigolzarri-Artaza
An Observational Study of Evidence-Based Therapies in Older Patients with Heart Failure with Reduced Ejection Fraction: Insights from a Dedicated Heart Failure Clinic
Reprinted from: *J. Clin. Med.* **2024**, *13*, 7171, https://doi.org/10.3390/jcm13237171 . . . . **164**

Luis Nieto Roca, Marcelino Cortés García, Jorge Balaguer Germán, Antonio José Bollas Becerra, José María Romero Otero, José Antonio Esteban Chapel, et al.
Use and Benefit of Sacubitril/Valsartan in Elderly Patients with Heart Failure with Reduced Ejection Fraction
Reprinted from: *J. Clin. Med.* **2024**, *13*, 4772, https://doi.org/10.3390/jcm13164772 . . . . **180**

Antoniu Octavian Petriş, Călin Pop and Diana Carmen Cimpoeşu
The Five Pillars of Acute Right Ventricular Heart Failure Therapy: Can We Keep the Pediment in Balance?
Reprinted from: *J. Clin. Med.* **2024**, *13*, 6949, https://doi.org/10.3390/jcm13226949 . . . . **192**

Josko Bulum, Marcelo B. Bastos, Ota Hlinomaz, Oren Malkin, Tomasz Pawlowski, Milan Dragula and Robert Gil
Pulsatile Left Ventricular Assistance in High-Risk Percutaneous Coronary Interventions: Short-Term Outcomes
Reprinted from: *J. Clin. Med.* **2024**, *13*, 5357, https://doi.org/10.3390/jcm13185357 . . . . **201**

Michele D'Alonzo, Amedeo Terzi, Massimo Baudo, Mauro Ronzoni, Nicola Uricchio, Claudio Muneretto and Lorenzo Di Bacco
Clinical Outcomes of Cardiac Transplantation in Heart Failure Patients with Previous Mechanical Cardiocirculatory Support
Reprinted from: *J. Clin. Med.* **2025**, *14*, 275, https://doi.org/10.3390/jcm14010275 . . . . **215**

Pupalan Iyngkaran, David Smith, Craig McLachlan, Malcolm Battersby, Maximilian de Courten and Fahad Hanna
Evaluating a New Short Self-Management Tool in Heart Failure Against the Traditional Flinders Program
Reprinted from: *J. Clin. Med.* **2024**, *13*, 6994, https://doi.org/10.3390/jcm13226994 . . . . **226**

About the Editors

Cristina Tudoran

Assistant professor, MD, PhD, Dr. Habil Cristina Tudoran is a senior physician in cardiology who works in the Cardiology Clinic of the County Emergency Hospital "Pius Brinzeu" Timisoara and at the University of Medicine and Pharmacy "Victor Babes" Timisoara. She completed her PhD thesis in 2013 with "magna cum laude" and, since then, has continued her research on cardiovascular alterations in patients with various pathologies. In 2020, during the COVID-19 pandemic, her interest shifted toward investigating cardiac abnormalities in patients recovering from an acute COVID-19 infection as well as during long-term follow-up. She published her first article on this topic in the *Journal of Clinical Medicine* at the beginning of 2021, shortly after the post-acute COVID-19 syndrome was first mentioned in the medical literature. Dr. Cristina Tudoran continued her research on cardiovascular abnormalities encountered in previously healthy individuals recovering from a SARS-CoV-2 infection and published over 17 articles on this topic.

Her research allowed her to fulfill the criteria for Dr. habilitatus and to obtain her habilitation degree from the Romanian Ministry of Education in 2023. She serves as PhD coordinator at the University of Medicine and Pharmacy "Victor Babes" Timisoara.

She published 61 articles in Clarivate-indexed journals, has an H-index of 16, and served as guest editor in 10 Special Issues in various ISI-indexed journals. She is an editorial board member of *Frontiers in Cardiovascular Medicine*.

She is a member of the Romanian and European Society of Cardiology.

Larisa Anghel

Dr. Larisa Anghel is a highly accomplished academic, clinician, and researcher, serving as a Senior Lecturer at the "Grigore T. Popa" University of Medicine and Pharmacy in Iași, Romania, and a specialist in cardiology. With a specialty in Cardiology, she has made significant contributions to this field, with over 48 ISI-indexed articles published, more than 1800 citations, and a H-index of 10. She has also authored one book and co-authored more than 55 book chapters, showcasing her commitment to advancing knowledge in cardiovascular medicine. Her research interests include emergency cardiology, heart failure, coronary artery disease, and arterial hypertension, with significant contributions as a reviewer and editor for leading international journals. Her extensive academic work highlights her expertise and dedication to both research and education in cardiology.

In her clinical role at the "Prof. Dr. George I.M. Georgescu" Institute of Cardiovascular Diseases in Iași, Dr. Anghel works in the Cardiac Intensive Care Unit, specializing in patient diagnostics, treatment, and intensive care management. She has also demonstrated a passion for education, mentoring undergraduate theses and conducting practical training for medical professionals. With her strong communication, organizational skills, and multidisciplinary expertise, Dr. Anghel continues to drive innovation in cardiology through education, clinical care, and research.

Preface

Heart failure remains one of the most pressing challenges in modern medicine, affecting millions worldwide and burdening healthcare systems. As clinicians and researchers, we are continuously striving to improve the outcomes for these patients. This reprint, Clinical Management of Patients with Heart Failure, seeks to provide healthcare professionals, researchers, and clinicians with a deeper understanding of the multifaceted aspects of heart failure management, from pathophysiology to cutting-edge therapeutic approaches. Additionally, this Special Issue explores the role of emerging therapies, personalized medicine, and multidisciplinary care in tackling the challenges posed by this complex condition.

The work presented here reflects collective dedication to improving quality of life for patients with heart failure, and each contribution has been meticulously reviewed by experts in the field, ensuring that only the most relevant and impactful findings are included. These articles not only highlight the advancements in heart failure treatment but also reflect the ongoing challenges and opportunities for improvement in clinical outcomes. The diverse approaches, from mechanical circulatory support to evidence-based drug therapy, offer new hope for patients with heart failure and will help guide clinicians in delivering the highest standards of care.

This reprint has been curated with contributions from renowned experts in the field, whose research and clinical expertise have significantly shaped current understandings and practices in heart failure management. Their collective efforts, along with those of the many dedicated professionals, reflect an ongoing commitment to advancing the field and are critical in driving forward the next generation of heart failure treatments and care strategies.

We would like to express our sincere gratitude to the contributing authors, reviewers, and editorial team for their invaluable support and expertise. Their dedication to heart failure research and patient care is evident in the quality of work presented in this Special Issue. The collaboration between researchers, clinicians, and healthcare teams remains central to advancing the field of heart failure management, and we hope this collection will inspire continued progress in heart failure management and foster further dialogue and innovation in the years to come. Our collective efforts—rooted in empathy, expertise, and collaboration—are crucial to improving outcomes, easing suffering, and ultimately offering hope for a better quality of life for patients with heart failure. With dedication and innovation, we can move closer to transforming the lives of those affected by this challenging condition, empowering them to not just survive but thrive.

Cristina Tudoran and Larisa Anghel
Guest Editors

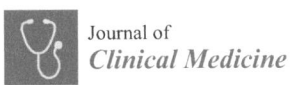

Review

Biomarkers in Heart Failure with Preserved Ejection Fraction: A Perpetually Evolving Frontier

Ana-Maria Vrabie [1,2,*], Stefan Totolici [1,2], Caterina Delcea [1,2] and Elisabeta Badila [1,2]

1. Cardio-Thoracic Pathology Department, "Carol Davila" University of Medicine and Pharmacy, 050474 Bucharest, Romania; stefan.totolici@drd.umfcd.ro (S.T.); caterina.delcea@umfcd.ro (C.D.); elisabeta.badila@umfcd.ro (E.B.)
2. Cardiology Department, Colentina Clinical Hospital, 020125 Bucharest, Romania
* Correspondence: ana-maria.vrabie@drd.umfcd.ro; Tel.: +40-730927510

Abstract: Heart failure with preserved ejection fraction (HFpEF) represents a complex clinical syndrome, often very difficult to diagnose using the available tools. As the global burden of this disease is constantly growing, surpassing the prevalence of heart failure with reduced ejection fraction, during the last few years, efforts have focused on optimizing the diagnostic and prognostic pathways using an immense panel of circulating biomarkers. After the paradigm of HFpEF development emerged more than 10 years ago, suggesting the impact of multiple comorbidities on myocardial structure and function, several phenotypes of HFpEF have been characterized, with an attempt to find an ideal biomarker for each distinct pathophysiological pathway. Acknowledging the limitations of natriuretic peptides, hundreds of potential biomarkers have been evaluated, some of them demonstrating encouraging results. Among these, soluble suppression of tumorigenesis-2 reflecting myocardial remodeling, growth differentiation factor 15 as a marker of inflammation and albuminuria as a result of kidney dysfunction or, more recently, several circulating microRNAs have proved their incremental value. As the number of emerging biomarkers in HFpEF is rapidly expanding, in this review, we aim to explore the most promising available biomarkers linked to key pathophysiological mechanisms in HFpEF, outlining their utility for diagnosis, risk stratification and population screening, as well as their limitations.

Keywords: heart failure with preserved ejection fraction; HFpEF; biomarkers; natriuretic peptides; troponins; diagnostic biomarkers; prognostic biomarkers

Citation: Vrabie, A.-M.; Totolici, S.; Delcea, C.; Badila, E. Biomarkers in Heart Failure with Preserved Ejection Fraction: A Perpetually Evolving Frontier. *J. Clin. Med.* **2024**, *13*, 4627. https://doi.org/10.3390/jcm13164627

Academic Editor: Christian Sohns

Received: 29 June 2024
Revised: 28 July 2024
Accepted: 5 August 2024
Published: 7 August 2024

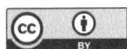

Copyright: © 2024 by the authors. Licensee MDPI, Basel, Switzerland. This article is an open access article distributed under the terms and conditions of the Creative Commons Attribution (CC BY) license (https:// creativecommons.org/licenses/by/ 4.0/).

1. Introduction

Heart failure (HF) is a complex clinical syndrome, resulting from a structural or functional abnormality of the heart, which leads to the classic cardinal symptoms of dyspnea, oedema and fatigue, usually accompanied by other signs, such as elevated jugular venous pressure and pulmonary crackles. At present, based on the measurement of left ventricular ejection fraction (LVEF), three distinct phenotypes are described: HF with reduced ejection fraction (HFrEF), defined as LVEF $\leq$ 40%; HF with mildly reduced ejection fraction (HFmrEF), with LVEF between 41% and 49%; and HF with preserved ejection fraction (HFpEF), with LVEF $\geq$ 50% [1]. HFpEF accounts for more than half of all cases of HF, representing one of the major public health problems worldwide [2,3]. Moreover, the diagnosis of HFpEF is often challenging, as signs and symptoms may be subtle or attributable to other comorbidities. As the incidence of this disease is continuously growing, with long-term mortality and re-hospitalization rates similar to HFrEF, major interests have risen regarding the optimal diagnostic and prognostic algorithms [4]. Ever since the concept of HFpEF as the result of a systemic proinflammatory state induced by multiple associated comorbidities emerged, major interests have focused on understanding the various pathophysiological mechanisms that lead to this complex syndrome [5]. The attempts to characterize each pathway by certain biomarkers have paved the way for a new field of research, leading to the discovery of hundreds of potential biomarkers in HFpEF. Most of the research efforts have mainly centered on HFrEF, demonstrating the incremental clinical utility of several biomarkers. The heterogeneous nature of HFpEF makes it difficult to find a single, ideal biomarker of diagnostic and prognostic value. This review aims to characterize the most promising biomarkers that demonstrated value in refining the diagnosis, risk stratification and monitoring response to treatment in patients with HFpEF (Figure 1). For this general review, we retrieved the most relevant studies from PubMed, searching for the literature in English, involving human subjects and published mainly from 2020 until 1 June 2024. We also included some older research articles that were considered relevant to the content of our review, such as landmark studies or those related to pathophysiological mechanisms in HFpEF. We excluded studies that referred only to HFrEF. Terms related to "Heart Failure with Preserved Ejection Fraction", "Diastolic Dysfunction", "Heart Failure, Diastolic", "Biomarkers" and names of each specific biomarker were used for the selection of qualified studies that analyzed the prognostic and diagnostic values of circulating biomarkers, as well as their utility for treatment monitoring in specific cases.

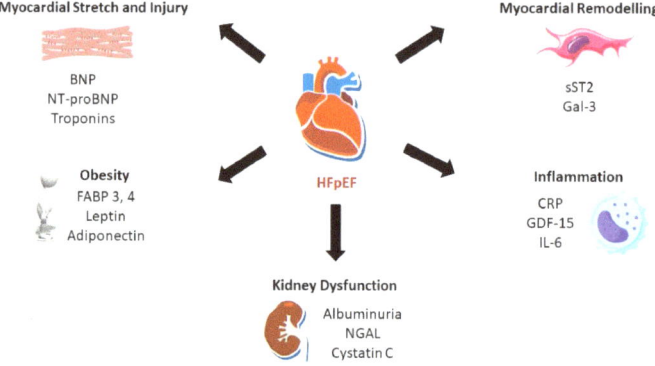

Figure 1. Multiple pathophysiological mechanisms involved in HFpEF and their representative biomarkers. Abbreviations: BNP, brain natriuretic peptide; NT-proBNP, N-terminal pro-B-type natriuretic peptide; FABP 3, 4, fatty acid binding protein 3, 4; NGAL, neutrophil gelatinase-associated lipocalin; CRP, C-reactive protein; GDF-15, growth differentiation factor 15; IL-6, interleukin-6; sST2, soluble suppression of tumorigenicity-2; Gal-3, galectin 3.

2. Pathophysiological Relevance of Circulating Biomarkers

It has long been suggested that myocardial remodeling and dysfunction in HFpEF evolve from a combination of multiple risk factors and comorbidities found in these patients, such as advanced age, obesity, hypertension, diabetes mellitus, chronic kidney disease (CKD) or chronic obstructive pulmonary disease (COPD) [6,7]. The systemic proinflammatory state induced by these coexisting factors leads to alterations in the coronary microvasculature, promoting cardiomyocyte hypertrophy and increased collagen deposition [5]. Moreover, the metabolic syndrome (MetS) and each risk factor for MetS generate changes in LV geometry, leading to the development of diastolic dysfunction [8]. Incriminated pathophysiological mechanisms are cardiomyocyte apoptosis caused by lipotoxicity, increased oxidative stress determined by hyperglycemia and lipoapoptosis triggered by excessive lipid accumulation in the myocardial cells [9–12]. These changes will further result in the complex remodeling of the left ventricle characteristic of the HFpEF phenotype, which is distinct from other forms of HF. This paradigm has led to the study of an extensive array of biomarkers associated with distinct pathophysiological mechanisms in HFpEF, including myocardial remodeling, systemic inflammation, myocyte death, oxidative stress, obesity and anemia.

Currently, only the biomarkers that reflect myocardial stretch, namely the natriuretic peptides (NPs), fulfill the criteria for an ideal biomarker, although their measurement demonstrated several limitations that seriously affect their performance [13,14]. Among the biomarkers that reflect myocardial injury, cardiac troponins demonstrated strong prognostic significance in both acute and chronic HFpEF [15–17]. Apart from their utility in acute settings, their levels also rise in chronic cardiovascular (CV) conditions, as a consequence of a higher wall stress and impaired microvascular function in the myocardium, which makes them valuable biomarkers reflecting the severity of diastolic dysfunction [18,19]. In HFpEF, microvascular dysfunction is mediated by pro-inflammatory cytokines, leading to monocyte infiltration and differentiation into macrophages, amplifying the inflammatory response in the myocardium. Considering the biomarkers highly expressed in any state of systemic inflammation, growth differentiation factor 15 (GDF-15) showed the most promising results, identifying patients with an early stage of HFpEF and providing important prognostic information, independent of the other biomarkers [20–22]. Furthermore, other biomarkers play key roles in the process of myocardial remodeling by interacting with extracellular matrix proteins. Such is the case of galectin-3 (Gal-3), a protein that promotes myocyte hypertrophy and collagen deposition in HFpEF. Recent studies suggest the ability of this biomarker to identify individuals at high risk of developing HFpEF, as well as to predict adverse outcomes in both acute and chronic settings [23,24]. Similar findings are related to suppression of tumorigenicity-2 (ST2), an agent promoting inflammation and fibrosis, useful for risk stratification in HFpEF and monitoring treatment response [25,26]. Ultimately, circulating biomarkers reflecting kidney dysfunction and obesity are useful for detecting early stages of HFpEF and predicting negative outcomes in those with established disease.

Overall, the field of biomarkers is rapidly expanding and efforts are directed towards finding molecules that have both clinical and pathophysiological significance. In the following parts, we will present the clinical implications of the most promising biomarkers currently under study, with respect to their screening performance, diagnostic and prognostic ability in both acute and chronic settings and their potential usefulness for monitoring treatment response in HFpEF.

3. Myocardial Stretch and Injury

3.1. Natriuretic Peptides

The discovery of NPs laid the foundation for a revolutionary approach in patients with HF. From its initial identification in the porcine brain to a sophisticated biomarker involved in the pathophysiology of HF, brain natriuretic peptide (BNP) has demonstrated great value as a diagnostic and prognostic tool across the entire ejection fraction (EF) spectrum [27]. The NP system consists of three hormones. As the name suggests, atrial natriuretic peptide (ANP) is secreted primarily by the atria, while BNP, despite its name, is secreted by the ventricular myocardium in response to the increased myocardial wall stress [28]. C-type natriuretic peptide (CNP) is expressed at high levels in the bone, brain and vascular endothelium, with limited applicability in HF. The physiological role of NPs is related to their diuretic, natriuretic and vasodilatatory properties, acting as important regulators of blood pressure and circulating volume, thus counteracting the deleterious effects of the renin-angiotensin system (RAS) and the sympathetic nervous system. In addition, they exert anti-hypertrophic and anti-fibrotic properties in the myocardium and inhibit the proliferation of vascular smooth muscle cells [29,30]. Due to their longer plasma half-lives, BNP and its inactive metabolite N-terminal pro B-type natriuretic peptide (NT-proBNP) have been extensively studied, becoming the gold standard biomarkers in HF.

3.1.1. Screening

Studies suggest that measurement of NPs may identify patients at risk of developing HF, although the cut-offs used for risk prediction in the apparently healthy population are not well established. NP levels could be used to optimize medical treatment in patients at high risk of developing HF. As the PONTIAC study demonstrated, in patients with type 2 diabetes mellitus and a NT-proBNP level > 125 pg/mL, up-titration of RAS antagonists and beta-blockers significantly reduced the primary outcome of 2-year CV mortality and hospitalizations [31]. A strategy based on BNP screening was also assessed in another randomized trial encompassing more than 1300 patients with at least one risk factor of HF or CV comorbidity, with a follow-up of 4.2 years. Results suggested that BNP is a good risk predictor for HF and CV events, as the measurement of BNP levels enhanced treatment optimization and adoption of lifestyle measurements [32]. Another recent meta-analysis suggested a reasonable diagnostic performance of NPs for the detection of diastolic dysfunction and HFpEF, at a cost of significant heterogeneity among studies [33].

3.1.2. Diagnosis

The Breathing Not Properly trial was the first to evaluate the use of BNP as a diagnostic test in patients complaining of dyspnea. At a cut-off of 100 pg/mL, BNP had 90% sensitivity and 73% specificity for the diagnosis of HF [34]. Similar findings were reported from the N-terminal Pro-BNP Investigation of Dyspnea in the Emergency department (PRIDE) study, with NT-proBNP demonstrating high sensitivity and specificity for the diagnosis of acute HF at cut-offs above 450 pg/mL or 900 pg/mL for patients below or above 50 years, respectively [35]. Ever since, the measurement of NPs has become a central element in the diagnostic algorithm for acute and chronic HF, as stated in both the European and the American guidelines. Circulating levels of NPs seem to be more increased in HFrEF compared to HFpEF, although no cut-off can accurately discern between the two conditions [36]. Moreover, levels of NPs are influenced by a number of conditions and comorbidities, affecting the accuracy of HF diagnosis. NP levels become more increased in the elderly, possibly as a consequence of the decrease in renal function, so that different cut-offs should be applied according to the age group [13]. Among the comorbidities that lead to increased levels of NPs, atrial fibrillation, COPD, pulmonary hypertension (PH) and CKD are notable. These conditions are actually frequent in HF patients, affecting the diagnostic sensitivity of NPs. As a result, cut-offs for diagnosis of HFpEF need to be adjusted according to age, gender, race, ethnicity and the presence of comorbidities and on-going treatment with neprilysin inhibitors. On the contrary, obesity tends to lower NP levels, presumably attributable to an increased clearance by adipocyte NPs' receptors, although other mechanisms are incriminated [14,37].

3.1.3. Prognosis

NPs demonstrate significant prognostic implications, as demonstrated by several studies. BNP levels are strongly associated with all-cause mortality and HF hospitalizations across the entire HF phenotype [1,38]. At similar BNP levels, the prognosis of patients with HFpEF is as poor as those with HFrEF [36,39]. The same results are reported for NT-proBNP levels, which are associated with adverse events at 1-year follow-up for both HFpEF and HFrEF [40]. In the PARAGON-HF trial, NT-proBNP levels at screening were strongly associated with a risk of CV death and HF hospitalizations [41].

Changes in NP levels during hospitalizations are also important in risk stratification [1,38]. In a post hoc analysis of the SURVIVE trial, mortality at 30 and 180 days was significantly higher in the non-responders' group, defined as patients who did not achieve a reduction in BNP level by $\geq$30% from baseline to day 5 [42]. Similar results regarding longitudinal changes in NP values were reported by other studies [43–45].

Discharge NP concentrations are also associated with clinical outcomes in HF [1]. In a sub-analysis from the OPTIMIZE-HF (Organized Program to Initiate Lifesaving Treatment in Hospitalized Patients with Heart Failure) registry, discharge BNP was a better predictor of 1-year mortality rate and rehospitalizations than admission BNP or ratio of the discharge/admission BNP [46]. Another study concluded that the absolute value of BNP at discharge was a better predictor of 6-month mortality than baseline BNP or the reduction in BNP during hospitalization [47].

3.1.4. Treatment Response

Regarding the effect of treatment on outcomes across the spectrum of NP levels, a sub-analysis from the TOPCAT trial (Treatment of Preserved Cardiac Function Heart Failure with an Aldosterone Antagonist Trial) revealed a greater benefit of spironolactone in the group with lower levels of NPs as compared to higher levels [48]. The same results were reported from the I-PRESERVE trial (Irbesartan in Heart Failure with Preserved Ejection Fraction), where the angiotensin-receptor blocker significantly reduced outcomes in patients with lower levels of NPs, although treatment with irbesartan showed no benefit in the overall population of HFpEF [49]. This could be explained by the fact that higher NP levels are encountered in older patients, with more comorbidities and more advanced structural heart disease associated with HFpEF. These findings suggest that drug intervention in HFpEF might be beneficial earlier in the course of the disease. This hypothesis should be tested in specifically designed clinical trials, according to specific concentrations of NPs below which positive results become prominent. On the other hand, following an analysis from the EMPEROR-Preserved trial, treatment with empagliflozin resulted in a relative reduction in risk across all NT-proBNP concentrations, with greatest absolute reduction observed in the population with the highest concentrations [50]. Similarly, in the PARAGON-HF trial, modest overall treatment effects of sacubitril/valsartan were reported across the entire spectrum of baseline NT-proBNP. Patients who experienced the greatest reduction in NT-proBNP during treatment had better outcomes [41].

Considering an NP-guided management of patients with HFpEF, studies have been contradictory. A sub-analysis of the TIME-CHF trial (Trial of Intensified versus standard Medical therapy in Elderly patients with Congestive Heart Failure) compared a symptom-guided versus an NT-proBNP-guided therapy, revealing that the latter tended to worsen primary outcomes at 18 months [51]. Another meta-analysis confirmed that NP-guided therapy is not superior to guideline-directed therapy in acute or chronic HF, regardless of the EF [52]. Overall, evidence supporting an NP-guided strategy in HFpEF is lacking.

3.2. Troponins

Apart from acute coronary syndromes, troponin levels can be increased in several other conditions, such as myocarditis, pulmonary embolism or HF, particularly when measured using high-sensitivity (hs) assays. Previously, it has been hypothesized that troponins can also be released in the bloodstream in the absence of myocyte death, a term named "cytosolic pool" [19]. As a consequence, the mechanisms responsible for troponin release in HF involve both ischemic and non-ischemic processes [18,19]. The latter may be related to the increased wall stress caused by volume or pressure overload, a pro-inflammatory state caused by circulating cytokines, catecholamines and oxidative stress and impairment of diastolic function [19]. In HFpEF, troponin levels are directly correlated with LV filling pressures and diastolic dysfunction, especially during exercise [53].

3.2.1. Prognosis

Several studies outlined the prognostic utility of high-sensitivity cardiac troponin T (hs-cTnT) in HFrEF [54]. In a meta-analysis including 9289 patients, the majority with HFrEF, hs-cTnT at a cut-off of 18 ng/L emerged as a strong, independent predictor of all-cause mortality (HR, 1.48; 95% CI, 1.41–1.55), CV mortality (HR, 1.40; 95% CI, 1.33–1.48) and hospitalization (HR, 1.42; 95% CI, 1.36–1.49), over a median follow-up of 2.4 years [55]. Although troponin levels are more elevated in HFrEF as compared to HFpEF, studies indicate a prognostic role for troponins in HFpEF as well [56,57].

Acute HF

In acute decompensated HF, hs-cTn levels carry important prognostic information [15,58]. In a sub-analysis of the ADHERE trial, including more than 60,000 patients, approximately 40% of patients testing positive for troponin had an EF above 40%. Compared to patients with negative troponin levels, those with detectable levels had an increased risk of in-hospital mortality (8% vs. 2.7%, p value < 0.001), prolonged hospitalization (adjusted mean stay 6.6 days vs. 5.5 days, *p* value < 0.001) and requirement for cardiac procedures. This association was maintained after adjustment for other established risk factors associated with negative outcomes [59]. In another observational cohort study including more than 34,000 patients with acute decompensated HFpEF, troponin elevation was significantly associated with in-hospital, 30-day and 1-year mortality and prolonged hospitalization [60].

Chronic HF

Elevated hs-cTnI levels were associated with a composite endpoint of all-cause mortality and HF rehospitalization in a cohort of patients with chronic HF, after adjustment for other established prognostic variables such as age, sex, smoking, diabetes, renal function and NT-proBNP levels. When comparing the prognostic significance across the EF, both hs-cTnI and hs-cTnT were more strongly associated with composite adverse events in HFpEF (TnI: HR 2.32; 95% CI 1.60–3.36; TnT: HR 3.01; 95% CI 2.01–4.51) than in HFrEF (TnI: HR 1.29; 95% CI 1.16–1.42; TnT: HR 1.36; 95% CI 1.22–1.53) [17].

The prognostic utility of hs-cTn was also demonstrated in several major trials in HFpEF. In a sub-analysis from the EMPEROR-Preserved Trial, similarly to NT-proBNP concentrations, hs-cTnT levels were significantly associated with the primary endpoint of CV mortality and HF hospitalizations. No treatment heterogeneity was noted, with empagliflozin demonstrating a comparable reduction in events rate across all hs-cTnT quartiles, although patients with the highest baseline hs-cTnT had the greatest absolute risk reduction. In the placebo group, patients with higher hs-cTnT values had a 4-fold increased risk for the primary endpoint [50]. Comparably, in another analysis from EMPEROR-Preserved, has-cTnT alongside NT-proBNP were the major predictors of the primary outcome (CV mortality, HF hospitalization). Those with lowest values for NT-proBNP and hs-cTnT had a primary event rate of 2.2 per 100 patient-years, in contrast with 19.2 per 100 patient-years in patients with the highest values for both biomarkers [61]. A risk model combining hs-cTnT and NPs provided important complementary information of prognosis, with good prognostic capacity (*c*-statistics ranging from 0.71 to 0.75 for mortality and the composite endpoint of HF hospitalizations or CV mortality) [61]. In another post hoc analysis from the TOPCAT trial, higher levels of hs-cTnI were independently associated with an increased risk of CV mortality or HF hospitalization (HR, 1.42; 95% CI, 1.20–1.69; *p* value < 0.001 per doubling of hs-cTnI). No treatment heterogeneity was noted across hs-cTnI levels with regard to the primary composite endpoint [16].

3.2.2. Screening

The association between hs-cTn and incident HF has been insufficiently studied. In a community-based cohort of more than 8000 asymptomatic patients, no biomarker was significantly associated with an increased risk of developing HFpEF [62]. After 11.4 years follow-up, hs-cTnT and NT-proBNP were significant predictors for HFrEF and not HFpEF [63]. In a study including more than 22,000 patients, hs-cTn demonstrated a significant association with HFrEF (HR, 1.37; 95% CI, 1.29–1.46; *p* < 0.001), whereas for HFpEF, the association was also suggestive (HR, 1.11; 95% CI, 1.03–1.19; *p* = 0.008) [64]. In another retrospective analysis of the STOP-HF study, hs-cTnI at baseline and follow-up significantly predicted new-onset HFpEF [65].

4. Inflammation

Systemic inflammation plays a central role in the development and progression of HFpEF. Upregulation of inflammation in HFpEF leads to worse cardiac structural and functional abnormalities, demonstrated using a wide array of biomarkers. The most promising ones are illustrated in Table 1. The first trial to provide evidence supporting the relationship between inflammation and HF outcomes was the CANTOS trial, in which patients with a history of myocardial infarction and systemic inflammation were either assigned to receive an IL-1β blocker or placebo [66]. In a sub-analysis of this trial, canakinumab was found to reduce HF hospitalizations in a dose-dependent manner, generating the hypothesis that cytokine inhibition may improve HF outcomes [67].

Table 1. Summary of biomarker studies reflecting inflammation and their clinical utility in HFpEF.

Biomarker		Application to HFpEF	
GDF-15	Prognosis	Acute HF ○ Admission levels associated with 30-day all-cause mortality [20] ○ Levels measured in the first 48h predict HF rehospitalization at 1 year [68] ○ In a multi-marker strategy, predicts all-cause long-term mortality [69]	Chronic HF ○ Predicts all-cause mortality, outperforming NT-proBNP [70] ○ Predicts the composite of mortality or first HF hospitalization regardless of the EF [71] ○ Associated with all-cause mortality, especially in ischemic patients [21]
	Diagnosis and Screening	○ Levels significantly differed among 4 phenogroups of subjects with HF-like symptoms [72] ○ Ability to identify early stages of HFpEF [22]	
CRP	Prognosis	○ Associated with markers of HFpEF severity [73] ○ Levels > 2 mg/dL associated with HF hospitalizations and CV mortality [74] ○ High levels predict all-cause and CV mortality [75]	
IL-6	Prognosis	○ Associated with HFpEF severity [76] ○ Predicts all-cause and CV mortality in acute decompensated HFpEF [77]	
	Diagnosis	○ Levels associated with increased risk to develop HFpEF and not HFrEF [78]	

Abbreviations: GDF-15, growth differentiation factor 15; CRP, C-reactive protein; IL-6, interleukin-6; NT-proBNP, N-terminal pro-B-type natriuretic peptide; HF, heart failure; HFpEF, heart failure with preserved ejection fraction; HFrEF, heart failure with reduced ejection fraction; EF, ejection fraction; CV, cardiovascular.

4.1. GDF-15

In healthy states, GDF-15, a member of the transforming growth factor-β superfamily, is expressed at low levels by various cell types, such as cardiomyocytes, adipocytes, vascular smooth muscle cells and macrophages [79]. Overexpression of GDF-15 is triggered by inflammation, oxidative stress, tissue injury and hypoxia. As a result, this biomarker is secreted in various pathological conditions, including numerous solid cancers, metabolic conditions such as anorexia or cachexia and autoimmune diseases [79–81] [82,83]. In HF, the expression of GDF-15 is associated with ischemia, neurohormonal activation, pro-inflammatory cytokines and mechanical strain [84]. Concentrations of GDF-15 increase in various CV conditions, including acute and chronic HF, atrial fibrillation and acute coronary syndromes.

4.1.1. Prognosis

The prognostic value of GDF-15 has been demonstrated in patients with HFrEF. In several studies, GDF-15 was shown to predict mortality and HF hospitalizations [85–87]. The diagnostic and prognostic utility of GDF-15 in HFpEF have also been studied in the last few years.

Acute HF

Regardless of the EF, admission GDF-15 levels were associated with all-cause mortality at 30 days in a prospective study including patients admitted for acute HF. In addition, reduction in GDF-15 levels between admission and discharge was associated with a lower rehospitalization rate [20]. In another study including patients hospitalized for acute HFpEF, GDF-15 measured within 48 h of admission independently predicted HF rehospitalization at 1 year, outperforming the prognostic value of NT-proBNP [68]. In another prospective study including 380 hospitalized patients with decompensated HFpEF, a multi-biomarker model was assessed for the ability to predict mortality at 2 years. GDF-15 was among the biomarkers independently associated with the primary endpoint, alongside NT-proBNP, hs-cTnT, TNFα and other biomarkers of extracellular matrix turnover [69].

Chronic HF

In a prospective study including 311 patients with HFpEF and HFmrEF, GDF-15 concentration but not NT-proBNP was an independent predictor of all-cause mortality, with an area under receiver operating characteristic curve (AUC) of 0.797 for the model including NT-proBNP versus an AUC of 0.819 for the overall model including GDF-15 (p value 0.016) [70]. In another prospective study comparing plasma GDF-15 levels in patients with HFrEF versus HFpEF, GDF-15 remained a significant predictor for the composite outcome of mortality or first HF hospitalization across both HF phenotypes. Median GDF-15 baseline values were similarly increased in both groups. When added to established clinical predictors, such as hs-cTnT and NT-proBNP, GDF-15 increased the AUC from 0.720 to 0.740 (p value < 0.019) [71]. In a randomized controlled trial assessing an antifibrotic agent versus placebo in patients with HFpEF, although no influence of treatment on changes in GDF-15 levels was noticed, changes in multiple variables were associated with an increase in GDF-15 over 1 year. These included increased NT-proBNP levels, anemia, diastolic dysfunction and right ventricular dilation, factors known to be associated with worse prognosis in HFpEF [88]. This suggests that GDF-15 may not be involved in myocardial fibrosis in patients with HFpEF but more probably with an inflammatory state. A recent meta-analysis assessed the prognostic value of GDF-15 in more than 6000 patients with chronic HF, regardless of the EF. A 6% increase in risk of all-cause mortality was noted for every 1 LnU increase in baseline GDF-15 concentration after multivariable adjustment (HR 1.06, 95% CI 1.03–1.10, p value < 0.001). In addition, the association of GDF-15 with all-cause mortality was more significant among ischemic HF patients [21].

Similarly to NP levels, aging increases concentrations of GDF-15 in healthy individuals [89]. However, one major distinction between these two biomarkers seems to be related to atrial fibrillation, a frequent comorbidity encountered in HFpEF. In a sub-analysis from the ARISTOTLE trial, including more than 18,000 patients with atrial fibrillation randomized to either apixaban or warfarin, GDF-15 predicted major bleeding events, stroke or systemic embolism and mortality, independently of NT-proBNP or hs-cTnI [90]. Concordantly, in a nested prospective biomarker study of the ENGAGE AF-TIMI 48 trial, including 8705 patients, elevated GDF-15 was independently associated with higher rates of stroke and major bleeding. The novel ABC-bleeding score, which included GDF-15 and hs-cTnT, outperformed the HAS-BLED score, serving to stratify patients who would benefit more from treatment with edoxaban compared to warfarin [91]. In another study of 1941 patients, comparing NT-proBNP and GDF-15 levels in patients with atrial fibrillation versus sinus rhythm, GDF-15 levels were not significantly influenced by the presence of atrial fibrillation, after adjustment for clinical confounders [92]. This would represent a major benefit for the assessment of patients with both HFpEF and atrial fibrillation, as levels of NT-proBNP are severely influenced by the presence of this arrhythmia.

4.1.2. Diagnosis and Screening

A prospective study including 507 patients referred for cardiac-related symptoms, without a history of HF or other CV diseases, identified distinct phenogroups using the HFA-PEFF score. Each phenogroup was further analyzed for its association with distinct biomarkers [72]. GDF-15 was among the biomarkers that significantly differed among the four clusters, enabling us to hypothesize that distinct circulating biomarker profiles might aid in understanding the pathophysiological mechanisms of HF development and help us classify distinct HFpEF phenotypes, which could benefit from early intervention. The ability of GDF-15 to identify patients at an early stage of HF was also assessed in another prospective cohort study of more than 2000 patients. GDF-15 was the strongest predictor of HF hospitalization and all-cause mortality (HR 2.12, 95% CI 1.71 to 2.63; $p < 0.0001$), whereas a multivariable prediction model incorporating GDF-15 performed better than the one without GDF-15 [22].

4.2. C-Reactive Protein

Increased C-reactive protein (CRP) levels are associated with many comorbidities leading to HFpEF. As inflammation is postulated to play an important role in the pathophysiology of HFpEF, CRP could be used as a surrogate biomarker to express this state. CRP is associated with markers of HF severity, including NT-proBNP values and NYHA class, and can be used to predict negative outcomes in patients with HFpEF [73]. In a subset of patients from the TOPCAT study, hs-CRP above 2 mg/L was associated with an increased risk of adverse events, including HF hospitalizations and CV mortality. Compared to patients with low levels of hs-CRP, those with high levels had more frequent hospitalizations, an increased prevalence of COPD and a higher BMI [74]. Another meta-analysis underlined the prognostic association between higher levels of CRP and an increased risk of CV and all-cause mortality in patients with HFpEF [75].

4.3. Interleukin-6

As with the other biomarkers of inflammation, it has been suggested that Interleukin-6 (IL-6) could play a major role in HF. In a subset of patients from the PREVEND cohort, IL-6 was independently associated with an increased risk of developing HFpEF and not HFrEF [78]. Increased IL-6 levels are associated with symptom severity, worse renal function, poor exercise capacity and excess body fat [76]. Moreover, in patients recently hospitalized with decompensated HFpEF, IL-6 was independently associated with CV and all-cause mortality [77]. Data from the CANTOS trial suggest that the magnitude of risk reduction observed in patients receiving canakinumab was directly related to the magnitude of IL-6 reduction, with greater benefits observed in patients who achieved greater than median reductions in IL-6 [93]. Further trials will need to assess the benefits of direct inhibition of IL-6 on CV outcomes in patients with HF.

5. Cardiac Remodeling

Although studies have evaluated many biomarkers that reflect extracellular matrix and myocardial fibrosis, including pro-collagen propeptides, matrix metalloproteinases and tissue inhibitors of metalloproteinases, two particular biomarkers have provided the most convincing results in patients with HFpEF (Table 2).

Table 2. Summary of biomarker studies reflecting myocardial remodeling and their clinical utility in HFpEF.

Biomarker		Application to HFpEF	
		Acute HF	Chronic HF
Gal-3	Prognosis	o After an ACS, high levels predict HF development and rehospitalization [94–96] o High levels on admission predict all-cause mortality [23,97,98]	o Repeated measures at baseline, 3 and 6 months associated with all-cause mortality and HF hospitalizations [99] o Levels associated with long-term adverse outcomes: CV and all-cause mortality, HF hospitalizations [24]
	Diagnosis	o High levels associated with the severity of diastolic dysfunction and an increased risk of new-onset HFpEF [24,100]	
	Treatment response	o Baseline pre-treatment levels could modify response to treatment with ARNI, assessed by a reduction in left atrial volume [101] o Possible benefit for patients with high levels, treated with spironolactone [26]	
sST-2		Acute HF	Chronic HF
	Prognosis	o Can predict all-cause mortality at 1 year [102] o Repeated measurements during follow-up predict all-cause mortality and HF hospitalization, regardless of NT-proBNP [103] o Admission and discharge levels predict negative outcomes [104]	o Independent predictor of all-cause and CV mortality [105] o Association with long-term all-cause mortality, CV mortality and HF hospitalizations [106] o Enhanced risk stratification when added to NT-proBNP, hs-cTn and other biomarkers [102,107]
	Treatment response	o Treatment with spironolactone is associated with better 30-day outcomes in patients with acute HF and increased levels of ST-2 [26] o For patients with sST-2 < 33 ng/mL, treatment with ARNI leads to a reduction in left atrial volume [101]	

Abbreviations: Gal-3, galectin 3; sST2, soluble suppression of tumorigenicity-2; hs-cTn, high-sensitivity cardiac troponin; ACS, acute coronary syndrome; ARNI, angiotensin receptor neprilysin inhibitor.

5.1. Galectin-3

Gal-3 is a galactoside-binding protein from the lectin family, widely expressed in human tissues and responsible for fibroblast activation, which leads to fibrous remodeling in various organs. In the pathophysiology of HF, overexpression of Gal-3 promotes fibrosis, inflammation and cardiac remodeling, influencing progression from subclinical cardiac disease to the development of HFpEF.

5.1.1. Prognosis

Acute HF

In acute HF, Gal-3 is an important prognostic biomarker. In a recent study including patients with ST-segment elevation myocardial infarction (STEMI) who underwent primary percutaneous coronary intervention, high Gal-3 concentrations were associated with HF development and rehospitalization both at 1 and 2 years [94]. Other studies support the association of Gal-3 with adverse cardiac remodeling and HF development after an acute coronary syndrome [95,96]. In a meta-analysis of 13 studies, higher serum Gal-3 levels on admission were independently associated with an increased risk of all-cause mortality (adjusted RR, 1.58; 95% CI, 1.33 to 1.88; $p < 0.001$) and CV mortality (adjusted RR, 1.29; 95% CI, 1.01 to 1.65; $p = 0.04$) in patients with acute HF, although significant heterogeneity was reported among studies [23]. Measurement of Gal-3 can also help predict short-term mortality in patients with acute HF, independently of NT-proBNP levels [97,98].

Chronic HF

The prognostic value of Gal-3 in chronic HFpEF has also been suggested. In two large cohort trials, repeated measures of Gal-3 at baseline and 3 or 6 months provided significant prognostic value. Increasing levels of Gal-3 were independently associated with all-cause mortality and HF hospitalizations [99]. A recent meta-analysis illustrated the association between Gal-3 levels and a high risk of long-term adverse outcomes in patients with HFpEF, including all-cause mortality (HR: 1.55; 95% CI: 1.27–1.87; $p = 0.138$, $I^2 = 42\%$), the composite of all-cause death and HF hospitalization (HR: 1.50; 95% CI: 1.30–1.74; $p = 0.001$, $I^2 = 61\%$) and CV death and HF hospitalizations (HR: 1.71; 95% CI: 1.51–1.94; $p = 0.036$, $I^2 = 58\%$) [24].

Similar to NT-proBNP, a potential link between serum levels of Gal-3 and renal dysfunction has been suggested [108]. In the RELAX trial, Gal-3 was associated with the severity of renal dysfunction but not with other pathophysiological mechanisms, assessed by biomarkers of fibrosis, inflammation or neurohormonal activation [109]. In a study including patients with acute HF, higher Gal-3 values were associated with renal dysfunction and renal tubular damage, predicting worse outcomes. After multivariable adjustment, Gal-3 remained associated with mortality during hospitalization [110]. This evidence supports the need to adjust for renal function when quantifying disease severity in HFpEF using Gal-3 levels.

5.1.2. Treatment Response

The interaction between Gal-3 and response to treatment in HFpEF was also investigated. In a sub-analysis of the PARAMOUNT trial, levels of Gal-3 correlated with the severity of HFpEF, whereas baseline pre-treatment Gal-3 might have modified the response to treatment with the angiotensin receptor neprilysin inhibitor [101]. This was assessed by a reduction in left atrial volume but not in NT-proBNP, so that a definite conclusion cannot be established. Interaction between Gal-3 levels and response to spironolactone has been evaluated in the Aldo-DHF trial. Although Gal-3 levels were not influenced by treatment, increasing levels at 6 or 12 months were associated with all-cause mortality and hospitalization, independently of NT-proBNP or treatment arm [111]. Moreover, in a secondary analysis of the COACH trial, which enrolled patients with acute HF irrespective of the EF, treatment with spironolactone seemed to be more beneficial to patients with elevated Gal-3 levels, among other biomarkers [26]. These data suggest that Gal-3 is probably more useful as a diagnostic or prognostic tool, rather than a biomarker of therapy response.

5.1.3. Diagnosis

The diagnostic utility of Gal-3 has been suggested in several studies, where higher levels of Gal-3 were associated with the severity of diastolic dysfunction and an increased risk of new-onset HFpEF [24,100]. Gal-3 can be used to identify individuals at risk of developing HFpEF and could be useful for phenotyping, especially in cases where fibrosis plays a major contribution to the pathology of HF. However, when comparing patients with HFpEF versus HFrEF, no significant difference is reported in serum Gal-3 levels [112].

5.2. Soluble ST2

Interleukin-1 receptor-like 1, commonly known in the literature as ST2, is a member of the interleukin-1 receptor family and presents as two isoforms: a soluble form—soluble ST2 (sST2)—and a transmembrane form—ST2 ligand (ST2L). Both of them bind to IL-33, which acts as either a pro- or anti-inflammatory cytokine, depending on co-stimulatory factors. The complex ST2L/IL-33 has a cardioprotective effect, limiting cardiomyocyte apoptosis, fibrosis and cardiac hypertrophy, whereas sST2 acts as a decoy receptor for IL-33, preventing its beneficial effects and leading to cardiac fibrosis, ventricular remodeling and negative cardiac outcomes [113].

Although cardiomyocytes and fibroblasts are important sources of sST2 in response to mechanical strain, in patients with HF, sST2 is secreted in large quantities from the lungs, specifically from alveolar epithelial cells. Experimental studies suggest that sST2 is involved in the pathophysiology of HF, being related to the presence and severity of pulmonary congestion [114]. sST2 measurement may offer some advantage compared to NT-proBNP, as circulating levels seem not to be affected by age, kidney function or obesity.

5.2.1. Prognosis

The prognostic utility of sST2 in HFrEF, beyond NT-proBNP or hs-cTn, has been extensively studied [25,115,116]. In patients with HFpEF, sST2 is associated with pro-inflammatory comorbidities, as evidence from the RELAX trial suggests. In this trial, higher sST2 levels were significantly associated with hypertension, diabetes mellitus, atrial fibrillation, renal dysfunction, systemic congestion and right ventricular dysfunction, among others [117]. In addition, sST2 concentrations are associated with multiple echocardiographic abnormalities, including biventricular size, LVEF and RV systolic pressure [118].

Acute HF

Results from the PRIDE study revealed that concentrations of ST2 strongly predicted 1-year mortality in patients with acute HF (HR 9.3, 95% CI 1.3 to 17.8; $p = 0.03$) [102]. In the TRIUMPH cohort study, including 496 patients with acute HF, baseline ST2 was independently associated with an increased risk of the composite endpoint of all-cause mortality and HF hospitalization (per log unit, HR 1.30, 95% CI 1.08 to 1.56; $p = 0.005$). Repeated measurements of sST2 during follow-up strongly predicted outcome, regardless of NT-proBNP levels (per log unit, HR 1.85; 95% CI: 1.02 to 3.33; $p = 0.044$) [103]. In another prospective cohort study of 331 patients with acute HF, after a median follow-up of 21 months, higher sST2 levels were independently associated with CV mortality (per log unit, HR 2.174; 95% CI 1.012–4.67; $p = 0.047$) [119]. A meta-analysis including 10 studies, with a population of 4835 patients, revealed that both admission and discharge sST2 were predictive of all-cause death, CV death and the composite of all-cause death or HF hospitalization. Discharge sST2 levels were predictive of HF hospitalization during a median follow-up of 13.5 months [104].

Chronic HF

In a prospective cohort study of 193 patients, sST2 was correlated with the composite endpoint of death or HF hospitalization. This association was stronger in patients with HFpEF (per log unit, HR: 6.62, 95% CI 1.04–42.28, $p = 0.046$) compared to HFrEF (HR 3.51; 95% CI 1.05–11.69, $p = 0.041$), although median values for sST2 were lower in the HFpEF group [120]. The first meta-analysis to assess the prognostic value of sST2 in chronic HF was performed in 2017, including seven studies with a total of 6372 patients. SST2 emerged as an independent predictor for both all-cause (HR 1.75; 95% CI: 1.37 to 2.22; $p < 0.001$) and CV mortality (HR 1.79; 95% CI: 1.22 to 2.63; $p < 0.001$) in outpatients with chronic HF, regardless of the EF [105]. Further on, another meta-analysis comprising 11 studies with 5121 patients evaluated the prognostic utility of sST2 in patients with chronic HF, regardless of the EF. Increased sST2 concentrations seemed to be associated with long-term all-cause mortality (HR: 1.03; 95% CI: 1.02–1.04; $p = 0.32$, $I^2 = 0\%$), long-term composite of CV mortality and HF hospitalizations (HR: 2.25; 95% CI: 1.82–2.79; $p = 0.47$, $I^2 = 0\%$) [106]. Another recent meta-analysis revealed that elevated levels of sST2 were associated with an increased risk of the composite endpoint of all-cause mortality and HF hospitalization (per log unit, HR: 6.52; 95% CI: 2.34, 18.19; $p = 0.985$, $I^2 = 0\%$), after multivariable adjustment [121]. Several studies support the addition of sST2 alongside NT-proBNP, hs-cTn or other biomarkers in key pathophysiological domains for an enhanced stratification of prognosis in patients with either acute or chronic HFpEF [102,107].

5.2.2. Treatment Response

Regarding the association between treatment and circulating levels of ST2, in a secondary analysis of the COACH trial, treatment with spironolactone was associated with favorable 30-day outcomes in patients with acute HF, especially in those with elevated ST-2 [26]. Data from the PARAMOUNT trial revealed that, in addition to Gal-3, sST2 was associated with the severity of HFpEF syndrome, although baseline levels of sST2 did not modify the response to Sacubitril/Valsartan. However, as in the case of Gal-3, patients with sST2 values less than the median of 33 ng/mL had a reduction in left atrial volume, which may signify a structural response to treatment [101].

5.2.3. Diagnosis

The diagnostic performance of sST2 for HFpEF is overall poor when compared to NT-proBNP, although in several studies, median sST2 values were significantly higher in patients with HFpEF compared to controls [122,123]. However, since sST2 is not specific for HF, it currently has no utility in diagnosing HFpEF [121]. A meta-analysis concluded that sST2 may have some diagnostic utility in HF (sensitivity 0.72; specificity 0.65, OR 3.63; AUC 0.75), although the high heterogeneity among studies and the inclusion of case–control studies causing selection bias should be taken into account [124].

6. Kidney Dysfunction

6.1. Worsening Renal Function

Renal dysfunction is one of the most frequent comorbidities in patients with HFpEF, associated with echocardiographic and biomarker profiles of more advanced disease [125]. Worsening renal function (WRF) during hospitalizations for acute decompensated HFpEF is related to multiple pathophysiological mechanisms, such as kidney venous congestion, hypoperfusion, inflammation or treatment reactions and is associated with adverse outcomes [126]. Several studies evaluated the impact of WRF, measured by an absolute increase in serum creatinine ≥ 0.3 mg/dL, on all-cause mortality or HF rehospitalizations, proving an independent prognostic association [127–129].

6.2. Albuminuria

Albuminuria is one of the earliest markers of kidney disease, denoting underlying glomerular structural damage. It is usually quantified by measuring the urinary albumin-creatinine ratio (UACR) in a spot urine, with microalbuminuria defined as a UACR between 30 and 300 mg/g and macroalbuminuria > 300 mg/g [130]. Albuminuria is known to be associated with an increased CV risk in the general population, as well as an increased risk for CKD, regardless of other risk factors. The reciprocal pathological mechanisms of cardiac and renal dysfunction, known as cardio-renal syndromes, are illustrated by this biomarker that mirrors both diseases. Studies have documented the association between albuminuria and the development of coronary artery disease, stroke, peripheral arterial disease, microvascular dysfunction, HF and atrial fibrillation [131].

UACR is a strong predictor of adverse outcomes in HF across the entire range of LVEF [132]. In patients with HFpEF, albuminuria was independently associated with lower global longitudinal strain, increased LV and RV remodeling and worse RV systolic function. The same study demonstrated that higher UACR predicted worse outcomes in a stepwise manner across the quartiles, although the association was attenuated after adjustment for BNP levels [133]. Moreover, another recent study demonstrated that in patients with new-onset or worsening HF with both reduced and preserved EF, albuminuria was strongly associated with clinical, echocardiographic and serum markers of congestion. In addition, albuminuria independently predicted higher mortality and HF hospitalization rates [134]. In acute decompensated HF, UACR in combination with BNP levels enabled a more accurate prediction of HF rehospitalizations than BNP alone [135]. Results from the TOPCAT study revealed that albuminuria was independently associated with worse CV outcomes, while treatment with spironolactone significantly reduced UACR at 1-year follow-up compared with placebo. A reduction in UACR by 50% was independently associated with a reduction in adverse outcomes [136]. Another prespecified analysis of the FIGARO-DKD trial suggested that albuminuria screening and early initiation of treatment with finerenone in patients with CKD and type 2 diabetes reduced the incidence of new-onset HF [137]. Overall, current evidence suggests that albuminuria in patients with HFpEF portends adverse prognosis, although the underlying mechanisms are incompletely elucidated. Incorporating UACR measurement in clinical practice is useful for an enhanced risk stratification and probably for monitoring treatment efficacy, although more trials are needed to assess the influence of therapy, especially sodium glucose cotransporter-2 (SGLT2) inhibitors, on albuminuria in patients with HFpEF.

6.3. NGAL

Neutrophil gelatinase-associated lipocalin (NGAL) is a predictor of acute kidney injury (AKI), as its plasma and urine levels rise before an increase in creatinine becomes apparent [138]. Its potential role in the prognostic stratification of patients with HF became a subject of interest in the past few years. However, evidence supporting its prognostic value is not conclusive. One study investigating the prognostic role of urinary NGAL (uNGAL) in patients with acute decompensated HF revealed that an elevated level of uNGAL on the first day of admission was independently associated with the primary endpoint (all-cause mortality, CV death and HF readmission) and with the development of AKI [139].

In another prospective cohort study including 927 patients hospitalized with acute HF, admission and peak values of serum NGAL (sNGAL), uNGAL, uNGAL/urine creatinine ratio were compared to admission and peak serum creatinine. Other studies support the prognostic value of NGAL in acute HF [140,141]. However, neither was superior to serum creatinine in predicting the composite endpoint of mortality, HF rehospitalization or initiation of renal replacement therapy [142]. A sub-analysis from the TOPCAT trial revealed that, although NGAL tended to predict mortality or HF hospitalizations, after multivariable correction, it did not meet significance [107]. A recent meta-analysis revealed that elevated sNGAL was associated with higher mortality or the composite outcome of mortality and rehospitalizations in patients with HF [143].

6.4. Cystatin C

Cystatin C (CysC) is a valuable alternative marker used for estimating kidney function, as represented by GFR. Its limited relationship to muscle mass and diet confers CysC an advantage over serum creatinine. In HFpEF, several studies suggest a potential role of CysC in risk stratification. The estimated GFR using CysC is significantly associated with worse diastolic function and adverse outcomes [144]. Serum CysC on admission is a strong predictor of all-cause mortality and HF readmission at 1 year, independently of NT-proBNP [145]. The same results are confirmed in a recent meta-analysis, demonstrating that CysC is an independent predictor of adverse outcomes in patients with HF, in addition to sNGAL [146]. With a clearance entirely dependent on GFR, CysC may be a good prognostic biomarker in both acute and chronic HFpEF, superior to creatinine.

7. Obesity

7.1. Fatty Acid Binding Protein 3 and 4

Fatty Acid Binding Protein 4 (FABP-4), a lipid chaperone found in adipocytes, appears to exert cardio-depressant effects, potentially leading to systolic dysfunction in obese patients [147]. A possible pathophysiological link exists between FABP-4 and HFpEF, as it is a marker of high metabolic risk, contributing to endothelial dysfunction through a pro-inflammatory cascade [148]. FABP-4 can also predict negative outcomes in patients with HFpEF. A prospective study revealed that in HFpEF, FABP-4 levels are associated with parameters of cardiac remodeling, diastolic and systolic dysfunction, predicting all-cause mortality or HF hospitalizations during a mean follow-up of 9.1 months [149]. Fatty Acid Binding Protein 3 (FABP-3) is another cytoplasmic protein found predominantly in the heart, with a crucial role in cardiac lipid transportation in myocardial metabolism. FABP-3 can also be used as a prognostic biomarker in HFpEF, with serum levels being independently associated with subsequent CV events [150,151]. In addition, both FABP-3 and FABP-4 were associated with all-cause and CV mortality in a group of patients with chronic HF and associated type 2 diabetes mellitus [152].

7.2. Leptin

Leptin is excreted from the adipose tissue and is involved in modulating food intake. It has complex CV effects, protecting against LV hypertrophy, promoting weight reduction and thus acting against the development of HF [153]. The role of leptin in the development of HF is intriguing, as it is associated with both protective and risk factors [154]. It has been suggested that increased leptin levels are associated with better outcomes in HFrEF but not in HFpEF, according to one study [155]. However, in another cross-sectional study including black women with preserved EF, higher leptin levels were associated with lower myocardial stiffness and LV mass index in obese patients, conferring a possible protective effect against the development of HFpEF [156]. These results need to be further confirmed in larger studies, taking into account the variability of racial or ethnic populations.

7.3. Adiponectin

Adiponectin is an anti-inflammatory cytokine derived from the adipose tissue, exerting cardio-protective effects via increasing insulin sensitivity and lipid regulation. This "rescue hormone" exerts anti-apoptotic, antioxidant and anti-fibrotic effects, protecting against the development of CV disease. The role of adiponectin in HF is controversial. In HFrEF, increased levels are paradoxically associated with the severity of the disease, as well as a higher NYHA class, probably related to adiponectin resistance in the myocardium. Patients with increased concentrations of adiponectin have a poor prognosis and a higher risk of mortality, particularly those with reduced muscle mass and cachexia [157,158]. In patients with chronic HF, baseline adiponectin levels are associated with mortality, while increasing levels over 3 months are associated with worse outcomes than stable levels [159]. In contrast, low levels of adiponectin are associated with the obesity-HFpEF phenotype, especially in women [160]. In a preclinical model of hypertension-related HFpEF, low levels of adiponectin exacerbated cardiac remodeling, diastolic dysfunction and pulmonary congestion [161].

8. Other Biomarkers

8.1. Antigen Carbohydrate 125

Antigen Carbohydrate 125 (CA 125) is a plasma biomarker traditionally used for the evaluation, risk stratification and monitoring of patients with ovarian cancer. Elevated levels of CA 125 are identified in other non-malignant conditions, such as pulmonary diseases, cirrhosis or HFCARDI. Increasing evidence has emerged, suggesting that CA 125 can serve as a prognostic tool in the risk stratification of patients with both acute and chronic HF [162]. In HFpEF, evidence supports the potential value of CA 125 as a biomarker for the prediction of mortality and HF readmissions, outperforming the prognostic value of NT-proBNP in some studies [163–165]. A positive correlation between CA 125 levels and the presence of fluid overload, such as serous effusions and peripheral edema, has been described, making this glycoprotein a useful biomarker for extravascular congestion in HF [166]. Concentrations of CA 125 are also increased in inflammatory states, in association with different types of cytokines [167]. As a result, CA 125 correlates with parameters of disease severity and it can be useful in guiding decongestion therapy [168,169]. In contrast, a recent sub-analysis of the EMPEROR trials revealed that in patients without clinical evidence of congestion, CA 125 predicted the primary endpoint only in those with HFrEF and not among those with HFpEF. The beneficial effect of empagliflozin seemed to be attenuated in patients with lower baseline CA 125 levels [170]. In addition, the highest baseline CA 125 levels were independently associated with an increased rate of kidney function decline [171]. Future trials should focus more on the association of treatment with SGLT2 inhibitors and CA 125 levels in patients with HFpEF, as this was already suggested in those with HFrEF [172,173].

8.2. Iron Deficiency

Iron deficiency (ID), defined as ferritin < 100 or transferrin saturation < 20%, is highly prevalent in patients with HFpEF. Contributing factors include decreased iron absorption due to congestion, reduced availability of stored iron and nutritional deficiency. ID can impact exercise performance in patients with HF, affecting oxygen consumption leading to anaerobic metabolism. In a retrospective study of 212 patients, both anemia and ID, along with advanced age and CKD, were independently associated with all-cause mortality in HFpEF. Patients with ID expressed more severe HF symptoms and worse functional capacity compared to those without ID [174]. ID was associated with worse functional outcomes but not HF hospitalization or mortality in another meta-analysis [175]. The importance of correcting ID is currently not established in HFpEF, as opposed to HFrEF, and further trials are needed in this field.

8.3. Circulating microRNAs

The discovery of microRNAs (miRNAs) has opened a new door in the era of molecular biology. They represent small, non-coding, regulatory RNA molecules of 22 nucleotides that operate at the level of gene expression by targeting specific regions of messenger RNAs (mRNAs). They have been shown to be promising diagnostic and prognostic biomarkers for many diseases, including HF [176,177]. Distinct miRNAs have been associated with different pathophysiological pathways in HF. MiR-126 has major roles in maintaining endothelial homeostasis and decreased levels have been associated with microvascular endothelial dysfunction. Other miRNAs, such as miR-802 and miR-103/107, are involved in insulin sensitivity in models of diabetes and obesity [178]. In a recent case–control study including symptomatic patients with HF, 13 different miRNAs were differentially expressed in HFpEF compared to HFrEF, most of them being down-regulated, such as miR-21-5p, miR-20a-5p, miR-130a-3p, miR-103a-3p, miR-423-5p, miR-19b-3p, miR-301-3p, let-7d-5p, miR-335-5p, miR-128a-3p and miR-25-3p. These miRNAs correlated with echocardiographic and cardiac magnetic resonance imaging (MRI) parameters of HF, suggesting that miRNAs could be involved in myocardial remodeling [179]. Overall, the different miRNA profiles expressed in HFpEF and HFrEF support the different pathobiological mechanisms underlying these two entities. More research is needed in order to select specific circulating miRNAs to better serve as prognostic and diagnostic biomarkers of HFpEF.

8.4. Proteomics and Metabolomics

Proteomic profiling is a powerful tool that allows for a large-scale characterization of the entire protein phenotype in HF. Investigating the various patterns of proteome changes provides further evidence of the different pathogenic mechanisms involved in HF. A recent study identified 29 unique HFpEF-associated proteins related to remodeling, inflammation, fibrosis, kidney injury and lipid metabolism. Of those, AOC3, CLSTN2, Gal-9 and MATN2 were associated with HFpEF hospitalization, while 11 others, including CDH2, CSTB, KIM1, PARP-1 and SPINT2, were associated with all-cause mortality, independently of other clinical factors and NT-proBNP [180]. Another study identified novel proteins related to HFpEF subtypes, associated with platelet degranulation and microvascular dysfunction (e.g., Gal3bp, ITIH3 and von Willebrand factor) and angiogenesis (e.g., LRG1 and IGFALS) [181]. An advanced proteomic profile has the potential for establishing more precise diagnostic and prognostic CV care for patients with HFpEF.

Metabolic dysfunction plays an important role in the development of HFpEF. Patients with HFpEF display distinct metabolic profiles when compared to those with HFrEF, including markers of impaired lipid metabolism, increased oxidative stress and enhanced collagen synthesis [182]. As an example, in spite of a higher prevalence of obesity and diabetes in patients with HFpEF compared to HFrEF, metabolites of fatty acid oxidation were expressed in a lower proportion in the HFpEF myocardium [183]. Other biomarkers of interest reflecting different metabolomic pathways in HFpEF are low levels of serine, cAMP and lysophosphatidylcholine and high levels of cystine, kynurenine and acylcarnitine, among many others [184].

9. Future Directions

HFpEF represents a multisystem disorder, a combination of risk factors, cardiac and extra-cardiac mechanisms, which are expressed by specific circulating biomarkers. Regarding their diagnostic value, a comprehensive overview of current studies assessing novel biomarkers demonstrated a high risk of bias, impacting the reliability of their results and their clinical utility. The main study limitations referred to the use of a case–control design, exclusion of important subsets of the HFpEF population, the absence of external validation and the absence of reference standard tests to confirm the diagnosis of HFpEF [185]. In order to correctly assess the incremental diagnostic value of novel biomarkers and to ensure their clinical uptake in our daily practice, methodological well-designed studies are needed. Such trials should have a prospective design and enroll a large number of patients with HFpEF in order to cover the phenotypical heterogeneity of this syndrome.

Regarding their prognostic utility, the combination of several biomarkers encompassing different pathophysiological pathways of HFpEF may demonstrate better predictive value than using individual biomarkers alone. Several studies aimed to assess the utility of a multi-marker approach for a better risk stratification of HFpEF patients, but more research is needed in this field in order to find a predictive model that effectively discriminates for both mortality and morbidity in HFpEF.

The advent of advanced proteomics and metabolomics technologies has enabled the identification of distinct biomarker profiles in HFpEF as compared to HFrEF. Development of these molecular biology techniques allowed us to define specific "biomarker signatures" of the different HFpEF phenotypes, providing the opportunity to explore new pathophysiological mechanisms and explore the dynamic changes in biomarkers after treatment interventions. The potential of these novel biomarkers is promising, but external validation in large cohort studies is needed before using them in clinical practice.

10. Discussion

The burden of HFpEF is continuously growing, surpassing the prevalence of HFrEF over the past decades. As a result, defining a standardized diagnostic and prognostic approach becomes crucial. Currently, the diagnosis of HFpEF in the non-acute setting remains challenging, as patients may experience symptoms only during exertion. The current diagnostic algorithm proposed by the European Society of Cardiology performs well in diagnosing HFpEF, but many cases require costly, invasive tests to confirm the diagnosis, which may not be readily available in all centers [186]. Consequently, research efforts have lately focused on finding novel circulating biomarkers for the detection and risk stratification of HFpEF.

Currently, NPs remain the gold standard for the diagnosis and prognosis of HFpEF, although their concentrations are greatly impacted by many co-existing conditions. In addition, NPs reflect only one pathophysiological mechanism, which is insufficient to characterize the complex phenotypical spectrum of HFpEF. As stated above, myocardial dysfunction in HFpEF is the result of the interaction between CV, metabolic, renal, pulmonary and geriatric conditions, each in different proportions. The impact of systemic inflammation can be evaluated by measuring various biomarkers, among which GDF-15 demonstrated additional value in refining the diagnosis and prognosis of patients with HFpEF. In addition, biomarkers reflecting myocardial fibrosis, such as Gal-3 and sST2, as well as those reflecting obesity and CKD, are involved in the development and progression of HFpEF and can be used for optimal risk stratification.

Previous studies characterized distinct phenogroups of patients with HFpEF, with important differences in circulating biomarkers [72,187]. Creating distinct biomarker profiles in patients with HFpEF will also enable us to select those who may benefit from distinct targeted interventions, such as mineralocorticoid receptor antagonists, angiotensin-converting enzyme inhibitors or angiotensin receptor blockers [188]. Until recently, the development of effective drugs for the treatment of HFpEF has been unsatisfying, with SGLT2 inhibitors being the only drugs with demonstrated improvement in clinical outcomes. However, depending on the phenogroup, biomarkers may be used to initiate tailored medication and monitor treatment efficacy in the population of HFpEF. As a result, biomarkers in HFpEF represent a continuously expanding field, with research efforts guided towards finding the ones with additional screening, diagnostic, prognostic and therapeutic roles.

11. Conclusions

The pathophysiology of underlying HFpEF remains a subject of controversy, although it is likely driven by a combination of several comorbidities, leading to low-grade systemic inflammation, microvascular dysfunction and ultimately cardiac remodeling and fibrosis. Given that HFpEF presents with clinical heterogeneity, the study of different biomarkers reflecting distinct pathophysiological pathways could provide major insights into our understanding of this complex disease. Many biomarkers have demonstrated their diagnostic and prognostic utility, but their lack of specificity, high costs and the absence of standardized measurement techniques have limited their applicability in clinical practice. A strategy based not only on NPs but also on other cardiac and non-cardiac biomarkers reflecting the comorbidities of HFpEF is likely useful to define the different phenotypes, stratify risk for adverse events and monitor treatment efficacy.

Author Contributions: Conceptualization, writing—original draft preparation, A.-M.V. and S.T.; methodology, resources, supervision, E.B.; supervision, writing—review and editing, C.D. All authors have read and agreed to the published version of the manuscript.

Funding: This research received no external funding.

Data Availability Statement: The original contributions presented in the study are included in the article, further inquiries can be directed to the corresponding author.

Acknowledgments: Publication of this paper was supported by the University of Medicine and Pharmacy Carol Davila, through the institutional program "Publish not Perish".

Conflicts of Interest: The authors declare no conflicts of interest.

References

1. McDonagh, T.A.; Metra, M.; Adamo, M.; Gardner, R.S.; Baumbach, A.; Böhm, M.; Burri, H.; Butler, J.; Čelutkienė, J.; Chioncel, O.; et al. 2021 ESC Guidelines for the diagnosis and treatment of acute and chronic heart failure. *Eur. Heart J.* **2021**, *42*, 3599–3726. [CrossRef] [PubMed]
2. Owan, T.E.; Hodge, D.O.; Herges, R.M.; Jacobsen, S.J.; Roger, V.L.; Redfield, M.M. Trends in Prevalence and Outcome of Heart Failure with Preserved Ejection Fraction. *N. Engl. J. Med.* **2006**, *355*, 251–259. [CrossRef]
3. Tsao, C.W.; Lyass, A.; Enserro, D.; Larson, M.G.; Ho, J.E.; Kizer, J.R.; Gottdiener, J.S.; Psaty, B.M.; Vasan, R.S. Temporal Trends in the Incidence of and Mortality Associated with Heart Failure with Preserved and Reduced Ejection Fraction. *JACC Heart Fail.* **2018**, *6*, 678–685. [CrossRef] [PubMed]
4. Shah, K.S.; Xu, H.; Matsouaka, R.A.; Bhatt, D.L.; Heidenreich, P.A.; Hernandez, A.F.; Devore, A.D.; Yancy, C.W.; Fonarow, G.C. Heart Failure with Preserved, Borderline, and Reduced Ejection Fraction: 5-Year Outcomes. *J. Am. Coll. Cardiol.* **2017**, *70*, 2476–2486. [CrossRef] [PubMed]
5. Paulus, W.J.; Tschöpe, C. A Novel Paradigm for Heart Failure with Preserved Ejection Fraction. *J. Am. Coll. Cardiol.* **2013**, *62*, 263–271. [CrossRef] [PubMed]
6. Ovchinnikov, A.G.; Arefieva, T.I.; Potekhina, A.V.; Filatova, A.Y.; Ageev, F.T.; Boytsov, S.A. The Molecular and Cellular Mechanisms Associated with a Microvascular Inflammation in the Pathogenesis of Heart Failure with Preserved Ejection Fraction. *Acta Naturae* **2020**, *12*, 40–51. [CrossRef] [PubMed]
7. Triposkiadis, F.; Giamouzis, G.; Parissis, J.; Starling, R.C.; Boudoulas, H.; Skoularigis, J.; Butler, J.; Filippatos, G. Reframing the association and significance of co-morbidities in heart failure. *Eur. J. Heart Fail.* **2016**, *18*, 744–758. [CrossRef]
8. Lee, S.; Kim, H.; Kil Oh, B.; Choi, H.; Sung, K.; Kang, J.; Lee, M.Y.; Lee, J. Association between metabolic syndrome and left ventricular geometric change including diastolic dysfunction. *Clin. Cardiol.* **2022**, *45*, 767–777. [CrossRef]
9. Seferović, P.M.; Paulus, W.J. Clinical diabetic cardiomyopathy: A two-faced disease with restrictive and dilated phenotypes. *Eur. Heart J.* **2015**, *36*, 1718–1727. [CrossRef]
10. Singh, R.M.; Waqar, T.; Howarth, F.C.; Adeghate, E.; Bidasee, K.; Singh, J. Hyperglycemia-induced cardiac contractile dysfunction in the diabetic heart. *Heart Fail. Rev.* **2018**, *23*, 37–54. [CrossRef]
11. Maack, C.; Lehrke, M.; Backs, J.; Heinzel, F.R.; Hulot, J.-S.; Marx, N.; Paulus, W.J.; Rossignol, P.; Taegtmeyer, H.; Bauersachs, J.; et al. Heart failure and diabetes: Metabolic alterations and therapeutic interventions: A state-of-the-art review from the Translational Research Committee of the Heart Failure Association–European Society of Cardiology. *Eur. Heart J.* **2018**, *39*, 4243–4254. [CrossRef] [PubMed]
12. Marx, N.; Federici, M.; Schütt, K.; Müller-Wieland, D.; Ajjan, R.A.; Antunes, M.J.; Christodorescu, R.M.; Crawford, C.; Di Angelantonio, E.; Eliasson, B.; et al. 2023 ESC Guidelines for the management of cardiovascular disease in patients with diabetes. *Eur. Heart J.* **2023**, *44*, 4043–4140. [CrossRef] [PubMed]
13. Mueller, C.; McDonald, K.; de Boer, R.A.; Maisel, A.; Cleland, J.G.; Kozhuharov, N.; Coats, A.J.; Metra, M.; Mebazaa, A.; Ruschitzka, F.; et al. Heart Failure Association of the European Society of Cardiology practical guidance on the use of natriuretic peptide concentrations. *Eur. J. Heart Fail.* **2019**, *21*, 715–731. [CrossRef] [PubMed]
14. Bachmann, K.N.; Gupta, D.K.; Xu, M.; Brittain, E.; Farber-Eger, E.; Arora, P.; Collins, S.; Wells, Q.S.; Wang, T.J. Unexpectedly Low Natriuretic Peptide Levels in Patients with Heart Failure. *JACC Heart Fail.* **2021**, *9*, 192–200. [CrossRef] [PubMed]
15. Harrison, N.; Favot, M.; Levy, P. The Role of Troponin for Acute Heart Failure. *Curr. Heart Fail. Rep.* **2019**, *16*, 21–31. [CrossRef] [PubMed]
16. Myhre, P.L.; O'meara, E.; Claggett, B.L.; de Denus, S.; Jarolim, P.; Anand, I.S.; Beldhuis, I.E.; Fleg, J.L.; Lewis, E.; Pitt, B.; et al. Cardiac Troponin I and Risk of Cardiac Events in Patients with Heart Failure and Preserved Ejection Fraction. *Circ. Heart Fail.* **2018**, *11*, e005312. [CrossRef] [PubMed]
17. Gohar, A.; Chong, J.P.; Liew, O.W.; Ruijter, H.D.; de Kleijn, D.P.; Sim, D.; Yeo, D.P.; Ong, H.Y.; Jaufeerally, F.; Leong, G.K.; et al. The prognostic value of highly sensitive cardiac troponin assays for adverse events in men and women with stable heart failure and a preserved vs. reduced ejection fraction. *Eur. J. Heart Fail.* **2017**, *19*, 1638–1647. [CrossRef]
18. Jakubiak, G.K. Cardiac Troponin Serum Concentration Measurement Is Useful Not Only in the Diagnosis of Acute Cardiovascular Events. *J. Pers. Med.* **2024**, *14*, 230. [CrossRef] [PubMed]
19. Eggers, K.M.; Lindahl, B. Application of Cardiac Troponin in Cardiovascular Diseases Other Than Acute Coronary Syndrome. *Clin. Chem.* **2017**, *63*, 223–235. [CrossRef]
20. Kosum, P.; Mattanapojanat, N.; Kongruttanachok, N.; Ariyachaipanic, A.H. GDF-15: A novel biomarker of heart failure predicts 30-day all-cause mortality and 30-day HF rehospitalization in patients with acute heart failure syndrome. *Eur. Heart J.* **2022**, *43* (Suppl. S1), ehab849.057. [CrossRef]
21. Luo, J.-W.; Duan, W.-H.; Song, L.; Yu, Y.-Q.; Shi, D.-Z. A Meta-Analysis of Growth Differentiation Factor-15 and Prognosis in Chronic Heart Failure. *Front. Cardiovasc. Med.* **2021**, *8*, 630818. [CrossRef] [PubMed]
22. Bradley, J.; Schelbert, E.B.; Bonnett, L.J.; A Lewis, G.; Lagan, J.; Orsborne, C.; Brown, P.F.; Black, N.; Naish, J.H.; Williams, S.G.; et al. Growth differentiation factor-15 in patients with or at risk of heart failure but before first hospitalisation. *Heart* **2023**, *110*, 195–201. [CrossRef] [PubMed]
23. Chen, H.; Chen, C.; Fang, J.; Wang, R.; Nie, W. Circulating galectin-3 on admission and prognosis in acute heart failure patients: A meta-analysis. *Heart Fail. Rev.* **2020**, *25*, 331–341. [CrossRef] [PubMed]

24. Shi, Y.; Dong, G.; Liu, J.; Shuang, X.; Liu, C.; Yang, C.; Qing, W.; Qiao, W. Clinical Implications of Plasma Galectin-3 in Heart Failure with Preserved Ejection Fraction: A Meta-Analysis. *Front. Cardiovasc. Med.* **2022**, *9*, 854501. [CrossRef] [PubMed]
25. Dudek, M.; Kałużna-Oleksy, M.; Migaj, J.; Sawczak, F.; Krysztofiak, H.; Lesiak, M.; Straburzyńska-Migaj, E. sST2 and Heart Failure—Clinical Utility and Prognosis. *J. Clin. Med.* **2023**, *12*, 3136. [CrossRef] [PubMed]
26. Maisel, A.; Xue, Y.; van Veldhuisen, D.J.; Voors, A.A.; Jaarsma, T.; Pang, P.S.; Butler, J.; Pitt, B.; Clopton, P.; de Boer, R.A. Effect of Spironolactone on 30-Day Death and Heart Failure Rehospitalization (from the COACH Study). *Am. J. Cardiol.* **2014**, *114*, 737–742. [CrossRef] [PubMed]
27. Sudoh, T.; Kangawa, K.; Minamino, N.; Matsuo, H. A new natriuretic peptide in porcine brain. *Nature* **1988**, *332*, 78–81. [CrossRef] [PubMed]
28. Goetze, J.P.; Bruneau, B.G.; Ramos, H.R.; Ogawa, T.; de Bold, M.K.; de Bold, A.J. Cardiac natriuretic peptides. *Nat. Rev. Cardiol.* **2020**, *17*, 698–717. [CrossRef]
29. Yoshimura, M.; Yasue, H.; Ogawa, H. Pathophysiological significance and clinical application of ANP and BNP in patients with heart failure. *Can. J. Physiol. Pharmacol.* **2001**, *79*, 730–735. [CrossRef]
30. Nishikimi, T.; Kuwahara, K.; Nakao, K. Current biochemistry, molecular biology, and clinical relevance of natriuretic peptides. *J. Cardiol.* **2011**, *57*, 131–140. [CrossRef]
31. Huelsmann, M.; Neuhold, S.; Resl, M.; Strunk, G.; Brath, H.; Francesconi, C.; Adlbrecht, C.; Prager, R.; Luger, A.; Pacher, R.; et al. PONTIAC (NT-proBNP Selected PreventiOn of cardiac eveNts in a populaTion of dIabetic patients without A history of Cardiac disease). *J. Am. Coll. Cardiol.* **2013**, *62*, 1365–1372. [CrossRef] [PubMed]
32. Ledwidge, M.; Gallagher, J.; Conlon, C.; Tallon, E.; O'connell, E.; Dawkins, I.; Watson, C.; O'hanlon, R.; Bermingham, M.; Patle, A.; et al. Natriuretic Peptide–Based Screening and Collaborative Care for Heart Failure. *JAMA* **2013**, *310*, 66. [CrossRef] [PubMed]
33. Remmelzwaal, S.; van Ballegooijen, A.J.; Schoonmade, L.J.; Canto, E.D.; Handoko, M.L.; Henkens, M.T.H.M.; van Empel, V.; Heymans, S.R.B.; Beulens, J.W.J. Natriuretic peptides for the detection of diastolic dysfunction and heart failure with preserved ejection fraction—A systematic review and meta-analysis. *BMC Med.* **2020**, *18*, 290. [CrossRef] [PubMed]
34. McCullough, P.A.; Nowak, R.M.; McCord, J.; Hollander, J.E.; Herrmann, H.C.; Steg, P.G.; Duc, P.; Westheim, A.; Omland, T.; Knudsen, C.W.; et al. B-Type Natriuretic Peptide and Clinical Judgment in Emergency Diagnosis of Heart Failure. *Circulation* **2002**, *106*, 416–422. [CrossRef] [PubMed]
35. Januzzi, J.L., Jr.; Camargo, C.A.; Anwaruddin, S.; Baggish, A.L.; Chen, A.A.; Krauser, D.G.; Tung, R.; Cameron, R.; Nagurney, J.T.; Chae, C.U.; et al. The N-terminal Pro-BNP Investigation of Dyspnea in the Emergency department (PRIDE) study. *Am. J. Cardiol.* **2005**, *95*, 948–954. [CrossRef] [PubMed]
36. van Veldhuisen, D.J.; Linssen, G.C.; Jaarsma, T.; van Gilst, W.H.; Hoes, A.W.; Tijssen, J.G.; Paulus, W.J.; Voors, A.A.; Hillege, H.L. B-Type Natriuretic Peptide and Prognosis in Heart Failure Patients with Preserved and Reduced Ejection Fraction. *J. Am. Coll. Cardiol.* **2013**, *61*, 1498–1506. [CrossRef] [PubMed]
37. Wang, T.J.; Larson, M.G.; Levy, D.; Benjamin, E.J.; Leip, E.P.; Wilson, P.W.; Vasan, R.S. Impact of Obesity on Plasma Natriuretic Peptide Levels. *Circulation* **2004**, *109*, 594–600. [CrossRef] [PubMed]
38. Heidenreich, P.A.; Bozkurt, B.; Aguilar, D.; Allen, L.A.; Byun, J.J.; Colvin, M.M.; Deswal, A.; Drazner, M.H.; Dunlay, S.M.; Evers, L.R.; et al. 2022 AHA/ACC/HFSA Guideline for the Management of Heart Failure: A Report of the American College of Cardiology/American Heart Association Joint Committee on Clinical Practice Guidelines. *Circulation* **2022**, *145*, E895–E1032. [CrossRef] [PubMed]
39. Kasahara, S.; Sakata, Y.; Nochioka, K.; Yamauchi, T.; Onose, T.; Tsuji, K.; Abe, R.; Oikawa, T.; Sato, M.; Aoyanagi, H.; et al. Comparable prognostic impact of BNP levels among HFpEF, Borderline HFpEF and HFrEF: A report from the CHART-2 Study. *Heart Vessel* **2018**, *33*, 997–1007. [CrossRef]
40. Kang, S.-H.; Park, J.J.; Choi, D.-J.; Yoon, C.-H.; Oh, I.-Y.; Kang, S.-M.; Yoo, B.-S.; Jeon, E.-S.; Kim, J.-J.; Cho, M.-C.; et al. Prognostic value of NT-proBNP in heart failure with preserved versus reduced EF. *Heart* **2015**, *101*, 1881–1888. [CrossRef]
41. Cunningham, J.W.; Vaduganathan, M.; Claggett, B.L.; Zile, M.R.; Anand, I.S.; Packer, M.; Zannad, F.; Lam, C.S.; Janssens, S.; Jhund, P.S.; et al. Effects of Sacubitril/Valsartan on N-Terminal Pro-B-Type Natriuretic Peptide in Heart Failure with Preserved Ejection Fraction. *JACC Heart Fail.* **2020**, *8*, 372–381. [CrossRef] [PubMed]
42. Cohen-Solal, A.; Logeart, D.; Huang, B.; Cai, D.; Nieminen, M.S.; Mebazaa, A. Lowered B-Type Natriuretic Peptide in Response to Levosimendan or Dobutamine Treatment Is Associated with Improved Survival in Patients with Severe Acutely Decompensated Heart Failure. *J. Am. Coll. Cardiol.* **2009**, *53*, 2343–2348. [CrossRef] [PubMed]
43. Bettencourt, P.; Azevedo, A.; Pimenta, J.; Frio, F.; Ferreira, S.; Ferreira, A. N-Terminal–Pro-Brain Natriuretic Peptide Predicts Outcome After Hospital Discharge in Heart Failure Patients. *Circulation* **2004**, *110*, 2168–2174. [CrossRef] [PubMed]
44. Salah, K.; Stienen, S.; Pinto, Y.M.; Eurlings, L.W.; Metra, M.; Bayes-Genis, A.; Verdiani, V.; Tijssen, J.G.P.; Kok, W.E. Prognosis and NT-proBNP in heart failure patients with preserved versus reduced ejection fraction. *Heart* **2019**, *105*, 1182–1189. [CrossRef]
45. Michtalik, H.J.; Yeh, H.-C.; Campbell, C.Y.; Haq, N.; Park, H.; Clarke, W.; Brotman, D.J. Acute Changes in N-Terminal Pro-B-Type Natriuretic Peptide during Hospitalization and Risk of Readmission and Mortality in Patients with Heart Failure. *Am. J. Cardiol.* **2011**, *107*, 1191–1195. [CrossRef]
46. Kociol, R.D.; Horton, J.R.; Fonarow, G.C.; Reyes, E.M.; Shaw, L.K.; O'Connor, C.M.; Felker, G.M.; Hernandez, A.F. Admission, Discharge, or Change in B-Type Natriuretic Peptide and Long-Term Outcomes. *Circ. Heart Fail.* **2011**, *4*, 628–636. [CrossRef]

47. Omar, H.R.; Guglin, M. Discharge BNP is a stronger predictor of 6-month mortality in acute heart failure compared with baseline BNP and admission-to-discharge percentage BNP reduction. *Int. J. Cardiol.* **2016**, *221*, 1116–1122. [CrossRef]
48. Anand, I.S.; Claggett, B.; Liu, J.; Shah, A.M.; Rector, T.S.; Shah, S.J.; Desai, A.S.; O'meara, E.; Fleg, J.L.; Pfeffer, M.A.; et al. Interaction between Spironolactone and Natriuretic Peptides in Patients with Heart Failure and Preserved Ejection Fraction: From the TOPCAT Trial. *JACC Heart Fail.* **2017**, *5*, 241–252. [CrossRef]
49. Anand, I.S.; Rector, T.S.; Cleland, J.G.; Kuskowski, M.; McKelvie, R.S.; Persson, H.; McMurray, J.J.; Zile, M.R.; Komajda, M.; Massie, B.M.; et al. Prognostic Value of Baseline Plasma Amino-Terminal Pro-Brain Natriuretic Peptide and Its Interactions with Irbesartan Treatment Effects in Patients with Heart Failure and Preserved Ejection Fraction. *Circ. Heart Fail.* **2011**, *4*, 569–577. [CrossRef]
50. Januzzi, J.L.; Butler, J.; Zannad, F.; Filippatos, G.; Ferreira, J.P.; Pocock, S.J.; Sattar, N.; Verma, S.; Vedin, O.; Iwata, T.; et al. Prognostic Implications of N-Terminal Pro–B-Type Natriuretic Peptide and High-Sensitivity Cardiac Troponin T in EMPEROR-Preserved. *JACC Heart Fail.* **2022**, *10*, 512–524. [CrossRef]
51. Maeder, M.T.; Rickenbacher, P.; Rickli, H.; Abbühl, H.; Gutmann, M.; Erne, P.; Vuilliomenet, A.; Peter, M.; Pfisterer, M.; Rocca, H.B.; et al. N-terminal pro brain natriuretic peptide-guided management in patients with heart failure and preserved ejection fraction: Findings from the Trial of Intensified versus standard Medical therapy in Elderly patients with Congestive Heart Failure (TIME-CHF). *Eur. J. Heart Fail.* **2013**, *15*, 1148–1156. [CrossRef] [PubMed]
52. Khan, M.S.; Siddiqi, T.J.; Usman, M.S.; Sreenivasan, J.; Fugar, S.; Riaz, H.; Murad, M.; Mookadam, F.; Figueredo, V.M. Does natriuretic peptide monitoring improve outcomes in heart failure patients? A systematic review and meta-analysis. *Int. J. Cardiol.* **2018**, *263*, 80–87. [CrossRef] [PubMed]
53. Obokata, M.; Reddy, Y.N.; Melenovsky, V.; Kane, G.C.; Olson, T.P.; Jarolim, P.; Borlaug, B.A. Myocardial Injury and Cardiac Reserve in Patients with Heart Failure and Preserved Ejection Fraction. *J. Am. Coll. Cardiol.* **2018**, *72*, 29–40. [CrossRef] [PubMed]
54. Lokaj, P.; Spinar, J.; Spinarova, L.; Malek, F.; Ludka, O.; Krejci, J.; Ostadal, P.; Vondrakova, D.; Labr, K.; Spinarova, M.; et al. Prognostic value of high-sensitivity cardiac troponin I in heart failure patients with mid-range and reduced ejection fraction. *PLoS ONE* **2021**, *16*, e0255271. [CrossRef]
55. Aimo, A.; Januzzi, J.J.L.; Vergaro, G.; Ripoli, A.; Latini, R.; Masson, S.; Magnoli, M.; Anand, I.S.; Cohn, J.N.; Tavazzi, L.; et al. Prognostic Value of High-Sensitivity Troponin T in Chronic Heart Failure. *Circulation* **2018**, *137*, 286–297. [CrossRef]
56. Fudim, M.; Ambrosy, A.P.; Sun, J.L.; Anstrom, K.J.; Bart, B.A.; Butler, J.; AbouEzzeddine, O.; Greene, S.J.; Mentz, R.J.; Redfield, M.M.; et al. High-Sensitivity Troponin I in Hospitalized and Ambulatory Patients with Heart Failure with Preserved Ejection Fraction: Insights from the Heart Failure Clinical Research Network. *J. Am. Heart Assoc.* **2018**, *7*, e010364. [CrossRef]
57. Kim, B.S.; Kwon, C.H.; Chang, H.; Choi, J.-H.; Kim, H.-J.; Kim, S.H. The association of cardiac troponin and cardiovascular events in patients with concomitant heart failure preserved ejection fraction and atrial fibrillation. *BMC Cardiovasc. Disord.* **2023**, *23*, 273. [CrossRef] [PubMed]
58. Arenja, N.; Reichlin, T.; Drexler, B.; Oshima, S.; Denhaerynck, K.; Haaf, P.; Potocki, M.; Breidthardt, T.; Noveanu, M.; Stelzig, C.; et al. Sensitive cardiac troponin in the diagnosis and risk stratification of acute heart failure. *J. Intern. Med.* **2012**, *271*, 598–607. [CrossRef]
59. Peacock, W.F.I.; De Marco, T.; Fonarow, G.C.; Diercks, D.; Wynne, J.; Apple, F.S.; Wu, A.H. Cardiac Troponin and Outcome in Acute Heart Failure. *N. Engl. J. Med.* **2008**, *358*, 2117–2126. [CrossRef]
60. Pandey, A.; Golwala, H.; Sheng, S.; DeVore, A.D.; Hernandez, A.F.; Bhatt, D.L.; Heidenreich, P.A.; Yancy, C.W.; de Lemos, J.A.; Fonarow, G.C. Factors Associated with and Prognostic Implications of Cardiac Troponin Elevation in Decompensated Heart Failure with Preserved Ejection Fraction. *JAMA Cardiol.* **2017**, *2*, 136. [CrossRef]
61. Pocock, S.J.; Ferreira, J.P.; Packer, M.; Zannad, F.; Filippatos, G.; Kondo, T.; McMurray, J.J.; Solomon, S.D.; Januzzi, J.L.; Iwata, T.; et al. Biomarker-driven prognostic models in chronic heart failure with preserved ejection fraction: The EMPEROR–Preserved trial. *Eur. J. Heart Fail.* **2022**, *24*, 1869–1878. [CrossRef] [PubMed]
62. Brouwers, F.P.; van Gilst, W.H.; Damman, K.; Berg, M.P.v.D.; Gansevoort, R.T.; Bakker, S.J.; Hillege, H.L.; van Veldhuisen, D.J.; van der Harst, P.; de Boer, R.A.; et al. Clinical Risk Stratification Optimizes Value of Biomarkers to Predict New-Onset Heart Failure in a Community-Based Cohort. *Circ. Heart Fail.* **2014**, *7*, 723–731. [CrossRef] [PubMed]
63. Brouwers, F.P.; de Boer, R.A.; van der Harst, P.; Voors, A.A.; Gansevoort, R.T.; Bakker, S.J.; Hillege, H.L.; van Veldhuisen, D.J.; van Gilst, W.H. Incidence and epidemiology of new onset heart failure with preserved vs. reduced ejection fraction in a community-based cohort: 11-year follow-up of PREVEND. *Eur. Heart. J.* **2013**, *34*, 1424–1431. [CrossRef]
64. de Boer, R.A.; Nayor, M.; Defilippi, C.R.; Enserro, D.; Bhambhani, V.; Kizer, J.R.; Blaha, M.J.; Brouwers, F.P.; Cushman, M.; Lima, J.A.C.; et al. Association of Cardiovascular Biomarkers with Incident Heart Failure with Preserved and Reduced Ejection Fraction. *JAMA Cardiol.* **2018**, *3*, 215. [CrossRef] [PubMed]
65. Watson, C.J.; Gallagher, J.; Wilkinson, M.; Russell-Hallinan, A.; Tea, I.; James, S.; O'reilly, J.; O'connell, E.; Zhou, S.; Ledwidge, M.; et al. Biomarker profiling for risk of future heart failure (HFpEF) development. *J. Transl. Med.* **2021**, *19*, 61. [CrossRef]
66. Ridker, P.M.; Everett, B.M.; Thuren, T.; MacFadyen, J.G.; Chang, W.H.; Ballantyne, C.; Fonseca, F.; Nicolau, J.; Koenig, W.; Anker, S.D.; et al. Antiinflammatory Therapy with Canakinumab for Atherosclerotic Disease. *N. Engl. J. Med.* **2017**, *377*, 1119–1131. [CrossRef]

67. Everett, B.M.; Cornel, J.H.; Lainscak, M.; Anker, S.D.; Abbate, A.; Thuren, T.; Libby, P.; Glynn, R.J.; Ridker, P.M. Anti-Inflammatory Therapy with Canakinumab for the Prevention of Hospitalization for Heart Failure. *Circulation* **2019**, *139*, 1289–1299. [CrossRef] [PubMed]
68. Yin, D.; Yan, X.; Bai, X.; Tian, A.; Gao, Y.; Li, J. Prognostic value of Growth differentiation factors 15 in Acute heart failure patients with preserved ejection fraction. *ESC Heart Fail.* **2023**, *10*, 1025–1034. [CrossRef] [PubMed]
69. Gao, Y.; Bai, X.; Lu, J.; Zhang, L.; Yan, X.; Huang, X.; Dai, H.; Wang, Y.; Hou, L.; Wang, S.; et al. Prognostic Value of Multiple Circulating Biomarkers for 2-Year Death in Acute Heart Failure with Preserved Ejection Fraction. *Front. Cardiovasc. Med.* **2021**, *8*, 779282. [CrossRef]
70. Fernandez, A.B.M.; Ferrero-Gregori, A.; Garcia-Osuna, A.; Mirabet-Perez, S.; Pirla-Buxo, M.J.; Cinca-Cuscullola, J.; Ordonez-Llanos, J.; Minguell, E.R. Growth differentiation factor 15 as mortality predictor in heart failure patients with non-reduced ejection fraction. *ESC Heart Fail.* **2020**, *7*, 2223–2229. [CrossRef]
71. Chan, M.M.; Santhanakrishnan, R.; Chong, J.P.; Chen, Z.; Tai, B.C.; Liew, O.W.; Ng, T.P.; Ling, L.H.; Sim, D.; Leong, K.T.G.; et al. Growth differentiation factor 15 in heart failure with preserved vs. reduced ejection fraction. *Eur. J. Heart Fail.* **2016**, *18*, 81–88. [CrossRef] [PubMed]
72. Henkens, M.T.; van Ommen, A.; Remmelzwaal, S.; Valstar, G.B.; Wang, P.; Verdonschot, J.A.; Hazebroek, M.R.; Hofstra, L.; van Empel, V.P.; Beulens, J.W.; et al. The HFA-PEFF score identifies 'early-HFpEF' phenogroups associated with distinct biomarker profiles. *ESC Heart Fail.* **2022**, *9*, 2032–2036. [CrossRef] [PubMed]
73. Koller, L.; Kleber, M.; Goliasch, G.; Sulzgruber, P.; Scharnagl, H.; Silbernagel, G.; Grammer, T.; Delgado, G.; Tomaschitz, A.; Pilz, S.; et al. C-reactive protein predicts mortality in patients referred for coronary angiography and symptoms of heart failure with preserved ejection fraction. *Eur. J. Heart Fail.* **2014**, *16*, 758–766. [CrossRef] [PubMed]
74. Ferreira, J.P.; Claggett, B.L.; Liu, J.; Sharma, A.; Desai, A.S.; Anand, I.S.; O'Meara, E.; Rouleau, J.L.; De Denus, S.; Pitt, B.; et al. High-sensitivity C-reactive protein in heart failure with preserved ejection fraction: Findings from TOPCAT. *Int. J. Cardiol.* **2024**, *402*, 131818. [CrossRef] [PubMed]
75. Lakhani, I.; Wong, M.V.; Hung, J.K.F.; Gong, M.; Bin Waleed, K.; Xia, Y.; Lee, S.; Roever, L.; Liu, T.; Tse, G.; et al. Diagnostic and prognostic value of serum C-reactive protein in heart failure with preserved ejection fraction: A systematic review and meta-analysis. *Heart Fail. Rev.* **2021**, *26*, 1141–1150. [CrossRef] [PubMed]
76. Alogna, A.; Koepp, K.E.; Sabbah, M.; Netto, J.M.E.; Jensen, M.D.; Kirkland, J.L.; Lam, C.S.; Obokata, M.; Petrie, M.C.; Ridker, P.M.; et al. Interleukin-6 in Patients with Heart Failure and Preserved Ejection Fraction. *JACC Heart Fail.* **2023**, *11*, 1549–1561. [CrossRef] [PubMed]
77. Mooney, L.; Jackson, C.; McConnachie, A.; Myles, R.; McMurray, J.; Petrie, M.; Jhund, P.; Lang, N. Interleukin-6 and outcomes in patients recently hospitalized with heart failure and preserved ejection fraction. *Eur. Heart J.* **2021**, *42*, ehab724.0738. [CrossRef]
78. Chia, Y.C.; Kieneker, L.M.; van Hassel, G.; Binnenmars, S.H.; Nolte, I.M.; van Zanden, J.J.; van der Meer, P.; Navis, G.; Voors, A.A.; Bakker, S.J.L.; et al. Interleukin 6 and Development of Heart Failure with Preserved Ejection Fraction in the General Population. *J. Am. Heart Assoc.* **2021**, *10*, e018549. [CrossRef] [PubMed]
79. Wischhusen, J.; Melero, I.; Fridman, W.H. Growth/Differentiation Factor-15 (GDF-15): From Biomarker to Novel Targetable Immune Checkpoint. *Front. Immunol.* **2020**, *11*, 951. [CrossRef]
80. Johnen, H.; Lin, S.; Kuffner, T.; Brown, D.A.; Tsai, V.W.-W.; Bauskin, A.R.; Wu, L.; Pankhurst, G.; Jiang, L.; Junankar, S.; et al. Tumor-induced anorexia and weight loss are mediated by the TGF-β superfamily cytokine MIC-1. *Nat. Med.* **2007**, *13*, 1333–1340. [CrossRef]
81. Lerner, L.; Tao, J.; Liu, Q.; Nicoletti, R.; Feng, B.; Krieger, B.; Mazsa, E.; Siddiquee, Z.; Wang, R.; Huang, L.; et al. MAP3K11/GDF15 axis is a critical driver of cancer cachexia. *J. Cachexia Sarcopenia Muscle* **2016**, *7*, 467–482. [CrossRef] [PubMed]
82. Adela, R.; Banerjee, S.K. GDF-15 as a Target and Biomarker for Diabetes and Cardiovascular Diseases: A Translational Prospective. *J. Diabetes Res.* **2015**, *2015*, 1–14. [CrossRef] [PubMed]
83. Xie, S.; Lui, L.; Ma, R.; Graham, C.; Chan, P.; Chan, F.; Fung, E. Elevated GDF-15 levels may indicate malnutrition in chronic compensated heart failure with or without diabetes mellitus. *Eur. Heart J.* **2020**, *41*, ehaa946.1169. [CrossRef]
84. Wollert, K.C.; Kempf, T. Growth Differentiation Factor 15 in Heart Failure: An Update. *Curr. Heart Fail. Rep.* **2012**, *9*, 337–345. [CrossRef] [PubMed]
85. Bouabdallaoui, N.; Claggett, B.; Zile, M.R.; McMurray, J.J.; O'Meara, E.; Packer, M.; Prescott, M.F.; Swedberg, K.; Solomon, S.D.; Rouleau, J.L.; et al. Growth differentiation factor-15 is not modified by sacubitril/valsartan and is an independent marker of risk in patients with heart failure and reduced ejection fraction: The PARADIGM-HF trial. *Eur. J. Heart Fail.* **2018**, *20*, 1701–1709. [CrossRef] [PubMed]
86. Anand, I.S.; Kempf, T.; Rector, T.S.; Tapken, H.; Allhoff, T.; Jantzen, F.; Kuskowski, M.; Cohn, J.N.; Drexler, H.; Wollert, K.C. Serial Measurement of Growth-Differentiation Factor-15 in Heart Failure. *Circulation* **2010**, *122*, 1387–1395. [CrossRef]
87. Binder, M.S.; Yanek, L.R.; Yang, W.; Butcher, B.; Norgard, S.; Marine, J.E.; Kolandaivelu, A.; Chrispin, J.; Fedarko, N.S.; Calkins, H.; et al. Growth Differentiation Factor-15 Predicts Mortality and Heart Failure Exacerbation but Not Ventricular Arrhythmias in Patients with Cardiomyopathy. *J. Am. Heart Assoc.* **2023**, *12*, e8023. [CrossRef] [PubMed]
88. Lewis, G.A.; Rosala-Hallas, A.; Dodd, S.; Schelbert, E.B.; Williams, S.G.; Cunnington, C.; McDonagh, T.; Miller, C.A. Characteristics Associated with Growth Differentiation Factor 15 in Heart Failure with Preserved Ejection Fraction and the Impact of Pirfenidone. *J. Am. Heart Assoc.* **2022**, *11*, e024668. [CrossRef]

89. Conte, M.; Giuliani, C.; Chiariello, A.; Iannuzzi, V.; Franceschi, C.; Salvioli, S. GDF15, an emerging key player in human aging. *Ageing Res. Rev.* **2022**, *75*, 101569. [CrossRef]
90. Wallentin, L.; Hijazi, Z.; Andersson, U.; Alexander, J.H.; De Caterina, R.; Hanna, M.; Horowitz, J.D.; Hylek, E.M.; Lopes, R.D.; Åsberg, S.; et al. Growth Differentiation Factor 15, a Marker of Oxidative Stress and Inflammation, for Risk Assessment in Patients with Atrial Fibrillation. *Circulation* **2014**, *130*, 1847–1858. [CrossRef]
91. Berg, D.D.; Ruff, C.T.; Jarolim, P.; Giugliano, R.P.; Nordio, F.; Lanz, H.J.; Mercuri, M.F.; Antman, E.M.; Braunwald, E.; Morrow, D.A. Performance of the ABC Scores for Assessing the Risk of Stroke or Systemic Embolism and Bleeding in Patients with Atrial Fibrillation in ENGAGE AF-TIMI 48. *Circulation* **2019**, *139*, 760–771. [CrossRef]
92. Santema, B.T.; Chan, M.M.Y.; Tromp, J.; Dokter, M.; van der Wal, H.H.; Emmens, J.E.; Takens, J.; Samani, N.J.; Ng, L.L.; Lang, C.C.; et al. The influence of atrial fibrillation on the levels of NT-proBNP versus GDF-15 in patients with heart failure. *Clin. Res. Cardiol.* **2020**, *109*, 331–338. [CrossRef]
93. Ridker, P.M.; Libby, P.; MacFadyen, J.G.; Thuren, T.; Ballantyne, C.; Fonseca, F.; Koenig, W.; Shimokawa, H.; Everett, B.M.; Glynn, R.J. Modulation of the interleukin-6 signalling pathway and incidence rates of atherosclerotic events and all-cause mortality: Analyses from the Canakinumab Anti-Inflammatory Thrombosis Outcomes Study (CANTOS). *Eur. Heart J.* **2018**, *39*, 3499–3507. [CrossRef] [PubMed]
94. Köktürk, U.; Püşüroğlu, H.; Somuncu, M.U.; Akgül, Ö.; Uygur, B.; Özyılmaz, S.; Işıksaçan, N.; Sürgit, Ö.; Yıldırım, A. Short and Long-Term Prognostic Significance of Galectin-3 in Patients with ST-Elevation Myocardial Infarction Undergoing Primary Percutaneous Coronary Intervention. *Angiology* **2023**, *74*, 889–896. [CrossRef]
95. Grandin, E.W.; Jarolim, P.; A Murphy, S.; Ritterova, L.; Cannon, C.P.; Braunwald, E.; A Morrow, D. Galectin-3 and the Development of Heart Failure after Acute Coronary Syndrome: Pilot Experience from PROVE IT-TIMI 22. *Clin. Chem.* **2012**, *58*, 267–273. [CrossRef] [PubMed]
96. Agnello, L.; Bivona, G.; Sasso, B.L.; Scazzone, C.; Bazan, V.; Bellia, C.; Ciaccio, M. Galectin-3 in acute coronary syndrome. *Clin. Biochem.* **2017**, *50*, 797–803. [CrossRef]
97. Miró, Ò.; de la Presa, B.G.; Herrero-Puente, P.; Bonifacio, R.F.; Möckel, M.; Mueller, C.; Casals, G.; Sandalinas, S.; Llorens, P.; Martín-Sánchez, F.J.; et al. The GALA study: Relationship between galectin-3 serum levels and short- and long-term outcomes of patients with acute heart failure. *Biomarkers* **2017**, *22*, 731–739. [CrossRef]
98. van Kimmenade, R.R.; Jr, J.L.J.; Ellinor, P.T.; Sharma, U.C.; Bakker, J.A.; Low, A.F.; Martinez, A.; Crijns, H.J.; MacRae, C.A.; Menheere, P.P.; et al. Utility of Amino-Terminal Pro-Brain Natriuretic Peptide, Galectin-3, and Apelin for the Evaluation of Patients with Acute Heart Failure. *J. Am. Coll. Cardiol.* **2006**, *48*, 1217–1224. [CrossRef] [PubMed]
99. van der Velde, A.R.; Gullestad, L.; Ueland, T.; Aukrust, P.; Guo, Y.; Adourian, A.; Muntendam, P.; van Veldhuisen, D.J.; de Boer, R.A. Prognostic Value of Changes in Galectin-3 Levels over Time in Patients with Heart Failure. *Circ. Heart Fail.* **2013**, *6*, 219–226. [CrossRef]
100. Baccouche, B.M.; Rhodenhiser, E. Galectin-3 and HFpEF: Clarifying an Emerging Relationship. *Curr. Cardiol. Rev.* **2023**, *19*, 19–26. [CrossRef]
101. Zile, M.R.; Jhund, P.S.; Baicu, C.F.; Claggett, B.L.; Pieske, B.; Voors, A.A.; Prescott, M.F.; Shi, V.; Lefkowitz, M.; McMurray, J.J.; et al. Plasma Biomarkers Reflecting Profibrotic Processes in Heart Failure with a Preserved Ejection Fraction. *Circ. Heart Fail.* **2016**, *9*, e002551. [CrossRef] [PubMed]
102. Januzzi, J.L.; Peacock, W.F.; Maisel, A.S.; Chae, C.U.; Jesse, R.L.; Baggish, A.L.; O'Donoghue, M.; Sakhuja, R.; Chen, A.A.; van Kimmenade, R.R.; et al. Measurement of the Interleukin Family Member ST2 in Patients with Acute Dyspnea. *J. Am. Coll. Cardiol.* **2007**, *50*, 607–613. [CrossRef] [PubMed]
103. van Vark, L.C.; Lesman-Leegte, I.; Baart, S.J.; Postmus, D.; Pinto, Y.M.; Orsel, J.G.; Westenbrink, B.D.; Rocca, H.P.B.-L.; van Miltenburg, A.J.; Boersma, E.; et al. Prognostic Value of Serial ST2 Measurements in Patients with Acute Heart Failure. *J. Am. Coll. Cardiol.* **2017**, *70*, 2378–2388. [CrossRef] [PubMed]
104. Aimo, A.; Vergaro, G.; Ripoli, A.; Bayes-Genis, A.; Figal, D.A.P.; de Boer, R.A.; Lassus, J.; Mebazaa, A.; Gayat, E.; Breidthardt, T.; et al. Meta-Analysis of Soluble Suppression of Tumorigenicity-2 and Prognosis in Acute Heart Failure. *JACC Heart Fail.* **2017**, *5*, 287–296. [CrossRef] [PubMed]
105. Aimo, A.; Vergaro, G.; Passino, C.; Ripoli, A.; Ky, B.; Miller, W.L.; Bayes-Genis, A.; Anand, I.; Januzzi, J.L.; Emdin, M. Prognostic Value of Soluble Suppression of Tumorigenicity-2 in Chronic Heart Failure. *JACC Heart Fail.* **2017**, *5*, 280–286. [CrossRef] [PubMed]
106. Dong, G.; Chen, H.; Zhang, H.; Gu, Y. Long-Term and Short-Term Prognostic Value of Circulating Soluble Suppression of Tumorigenicity-2 Concentration in Chronic Heart Failure: A Systematic Review and Meta-Analysis. *Cardiology* **2021**, *146*, 433–440. [CrossRef] [PubMed]
107. Chirinos, J.A.; Orlenko, A.; Zhao, L.; Basso, M.D.; Cvijic, M.E.; Li, Z.; Spires, T.E.; Yarde, M.; Wang, Z.; Seiffert, D.A.; et al. Multiple Plasma Biomarkers for Risk Stratification in Patients with Heart Failure and Preserved Ejection Fraction. *J. Am. Coll. Cardiol.* **2020**, *75*, 1281–1295. [CrossRef] [PubMed]
108. Zamora, E.; Lupón, J.; de Antonio, M.; Galán, A.; Domingo, M.; Urrutia, A.; Troya, M.; Bayes-Genis, A. Renal function largely influences Galectin-3 prognostic value in heart failure. *Int. J. Cardiol.* **2014**, *177*, 171–177. [CrossRef] [PubMed]
109. AbouEzzeddine, O.F.; Haines, P.; Stevens, S.; Nativi-Nicolau, J.; Felker, G.M.; Borlaug, B.A.; Chen, H.H.; Tracy, R.P.; Braunwald, E.; Redfield, M.M. Galectin-3 in Heart Failure with Preserved Ejection Fraction. *JACC Heart Fail.* **2015**, *3*, 245–252. [CrossRef]

110. Horiuchi, Y.; Wettersten, N.; VAN Veldhuisen, D.J.; Mueller, C.; Filippatos, G.; Nowak, R.; Hogan, C.; Kontos, M.C.; Cannon, C.M.; Müeller, G.A.; et al. Galectin-3, Acute Kidney Injury and Myocardial Damage in Patients with Acute Heart Failure. *J. Card. Fail.* **2023**, *29*, 269–277. [CrossRef]
111. Edelmann, F.; Holzendorf, V.; Wachter, R.; Nolte, K.; Schmidt, A.G.; Kraigher-Krainer, E.; Duvinage, A.; Unkelbach, I.; Düngen, H.; Tschöpe, C.; et al. Galectin-3 in patients with heart failure with preserved ejection fraction: Results from the Aldo-DHF trial. *Eur. J. Heart Fail.* **2015**, *17*, 214–223. [CrossRef]
112. Rabkin, S.W.; Tang, J.K.K. The utility of growth differentiation factor-15, galectin-3, and sST2 as biomarkers for the diagnosis of heart failure with preserved ejection fraction and compared to heart failure with reduced ejection fraction: A systematic review. *Heart Fail. Rev.* **2021**, *26*, 799–812. [CrossRef]
113. Riccardi, M.; Myhre, P.L.; Zelniker, T.A.; Metra, M.; Januzzi, J.L.; Inciardi, R.M. Soluble ST2 in Heart Failure: A Clinical Role beyond B-Type Natriuretic Peptide. *J. Cardiovasc. Dev. Dis.* **2023**, *10*, 468. [CrossRef] [PubMed]
114. Pascual-Figal, D.A.; Pérez-Martínez, M.T.; Asensio-Lopez, M.C.; Sanchez-Más, J.; García-García, M.E.; Martinez, C.M.; Lencina, M.; Jara, R.; Januzzi, J.L.; Lax, A. Pulmonary Production of Soluble ST2 in Heart Failure. *Circ. Heart Fail.* **2018**, *11*, e005488. [CrossRef] [PubMed]
115. Emdin, M.; Aimo, A.; Vergaro, G.; Bayes-Genis, A.; Lupón, J.; Latini, R.; Meessen, J.; Anand, I.S.; Cohn, J.N.; Gravning, J.; et al. sST2 Predicts Outcome in Chronic Heart Failure Beyond NT−proBNP and High-Sensitivity Troponin T. *J. Am. Coll. Cardiol.* **2018**, *72*, 2309–2320. [CrossRef]
116. Lupón, J.; de Antonio, M.; Galán, A.; Vila, J.; Zamora, E.; Urrutia, A.; Bayes-Genis, A. Combined Use of the Novel Biomarkers High-Sensitivity Troponin T and ST2 for Heart Failure Risk Stratification vs. Conventional Assessment. *Mayo Clin. Proc.* **2013**, *88*, 234–243. [CrossRef] [PubMed]
117. AbouEzzeddine, O.F.; McKie, P.M.; Dunlay, S.M.; Stevens, S.R.; Felker, G.M.; Borlaug, B.A.; Chen, H.H.; Tracy, R.P.; Braunwald, E.; Redfield, M.M. Soluble ST2 in Heart Failure with Preserved Ejection Fraction. *J. Am. Heart Assoc.* **2017**, *6*, e004382. [CrossRef]
118. Shah, R.V.; Chen-Tournoux, A.A.; Picard, M.H.; van Kimmenade, R.R.J.; Januzzi, J.L. Serum Levels of the Interleukin-1 Receptor Family Member ST2, Cardiac Structure and Function, and Long-Term Mortality in Patients with Acute Dyspnea. *Circ. Heart Fail.* **2009**, *2*, 311–319. [CrossRef]
119. Wang, Z.; Pan, X.; Xu, H.; Wu, Y.; Jia, X.; Fang, Y.; Lu, Y.; Xu, Y.; Zhang, J.; Su, Y. Serum Soluble ST2 Is a Valuable Prognostic Biomarker in Patients with Acute Heart Failure. *Front. Cardiovasc. Med.* **2022**, *9*, 812654. [CrossRef]
120. Najjar, E.; Faxén, U.L.; Hage, C.; Donal, E.; Daubert, J.-C.; Linde, C.; Lund, L.H. ST2 in heart failure with preserved and reduced ejection fraction. *Scand. Cardiovasc. J.* **2019**, *53*, 21–27. [CrossRef]
121. Shi, Y.; Liu, J.; Liu, C.; Shuang, X.; Yang, C.; Qiao, W.; Dong, G. Diagnostic and prognostic value of serum soluble suppression of tumorigenicity-2 in heart failure with preserved ejection fraction: A systematic review and meta-analysis. *Front. Cardiovasc. Med.* **2022**, *9*, 937291. [CrossRef] [PubMed]
122. Sinning, C.; Kempf, T.; Schwarzl, M.; Lanfermann, S.; Ojeda, F.; Schnabel, R.B.; Zengin, E.; Wild, P.S.; Lackner, K.-J.; Munzel, T.; et al. Biomarkers for characterization of heart failure—Distinction of heart failure with preserved and reduced ejection fraction. *Int. J. Cardiol.* **2017**, *227*, 272–277. [CrossRef] [PubMed]
123. Wang, Y.-C.; Yu, C.-C.; Chiu, F.-C.; Tsai, C.-T.; Lai, L.-P.; Hwang, J.-J.; Lin, J.-L. Soluble ST2 as a Biomarker for Detecting Stable Heart Failure with a Normal Ejection Fraction in Hypertensive Patients. *J. Card. Fail.* **2013**, *19*, 163–168. [CrossRef] [PubMed]
124. Yang, C.; Fan, Z.; Wu, J.; Zhang, J.; Zhang, W.; Yang, J.; Yang, J. The Diagnostic Value of Soluble ST2 in Heart Failure: A Meta-Analysis. *Front. Cardiovasc. Med.* **2021**, *8*, 685904. [CrossRef]
125. Patel, R.B.; Mehta, R.; Redfield, M.M.; Borlaug, B.A.; Hernandez, A.F.; Shah, S.J.; Dubin, R.F. Renal Dysfunction in Heart Failure with Preserved Ejection Fraction: Insights from the RELAX Trial. *J. Card. Fail.* **2020**, *26*, 233–242. [CrossRef] [PubMed]
126. Kenneally, L.F.; Lorenzo, M.; Romero-González, G.; Cobo, M.; Núñez, G.; Górriz, J.L.; Barrios, A.G.; Fudim, M.; de la Espriella, R.; Núñez, J. Kidney function changes in acute heart failure: A practical approach to interpretation and management. *Clin. Kidney J.* **2023**, *16*, 1587–1599. [CrossRef]
127. Kang, J.; Park, J.J.; Cho, Y.; Oh, I.; Park, H.; Lee, S.E.; Kim, M.; Cho, H.; Lee, H.; Choi, J.O.; et al. Predictors and Prognostic Value of Worsening Renal Function during Admission in HFpEF Versus HFrEF: Data from the KorAHF (Korean Acute Heart Failure) Registry. *J. Am. Heart Assoc.* **2018**, *7*, e007910. [CrossRef] [PubMed]
128. Presume, J.; Cunha, G.J.; Rocha, B.M.; Landeiro, L.; Trevas, S.; Roldão, M.; Silva, M.I.; Madeira, M.; Maltês, S.; Rodrigues, C.; et al. Acute kidney injury patterns in acute heart failure: The prognostic value of worsening renal function and its timing. *Rev. Port. Cardiol.* **2023**, *42*, 423–430. [CrossRef]
129. Sawamura, A.; Kajiura, H.; Sumi, T.; Umemoto, N.; Sugiura, T.; Taniguchi, T.; Ohashi, M.; Asai, T.; Shimizu, K.; Murohara, T. Clinical Impact of Worsening Renal Function in Elderly Patients with Acute Decompensated Heart Failure. *Int. J. Heart Fail.* **2021**, *3*, 128. [CrossRef]
130. KDIGO Executive Committee. KDIGO 2024 Clinical Practice Guideline for the Evaluation and Management of Chronic Kidney Disease. *Kidney Int.* **2024**, *105*, S117–S314. [CrossRef]
131. Barzilay, J.I.; Farag, Y.M.K.; Durthaler, J. Albuminuria: An Underappreciated Risk Factor for Cardiovascular Disease. *J. Am. Heart. Assoc.* **2024**, *13*, e030131. [CrossRef]
132. Khan, M.S.; Shahid, I.; Anker, S.D.; Fonarow, G.C.; Fudim, M.; Hall, M.E.; Hernandez, A.; Morris, A.A.; Shafi, T.; Weir, M.R.; et al. Albuminuria and Heart Failure: JACC State-of-the-Art Review. *J. Am. Coll. Cardiol.* **2023**, *81*, 270–282. [CrossRef] [PubMed]

133. Katz, D.H.; Burns, J.A.; Aguilar, F.G.; Beussink, L.; Shah, S.J. Albuminuria Is Independently Associated with Cardiac Remodeling, Abnormal Right and Left Ventricular Function, and Worse Outcomes in Heart Failure with Preserved Ejection Fraction. *JACC Heart Fail.* **2014**, *2*, 586–596. [CrossRef] [PubMed]
134. Boorsma, E.M.; ter Maaten, J.M.; Damman, K.; van Essen, B.J.; Zannad, F.; van Veldhuisen, D.J.; Samani, N.J.; Dickstein, K.; Metra, M.; Filippatos, G.; et al. Albuminuria as a marker of systemic congestion in patients with heart failure. *Eur. Heart J.* **2023**, *44*, 368–380. [CrossRef] [PubMed]
135. Matsumoto, Y.; Orihara, Y.; Asakura, M.; Min, K.-D.; Okuhara, Y.; Azuma, K.; Nishimura, K.; Sunayama, I.; Kashiwase, K.; Naito, Y.; et al. Urine albumin-to-creatinine ratio on admission predicts early rehospitalization in patients with acute decompensated heart failure. *Heart Vessel* **2022**, *37*, 1184–1194. [CrossRef] [PubMed]
136. Selvaraj, S.; Claggett, B.; Shah, S.J.; Anand, I.; Rouleau, J.L.; O'meara, E.; Desai, A.S.; Lewis, E.F.; Pitt, B.; Sweitzer, N.K.; et al. Prognostic Value of Albuminuria and Influence of Spironolactone in Heart Failure with Preserved Ejection Fraction. *Circ. Heart Fail.* **2018**, *11*, e005288. [CrossRef] [PubMed]
137. Filippatos, G.; Anker, S.D.; Agarwal, R.; Ruilope, L.M.; Rossing, P.; Bakris, G.L.; Tasto, C.; Joseph, A.; Kolkhof, P.; Lage, A.; et al. Finerenone Reduces Risk of Incident Heart Failure in Patients with Chronic Kidney Disease and Type 2 Diabetes: Analyses from the FIGARO-DKD Trial. *Circulation* **2022**, *145*, 437–447. [CrossRef]
138. Shang, W.; Wang, Z. The Update of NGAL in Acute Kidney Injury. *Curr. Protein Pept. Sci.* **2017**, *18*, 1211–1217. [CrossRef] [PubMed]
139. Nakada, Y.; Kawakami, R.; Matsui, M.; Ueda, T.; Nakano, T.; Takitsume, A.; Nakagawa, H.; Nishida, T.; Onoue, K.; Soeda, T.; et al. Prognostic Value of Urinary Neutrophil Gelatinase-Associated Lipocalin on the First Day of Admission for Adverse Events in Patients with Acute Decompensated Heart Failure. *J. Am. Heart. Assoc.* **2017**, *6*, e004582. [CrossRef]
140. Maisel, A.S.; Mueller, C.; Fitzgerald, R.; Brikhan, R.; Hiestand, B.C.; Iqbal, N.; Clopton, P.; van Veldhuisen, D.J. Prognostic utility of plasma neutrophil gelatinase-associated lipocalin in patients with acute heart failure: The NGAL EvaLuation Along with B-type NaTriuretic Peptide in acutely decompensated heart failure (GALLANT) trial. *Eur. J. Heart Fail.* **2011**, *13*, 846–851. [CrossRef]
141. Alvelos, M.; Lourenço, P.; Dias, C.; Amorim, M.; Rema, J.; Leite, A.B.; Guimarães, J.T.; Almeida, P.; Bettencourt, P. Prognostic value of neutrophil gelatinase-associated lipocalin in acute heart failure. *Int. J. Cardiol.* **2013**, *165*, 51–55. [CrossRef] [PubMed]
142. Wettersten, N.; Horiuchi, Y.; van Veldhuisen, D.J.; Mueller, C.; Filippatos, G.; Nowak, R.; Hogan, C.; Kontos, M.C.; Cannon, C.M.; Müeller, G.A.; et al. Short-term prognostic implications of serum and urine neutrophil gelatinase-associated lipocalin in acute heart failure: Findings from the AKINESIS study. *Eur. J. Heart Fail.* **2020**, *22*, 251–263. [CrossRef] [PubMed]
143. Kumar, A. Novel kidney injury markers (NGAL and KIM-1) and outcomes in patients with heart failure—Systematic review and meta-analysis. In Proceedings of the Heart Failure Congress, Madrid, Spain, 21–24 May 2022.
144. Burns, J.A.; Trivedi, R.; Vaishnav, J.; Hahn, V.; Sharma, K. Cystatin C Predicts Adverse Outcomes in Heart Failure with Preserved Ejection Fraction. *J. Card. Fail.* **2022**, *28*, S80–S81. [CrossRef]
145. Carrasco-Sánchez, F.J.; Galisteo-Almeda, L.; Páez-Rubio, I.; Martínez-Marcos, F.J.; Camacho-Vázquez, C.; Ruiz-Frutos, C.; La Llave, E.P.-D. Prognostic Value of Cystatin C on Admission in Heart Failure with Preserved Ejection Fraction. *J. Card. Fail.* **2011**, *17*, 31–38. [CrossRef] [PubMed]
146. Kumar, A.; Chidambaram, V.; Geetha, H.S.; Majella, M.G.; Bavineni, M.; Pona, P.K.; Jain, N.; Sharalaya, Z.; Al'Aref, S.J.; Asnani, A.; et al. Renal Biomarkers in Heart Failure. *JACC Adv.* **2024**, *3*, 100765. [CrossRef] [PubMed]
147. Lamounier-Zepter, V.; Look, C.; Alvarez, J.; Christ, T.; Ravens, U.; Schunck, W.-H.; Ehrhart-Bornstein, M.; Bornstein, S.R.; Morano, I. Adipocyte Fatty Acid–Binding Protein Suppresses Cardiomyocyte Contraction. *Circ. Res.* **2009**, *105*, 326–334. [CrossRef]
148. Aragonès, G.; Ferré, R.; Lázaro, I.; Cabré, A.; Plana, N.; Merino, J.; Heras, M.; Girona, J.; Masana, L. Fatty acid-binding protein 4 is associated with endothelial dysfunction in patients with type 2 diabetes. *Atherosclerosis* **2010**, *213*, 329–331. [CrossRef] [PubMed]
149. Harada, T.; Sunaga, H.; Sorimachi, H.; Yoshida, K.; Kato, T.; Kurosawa, K.; Nagasaka, T.; Koitabashi, N.; Iso, T.; Kurabayashi, M.; et al. Pathophysiological role of fatty acid-binding protein 4 in Asian patients with heart failure and preserved ejection fraction. *ESC Heart Fail.* **2020**, *7*, 4256–4266. [CrossRef]
150. Kutsuzawa, D.; Arimoto, T.; Watanabe, T.; Shishido, T.; Miyamoto, T.; Miyashita, T.; Takahashi, H.; Niizeki, T.; Takeishi, Y.; Kubota, I. Ongoing myocardial damage in patients with heart failure and preserved ejection fraction. *J. Cardiol.* **2012**, *60*, 454–461. [CrossRef]
151. Rezar, R.; Jirak, P.; Gschwandtner, M.; Derler, R.; Felder, T.K.; Haslinger, M.; Kopp, K.; Seelmaier, C.; Granitz, C.; Hoppe, U.C.; et al. Heart-Type Fatty Acid-Binding Protein (H-FABP) and Its Role as a Biomarker in Heart Failure: What Do We Know So Far? *J. Clin. Med.* **2020**, *9*, 164. [CrossRef]
152. Rodríguez-Calvo, R.; Granado-Casas, M.; de Oca, A.P.-M.; Julian, M.T.; Domingo, M.; Codina, P.; Santiago-Vacas, E.; Cediel, G.; Julve, J.; Rossell, J.; et al. Fatty Acid Binding Proteins 3 and 4 Predict Both All-Cause and Cardiovascular Mortality in Subjects with Chronic Heart Failure and Type 2 Diabetes Mellitus. *Antioxidants* **2023**, *12*, 645. [CrossRef] [PubMed]
153. Shimada, Y.J. Is leptin protective against heart failure with preserved ejection fraction? A complex interrelationship among leptin, obesity, and left ventricular hypertrophy. *Hypertens. Res.* **2019**, *42*, 141–142. [CrossRef] [PubMed]
154. Vilariño-García, T.; Polonio-González, M.L.; Pérez-Pérez, A.; Ribalta, J.; Arrieta, F.; Aguilar, M.; Obaya, J.C.; Gimeno-Orna, J.A.; Iglesias, P.; Navarro, J.; et al. Role of Leptin in Obesity, Cardiovascular Disease, and Type 2 Diabetes. *Int. J. Mol. Sci.* **2024**, *25*, 2338. [CrossRef] [PubMed]

155. Faxén, U.L.; Hage, C.; Andreasson, A.; Donal, E.; Daubert, J.-C.; Linde, C.; Brismar, K.; Lund, L.H. HFpEF and HFrEF exhibit different phenotypes as assessed by leptin and adiponectin. *Int. J. Cardiol.* **2017**, *228*, 709–716. [CrossRef] [PubMed]
156. Kamimura, D.; Suzuki, T.; Wang, W.; Deshazo, M.; Hall, J.E.; Winniford, M.D.; Kullo, I.J.; Mosley, T.H.; Butler, K.R.; Hall, M.E. Higher plasma leptin levels are associated with reduced left ventricular mass and left ventricular diastolic stiffness in black women: Insights from the Genetic Epidemiology Network of Arteriopathy (GENOA) study. *Hypertens. Res.* **2018**, *41*, 629–638. [CrossRef] [PubMed]
157. Lei, X.; Qiu, S.; Yang, G.; Wu, Q. Adiponectin and metabolic cardiovascular diseases: Therapeutic opportunities and challenges. *Genes Dis.* **2023**, *10*, 1525–1536. [CrossRef] [PubMed]
158. Szabó, T.; Scherbakov, N.; Sandek, A.; Kung, T.; von Haehling, S.; Lainscak, M.; Jankowska, E.; Rudovich, N.; Anker, S.; Frystyk, J.; et al. Plasma adiponectin in heart failure with and without cachexia: Catabolic signal linking catabolism, symptomatic status, and prognosis. *Nutr. Metab. Cardiovasc. Dis.* **2014**, *24*, 50–56. [CrossRef] [PubMed]
159. Masson, S.; Gori, F.; Latini, R.; Milani, V.; Flyvbjerg, A.; Frystyk, J.; Crociati, L.; Pietri, S.; Vago, T.; Barlera, S.; et al. Adiponectin in chronic heart failure: Influence of diabetes and genetic variants. *Eur. J. Clin. Investig.* **2011**, *41*, 1330–1338. [CrossRef] [PubMed]
160. Oh, A.; Okazaki, R.; Sam, F.; Valero-Muñoz, M. Heart Failure with Preserved Ejection Fraction and Adipose Tissue: A Story of Two Tales. *Front. Cardiovasc. Med.* **2019**, *6*, 110. [CrossRef]
161. Sam, F.; Duhaney, T.-A.S.; Sato, K.; Wilson, R.M.; Ohashi, K.; Sono-Romanelli, S.; Higuchi, A.; De Silva, D.S.; Qin, F.; Walsh, K.; et al. Adiponectin Deficiency, Diastolic Dysfunction, and Diastolic Heart Failure. *Endocrinology* **2010**, *151*, 322–331. [CrossRef]
162. Núñez, J.; de la Espriella, R.; Miñana, G.; Santas, E.; Llácer, P.; Núñez, E.; Palau, P.; Bodí, V.; Chorro, F.J.; Sanchis, J.; et al. Antigen carbohydrate 125 as a biomarker in heart failure: A narrative review. *Eur. J. Heart Fail.* **2021**, *23*, 1445–1457. [CrossRef] [PubMed]
163. Miñana, G.; de la Espriella, R.; Palau, P.; Llácer, P.; Núñez, E.; Santas, E.; Valero, E.; Lorenzo, M.; Núñez, G.; Bodí, V.; et al. Carbohydrate antigen 125 and risk of heart failure readmissions in patients with heart failure and preserved ejection fraction. *Sci. Rep.* **2022**, *12*, 1344. [CrossRef] [PubMed]
164. Menghoum, N.; Badii, M.C.; Deltombe, M.; Lejeune, S.; Roy, C.; Vancraeynest, D.; Pasquet, A.; Gerber, B.L.; Horman, S.; Gruson, D.; et al. Carbohydrate antigen 125: A useful marker of congestion, fibrosis, and prognosis in heart failure with preserved ejection fraction. *ESC Heart Fail.* **2024**, *11*, 1493–1505. [CrossRef] [PubMed]
165. Hung, C.-L.; Hung, T.-C.; Liu, C.-C.; Wu, Y.-J.; Kuo, J.-Y.; Hou, C.J.-Y.; Yeh, H.-I. Relation of Carbohydrate Antigen-125 to Left Atrial Remodeling and its Prognostic Usefulness in Patients with Heart Failure and Preserved Left Ventricular Ejection Fraction in Women. *Am. J. Cardiol.* **2012**, *110*, 993–1000. [CrossRef] [PubMed]
166. Llàcer, P.; Bayés-Genís, A.; Núñez, J. Carbohydrate antigen 125 in heart failure. A New era in the monitoring and control of treatment. *Med. Clínica (Engl. Ed.)* **2019**, *152*, 266–273. [CrossRef] [PubMed]
167. Huang, F.; Chen, J.; Liu, Y.; Zhang, K.; Wang, J.; Huang, H. New mechanism of elevated CA125 in heart failure: The mechanical stress and inflammatory stimuli initiate CA125 synthesis. *Med. Hypotheses* **2012**, *79*, 381–383. [CrossRef] [PubMed]
168. Núñez, J.; Llàcer, P.; García-Blas, S.; Bonanad, C.; Ventura, S.; Núñez, J.M.; Sánchez, R.; Fácila, L.; de la Espriella, R.; Vaquer, J.M.; et al. CA125-Guided Diuretic Treatment Versus Usual Care in Patients with Acute Heart Failure and Renal Dysfunction. *Am. J. Med.* **2020**, *133*, 370–380.e4. [CrossRef]
169. Núñez, J.; Llàcer, P.; Bertomeu-González, V.; Bosch, M.J.; Merlos, P.; Montagud, V.; Bodí, V.; Bertomeu-Martínez, V.; Pedrosa, V.; Cordero, A.; et al. Carbohydrate Antigen-125–Guided Therapy in Acute Heart Failure. *JACC Heart Fail.* **2016**, *4*, 833–843. [CrossRef]
170. Ferreira, J.P.; Packer, M.; Sattar, N.; Butler, J.; Pocock, S.J.; Anker, S.D.; Maldonado, S.G.; Panova-Noeva, M.; Sumin, M.; Masson, S.; et al. Carbohydrate antigen 125 concentrations across the ejection fraction spectrum in chronic heart failure: The EMPEROR programme. *Eur. J. Heart Fail.* **2024**, *26*, 788–802. [CrossRef]
171. Januzzi, J.; Mohebi, R.; On Behalf of Emperor Committees and Investigators. CA-125 concentrations are associated with renal function decline but not congestion or prognosis in patients with chronic heart failure: Results from EMPEROR-POOLED. *Eur. Heart J.* **2023**, *44*, ehad655.914. [CrossRef]
172. Docherty, K.F.; McDowell, K.; Welsh, P.; Osmanska, J.; Anand, I.; de Boer, R.A.; Køber, L.; Kosiborod, M.N.; Martinez, F.A.; O'meara, E.; et al. Association of Carbohydrate Antigen 125 on the Response to Dapagliflozin in Patients with Heart Failure. *J. Am. Coll. Cardiol.* **2023**, *82*, 142–157. [CrossRef] [PubMed]
173. de la Espriella, R.; Miñana, G.; Santas, E.; Núñez, G.; Lorenzo, M.; Núñez, E.; Bayés-Genís, A.; Núñez, J. Effects of empagliflozin on CA125 trajectory in patients with chronic congestive heart failure. *Int. J. Cardiol.* **2021**, *339*, 102–105. [CrossRef]
174. Köseoğlu, F.D.; Özlek, B. Anemia and Iron Deficiency Predict All-Cause Mortality in Patients with Heart Failure and Preserved Ejection Fraction: 6-Year Follow-Up Study. *Diagnostics* **2024**, *14*, 209. [CrossRef] [PubMed]
175. Beale, A.L.; Warren, J.L.; Roberts, N.; Meyer, P.; Townsend, N.P.; Kaye, D. Iron deficiency in heart failure with preserved ejection fraction: A systematic review and meta-analysis. *Open Heart* **2019**, *6*, e001012. [CrossRef] [PubMed]
176. Parvan, R.; Hosseinpour, M.; Moradi, Y.; Devaux, Y.; Cataliotti, A.; da Silva, G.J.J. Diagnostic performance of microRNAs in the detection of heart failure with reduced or preserved ejection fraction: A systematic review and meta-analysis. *Eur. J. Heart Fail.* **2022**, *24*, 2212–2225. [CrossRef]
177. Figueiredo, R.; Adão, R.; Leite-Moreira, A.F.; Mâncio, J.; Brás-Silva, C. Candidate microRNAs as prognostic biomarkers in heart failure: A systematic review. *Rev. Port. Cardiol.* **2022**, *41*, 865–885. [CrossRef] [PubMed]

178. Rech, M.; Aizpurua, A.B.; van Empel, V.; van Bilsen, M.; Schroen, B. Pathophysiological understanding of HFpEF: microRNAs as part of the puzzle. *Cardiovasc. Res.* **2018**, *114*, 782–793. [CrossRef] [PubMed]
179. Paim, L.R.; da Silva, L.M.; Antunes-Correa, L.M.; Ribeiro, V.C.; Schreiber, R.; Minin, E.O.; Bueno, L.C.; Lopes, E.C.; Yamaguti, R.; Coy-Canguçu, A.; et al. Profile of serum microRNAs in heart failure with reduced and preserved ejection fraction: Correlation with myocardial remodeling. *Heliyon* **2024**, *10*, e27206. [CrossRef]
180. Regan, J.A.; Truby, L.K.; Tahir, U.A.; Katz, D.H.; Nguyen, M.; Kwee, L.C.; Deng, S.; Wilson, J.G.; Mentz, R.J.; Kraus, W.E.; et al. Protein biomarkers of cardiac remodeling and inflammation associated with HFpEF and incident events. *Sci. Rep.* **2022**, *12*, 20072. [CrossRef]
181. Chen, H.; Tesic, M.; Nikolic, V.N.; Pavlovic, M.; Vucic, R.M.; Spasic, A.; Jovanovic, H.; Jovanovic, I.; Town, S.E.L.; Padula, M.P.; et al. Systemic Biomarkers and Unique Pathways in Different Phenotypes of Heart Failure with Preserved Ejection Fraction. *Biomolecules* **2022**, *12*, 1419. [CrossRef]
182. De Jong, K.A.; Lopaschuk, G.D. Complex Energy Metabolic Changes in Heart Failure with Preserved Ejection Fraction and Heart Failure with Reduced Ejection Fraction. *Can. J. Cardiol.* **2017**, *33*, 860–871. [CrossRef] [PubMed]
183. Hahn, V.S.; Petucci, C.; Kim, M.-S.; Bedi, K.C.; Wang, H.; Mishra, S.; Koleini, N.; Yoo, E.J.; Margulies, K.B.; Arany, Z.; et al. Myocardial Metabolomics of Human Heart Failure with Preserved Ejection Fraction. *Circulation* **2023**, *147*, 1147–1161. [CrossRef] [PubMed]
184. Palazzuoli, A.; Tramonte, F.; Beltrami, M. Laboratory and Metabolomic Fingerprint in Heart Failure with Preserved Ejection Fraction: From Clinical Classification to Biomarker Signature. *Biomolecules* **2023**, *13*, 173. [CrossRef] [PubMed]
185. Henkens, M.T.; Remmelzwaal, S.; Robinson, E.L.; van Ballegooijen, A.J.; Aizpurua, A.B.; Verdonschot, J.A.; Raafs, A.G.; Weerts, J.; Hazebroek, M.R.; Wijk, S.S.; et al. Risk of bias in studies investigating novel diagnostic biomarkers for heart failure with preserved ejection fraction. A systematic review. *Eur. J. Heart Fail.* **2020**, *22*, 1586–1597. [CrossRef] [PubMed]
186. Pieske, B.; Tschöpe, C.; A de Boer, R.; Fraser, A.G.; Anker, S.D.; Donal, E.; Edelmann, F.; Fu, M.; Guazzi, M.; Lam, C.S.P.; et al. *How to Diagnose Heart Failure with Preserved Ejection Fraction: The HFA-PEFF Diagnostic Algorithm: A Consensus Recommendation from the Heart Failure Association (HFA) of the European Society of Cardiology (ESC)*; Oxford University Press: Oxford, UK, 2019. [CrossRef]
187. Cohen, J.B.; Schrauben, S.J.; Zhao, L.; Basso, M.D.; Cvijic, M.E.; Li, Z.; Yarde, M.; Wang, Z.; Bhattacharya, P.T.; Chirinos, D.A.; et al. Clinical Phenogroups in Heart Failure with Preserved Ejection Fraction. *JACC Heart Fail.* **2020**, *8*, 172–184. [CrossRef]
188. Sotomi, Y.; Hikoso, S.; Nakatani, D.; Okada, K.; Dohi, T.; Sunaga, A.; Kida, H.; Sato, T.; Matsuoka, Y.; Kitamura, T.; et al. Medications for specific phenotypes of heart failure with preserved ejection fraction classified by a machine learning-based clustering model. *Heart* **2023**, *109*, 1231–1240. [CrossRef]

Disclaimer/Publisher's Note: The statements, opinions and data contained in all publications are solely those of the individual author(s) and contributor(s) and not of MDPI and/or the editor(s). MDPI and/or the editor(s) disclaim responsibility for any injury to people or property resulting from any ideas, methods, instructions or products referred to in the content.

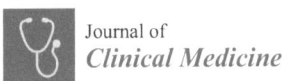

Article

The Role of High-Sensitivity Troponin T Regarding Prognosis and Cardiovascular Outcome across Heart Failure Spectrum

Andrea D'Amato [1,2,*,†], Paolo Severino [1,†], Silvia Prosperi [1], Marco Valerio Mariani [1], Rosanna Germanò [1], Andrea De Prisco [1], Vincenzo Myftari [1], Claudia Cestiè [1], Aurora Labbro Francia [1], Stefanie Marek-Iannucci [1], Leonardo Tabacco [1], Leonardo Vari [1], Silvia Luisa Marano [1], Gianluca Di Pietro [1], Carlo Lavalle [1], Gennaro Sardella [1], Massimo Mancone [1], Roberto Badagliacca [1], Francesco Fedele [3] and Carmine Dario Vizza [1]

1. Department of Clinical, Internal, Anaesthesiology and Cardiovascular Sciences, Sapienza University of Rome, Viale del Policlinico 155, 00161 Rome, Italy; paolo.severino@uniroma1.it (P.S.); silviapro@outlook.it (S.P.); marcoval.mariani@gmail.com (M.V.M.); rosanna.germano@gmail.com (R.G.); deprisco.1843735@studenti.uniroma1.it (A.D.P.); vincenzo.myftari@gmail.com (V.M.); claudia.cestie@gmail.com (C.C.); auro1298@gmail.com (A.L.F.); stefanie.marekiannucci@gmail.com (S.M.-I.); tabacco.1852080@studenti.uniroma1.it (L.T.); leonardovari98@gmail.com (L.V.); silviamarano35@gmail.com (S.L.M.); gianluca.dipietro@uniroma1.it (G.D.P.); carlo.lavalle@uniroma1.it (C.L.); gennaro.sardella@uniroma1.it (G.S.); massimo.mancone@uniroma1.it (M.M.); roberto.badagliacca@uniroma1.it (R.B.); dario.vizza@uniroma1.it (C.D.V.)
2. Department of Cardiology, Ospedale Fabrizio Spaziani, 03100 Frosinone, Italy
3. San Raffaele Cassino, 03043 Cassino, Italy; francesco.fedele@uniroma1.it
* Correspondence: andrea.damato@uniroma1.it
† These authors contributed equally to this work.

Abstract: Background: Cardiac troponin release is related to the cardiomyocyte loss occurring in heart failure (HF). The prognostic role of high-sensitivity cardiac troponin T (hs-cTnT) in several settings of HF is under investigation. The aim of the study is to assess the prognostic role of intrahospital hs-cTnT in patients admitted due to HF. **Methods:** In this observational, single center, prospective study, patients hospitalized due to HF have been enrolled. Admission, in-hospital peak, and discharge hs-cTnT have been assessed. Patients were followed up for 6 months. Cardiovascular (CV) death, HF hospitalization (HFH), and worsening HF (WHF) (i.e., urgent ambulatory visit/loop diuretics escalation) events have been assessed at 6-month follow up. **Results:** 253 consecutive patients have been enrolled in the study. The hs-cTnT median values at admission and discharge were 0.031 ng/mL (IQR 0.02–0.078) and 0.031 ng/mL (IQR 0.02–0.077), respectively. The risk of CV death/HFH was higher in patients with admission hs-cTnT values above the median ($p = 0.02$) and in patients who had an increase in hs-cTnT during hospitalization ($p = 0.03$). Multivariate Cox regression analysis confirmed that hs-cTnT above the median (OR: 2.06; 95% CI: 1.02–4.1; $p = 0.04$) and increase in hs-cTnT during hospitalization (OR:1.95; 95%CI: 1.006–3.769; $p = 0.04$) were predictors of CV death/HFH. In a subgroup analysis of patients with chronic HF, hs-cTnT above the median was associated with increased risk of CV death/HFH ($p = 0.03$), while in the subgroup of patients with HFmrEF/HFpEF, hs-cTnT above the median was associated with outpatient WHF events ($p = 0.03$). **Conclusions:** Inpatient hs-cTnT levels predict CV death/HFH in patients with HF. In particular, in the subgroup of chronic HF patients, hs-cTnT is predictive of CV death/HFH; while in patients with HFmrEF/HFpEF, hs-cTnT predicts WHF events.

Keywords: heart failure; biomarkers; high-sensitivity cardiac troponin T; hospitalization; cardiovascular mortality; worsening heart failure

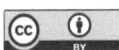

Citation: D'Amato, A.; Severino, P.; Prosperi, S.; Mariani, M.V.; Germanò, R.; De Prisco, A.; Myftari, V.; Cestiè, C.; Labbro Francia, A.; Marek-Iannucci, S.; et al. The Role of High-Sensitivity Troponin T Regarding Prognosis and Cardiovascular Outcome across Heart Failure Spectrum. *J. Clin. Med.* **2024**, *13*, 3533. https://doi.org/10.3390/jcm13123533

Academic Editors: Cristina Tudoran and Larisa Anghel

Received: 21 May 2024
Revised: 12 June 2024
Accepted: 14 June 2024
Published: 17 June 2024

Copyright: © 2024 by the authors. Licensee MDPI, Basel, Switzerland. This article is an open access article distributed under the terms and conditions of the Creative Commons Attribution (CC BY) license (https://creativecommons.org/licenses/by/4.0/).

1. Introduction

Heart failure (HF) is one of the main causes of morbidity and mortality worldwide [1]. It is a clinical syndrome caused by the incapacity of the heart to maintain normal systemic perfusion at normal intraventricular filling pressures. Once diagnosed, patients with HF have an average rate of one hospital readmission per year [1,2] and an estimated mortality rate of 67% within five years [3].

HF is characterized by variable periods of symptomatic stability, often interrupted by episodes of decompensated HF despite optimized therapy. The phases of clinical deterioration are increasingly recognized as a distinct phase in the history of HF, termed worsening HF (WHF) [4]. WHF is a condition of deterioration of clinical signs of HF, despite optimized medical management, requiring escalation of diuretic therapy, hospitalization or urgent ambulatorial visits [5]. The interesting and challenging aspect of this condition is that the culminating event of WHF is hospitalization, but the progressive worsening develops outside of the hospital, and it is often subclinical, manifesting itself with myocardial biomarkers increase, need for diuretic escalation, as well as symptoms and signs requiring urgent observation by a cardiologist in the outpatient setting. The early identification of patients in need of diuretic dose adjustments and ambulatory urgent visits may be crucial in the management of these patients in order to avoid hospitalization and related adverse events.

Besides echocardiographic parameters, natriuretic peptides (NPs) are fundamental to rule out the clinical condition of HF and to predict short-term mortality in patients hospitalized due to the latter [1,2]. The association between NPs and poor prognosis has been demonstrated [6]. High pre-discharge levels of brain natriuretic peptide (BNP) and N-terminal pro B-type natriuretic peptide (NT-proBNP) are associated with a high risk of cardiovascular (CV) death and hospital readmission [7]. Similar findings have been reported in the OPTIMIZE-HF registry [8]. In acute HF, congestion is the main factor influencing NP elevation. However, in chronic stable conditions, transmural wall stress is usually the main determinant of NP concentrations. On the other hand, the mechanism behind NP augmentation in HF with preserved ejection fraction (HFpEF) is less clear, since there is a reduction in wall stress due to the generally smaller size of the left ventricular chamber. Comorbidities, such as kidney disease or obesity, may also affect the concentration of NPs and thus the prognostic significance of these biomarkers [9].

NPs are sensitive prognostic markers in HF, but it may be important to identify alternative biomarkers for more accurate management and prognostic stratification of HF patients. Recently, the importance of the high-sensitivity cardiac troponin T (hs-cTnT) assay in the diagnosis and prognosis of HF has been demonstrated [10]. Troponins are part of the skeletal and cardiac myocyte contraction system. Different troponin isoforms are represented in the different muscle types. While troponin C is synthesized in equal manner in skeletal and cardiac myocytes, the troponin T and I isoforms are highly specific [11]. The latter are expressed especially in cardiac myocytes and are by far the most specific and sensitive indicators for the diagnosis of acute myocardial infarction (AMI) [12]. Myocyte damage induces troponin release into the circulation. The increase in hs-cTnT levels is directly related to the severity of myocyte damage, making troponins quantitative markers of heart tissue damage [13]. Molecular events such as cardiomyocyte death and apoptosis also take place during chronic disease, and high hs-cTnT levels are representative of the long-standing cardiac damage occurring in HF. In fact, in patients with dilatative cardiomyopathy, higher hs-cTnT levels were found to be predictive of a deterioration in clinical conditions [14]. Setsuka et al. [15] have shown that higher troponin levels are found in severe HF, with advanced New York Heart Association (NYHA) class, and in patients who developed complications and HF exacerbation. Various studies have investigated the predictive power of troponin levels in HF patients, showing a higher incidence of major CV events in patients with higher troponin levels [16]. These studies mainly included patients with HF with reduced ejection fraction (HFrEF) and had major CV events as their main endpoints. Evidence regarding the role of cardiac troponins in HF subpopulations is lacking. Furthermore, the prognostic role of cardiac troponins in terms of WHF events (i.e., the need for diuretic escalation or urgent ambulatory visits due to HF) has not been investigated yet.

The aim of the current study was to assess the role of inpatient cardiac hs-cTnT regarding the identification of HF patients at higher risk of adverse events, including CV mortality, HFH and WHF events, with special focus on the different subgroups of HF.

2. Methods

This was an observational, prospective, single center study, enrolling patients with a diagnosis of HF who have been consecutively admitted to the Department of Clinical, Internal, Anesthesiology and Cardiovascular Sciences at Policlinico Umberto I, Sapienza University of Rome. Inclusion criteria were the following: (I) written, signed and dated informed consent; (II) age above 18 years; (III) diagnosis of HF according to the Guidelines [1]. Exclusion criteria were the following: (I) presence of any condition representing the main cause of hs-cTnT increase beyond HF; (II) planned or history of heart transplantation or ventricular assist device (VAD); (III) end-stage kidney failure and/or dialysis; (IV) any condition limiting life expectancy less than one year; (V) pregnancy or nursing; (VI) non-compliance with the study protocol.

Patients enrolled constituted one study group.

The following parameters were collected: (i) clinical parameters (past medical history, physical examination, electrocardiogram, arterial blood pressure, NYHA class, and pharmacological therapy); (ii) echocardiographic parameters (ventricular chambers size, systolic and diastolic function, and valve disease and severity); (iii) laboratory parameters (hs-cTnT, blood cell count, creatinine, electrolytes, alanine aminotransferase, and aspartate aminotransferase). Specifically, the admission, peak, and discharge values of hs-cTnT were recorded. Moreover, the delta between admission and peak values of hs-cTnT was calculated. An increase in hs-cTnT during an in-hospital stay was defined as a delta of at least 0.014 ng/mL, between the admission and peak hs-cTnT values (representing the upper reference limit of hs-cTnT). The assay Elecsys® (Roche Diagnostics International Ltd., Rotkreuz, Switzerland) for hs-cTnT has been used.

Over a follow-up period of 6 months after the index hospitalization, CV death, HFH, and urgent ambulatory visits/need of loop diuretic escalation were investigated in the outpatient HF clinic.

Specific subgroup analyses according to LVEF values and clinical presentation of HF were performed in order to define the prognostic role of hs-cTnT in terms of CV death, HFH, and urgent ambulatory visits/need of loop diuretic escalation.

Data were collected in a dedicated Excel Database (Version 2405 Build 16.0.17628.20006; 64 bit). The study was conducted according to the Helsinki Declaration. The study protocol was approved by the Ethical Committee of Policlinico Umberto I in Rome (rif.7068, approved on 8 May 2023).

Statistical Analysis

The normal distribution of continuous variables was assessed with the Kolmogorov–Smirnov test. Continuous variables were expressed as mean and standard deviation, whereas median and first and third quartiles were used for non-normally distributed data. Categorical data were described as numbers and percentages. Student's t-test, the Mann–Whitney test, the χ^2 test, and the Fisher exact test were used for comparisons, as needed. The Kaplan–Meier method was used to estimate the cumulative event rates of study outcomes in the overall population, categorized based on admission troponin (above or below the median value of the studied population) and on the basis of the trend in troponin values during the hospitalization (patients with an increase or decrease in troponin values). Kaplan–Meier analysis was used to analyze the differences in clinical outcome rates in subgroups of patients with HFpEF and HF with mildly reduced ejection fraction (HFmrEF), and in patients with chronic HF presentation. The differences in each group were compared using log-rank tests. Univariate and multivariate Cox regression analyses were performed to obtain the odds ratios (ORs) of the associations among hs-cTnT with the endpoints. All the associations among variables and the composite endpoints with a *p*-value < 0.1 at univariate analysis were included at multivariate analysis. At multivariate analysis, variables potentially associated with the composite outcomes of CV death and HFH have been considered. For all tests, a *p*-value < 0.05 was considered statistically significant.

The statistical analysis was performed using SPSS version 27.0 for Mac (IBM Software, Inc., Armonk, NY, USA).

3. Results

A total of 253 consecutive patients were enrolled from October 2022 to April 2023 and they were followed-up for a period of 6 months.

The baseline features of the patient population are listed in Table 1. The types of admission and discharge therapies for the total population have been represented in Figure 1. The occurrence of each outcome in the total population has been represented in Figure 2.

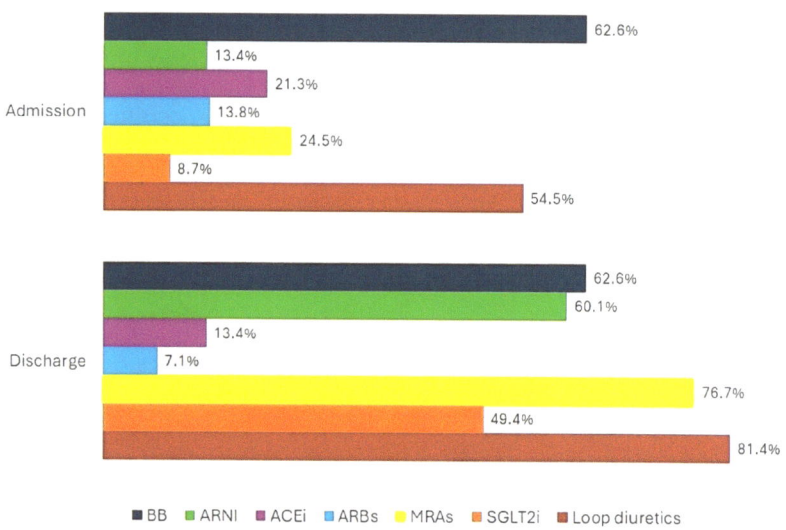

Figure 1. Percentage of total population on treatment with heart failure disease modifying drugs and loop diuretics at hospital admission and discharge. HF—heart failure; BB—beta blocker; ARNI—angiotensin receptor/neprilysin inhibitor; ACEi—angiotensin-converting enzyme inhibitor; ARBs—angiotensin receptor blockers; MRAs—mineralocorticoid receptor antagonists; SGLT2i—sodium glucose cotransporter 2 inhibitor.

Considering the total population, the composite of CV death and HFH was significantly higher in patients with hs-cTnT levels at admission above the median (23 vs. 13; 19.8% vs. 9.5%; $p = 0.02$) and in patients with a significant increase in hs-cTnT during hospitalization (20 vs. 16; 20% vs. 10.5%; $p = 0.03$) (Tables 2 and 3).

Kaplan–Meier survival analysis (Figure 3A,B) demonstrated that patients with admission hs-cTnT levels above the median value and patients with an increase in hs-cTnT during in-hospital stays experienced more commonly the composite outcome CV death and HFH (log-rank p-value = 0.02 and p-value = 0.03, respectively).

Cox regression analysis showed that an admission hs-cTnT above the median and an in-hospital increase in hs-cTnT represent an independent predictor of the composite of CV death and HFH at 6-month follow-up (Tables 4 and 5).

The subgroup analysis, considering patients with chronic HF, demonstrated that the risk of the composite of CV death and HFH was significantly higher in patients with an admission hs-cTnT above the median value compared to patients with an admission hs-cTnT below the median value (7 vs. 2; 14.9% vs. 3.3%; $p = 0.04$) (Table 6).

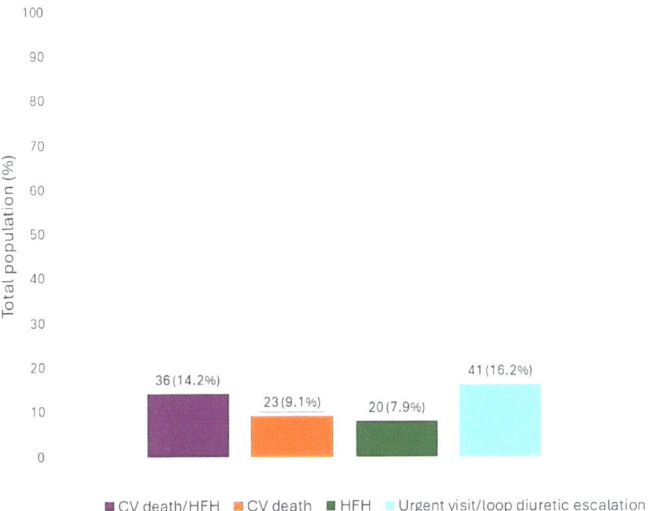

Figure 2. Total number and percentage rate of adverse events in the total population at 6-month follow-up. CV—cardiovascular; HFH—heart failure hospitalization.

Table 1. Baseline features of the study population at hospital admission.

Variable	Total Population (N = 253)
Age, years (IQR)	73 (64.5–80)
Male sex, n (%)	177 (70)
Arterial hypertension, n (%)	195 (77.1)
Diabetes mellitus, n (%)	72 (28.5)
Dyslipidemia, n (%)	133 (52.6)
Family history of CVD, n (%)	66 (26.1)
COPD, n (%)	67 (26.5)
Smoking habit, n (%)	96 (37.9)
Ischemic, n (%)	138 (54.5)
Hypertensive, n (%)	35 (13.8)
Idiopathic, n (%)	29 (11.5)
Valvular, n (%)	29 (11.5)
Inflammatory/drug induced, n (%)	22 (8.7)
Acute presentation, n (%)	146 (57.7)
Chronic presentation, n (%)	107 (42.3)
eGFR, mL/min/m^2 (IQR)	64 (46–81.7)
Hemoglobin, g/dL (IQR)	12.9 (10.9–14.3)
K$^+$, mmol/L (IQR)	4 (3.68–4.33)
Admission hs-cTnT, ng/mL (IQR)	0.031 (0.02–0.078)
Discharge hs-cTnT, ng/mL (IQR)	0.031 (0.02–0.077)
hs-cTnT peak, ng/mL (IQR)	0.042 (0.023–0.121)

Table 1. Cont.

Variable	Total Population (N = 253)
hs-cTnT delta peak-admission, ng/mL (IQR)	0.001 (0–0.026)
HFrEF, n (%)	199 (78.7)
HFmrEF/HFpEF, n (%)	54 (21.3)
LVEF, % (IQR)	32 (25–40)
LVEDD, mm (IQR)	58 (52–64)
IVS, mm (IQR)	11 (9–12)
PW, mm (IQR)	10 (9–10.5)
Basal RVEDD, mm (IQR)	36 (31–44)
TAPSE, mm (IQR)	18 (15–20)
Median NYHA, class (IQR)	3 (2–3)

IQR—interquartile range; CVD—cardiovascular disease; COPD—chronic obstructive pulmonary disease; eGFR—estimated glomerular filtration rate; K$^+$—potassium; hs-cTnT—high-sensitivity T troponin; HFrEF—heart failure with reduced ejection fraction; HFmrEF—heart failure with mildly reduced ejection fraction; HFpEF—heart failure with preserved ejection fraction; LVEF—left ventricular ejection fraction; LVEDD—left ventricular end diastolic diameter; IVS—interventricular septum; PW—posterior wall; RVEDD—right ventricular end diastolic diameter; TAPSE—tricuspid annular plane systolic excursion; NYHA—New York Heart Association.

Table 2. Relationship between high-sensitivity T troponin at admission and the occurrence of each outcome in the total population.

Variable	hs-cTnT below Median Value	hs-cTnT above Median Value	p Value
CV death/HFH, n (%)	13 (9.5)	23 (19.8)	0.02
CV death, n (%)	8 (5.8)	15 (12.9)	0.05
HFH, n (%)	9 (6.6)	11 (9.5)	0.4
Urgent visit/loop diuretic escalation, n (%)	21 (15.3)	20 (17.2)	0.68

CV—cardiovascular; HFH—heart failure hospitalization; hs-cTnT—high-sensitivity T troponin.

Table 3. Relationship between high-sensitivity T troponin increase during hospitalization and the occurrence of each outcome in the total population.

Variable	No hs-cTnT Increase	hs-cTnT Increase	p Value
CV death/HFH, n (%)	16 (10.5)	20 (20)	0.03
CV death, n (%)	10 (6.5)	13 (13)	0.08
HFH, n (%)	11 (7.2)	9 (9)	0.6
Urgent visit/loop diuretic escalation, n (%)	28 (18.3)	13 (13)	0.26

CV—cardiovascular; HFH—heart failure hospitalization; hs-cTnT—high-sensitivity T troponin.

Kaplan–Meier survival analysis evidenced that an admission hs-cTnT above the median value in the subgroup of patients with chronic HF is associated with an increased risk of CV death and HFH (log rank $p = 0.03$) at 6-month follow-up (Figure 3C).

The baseline features of patients according to LVEF values have been reported in Table 7.

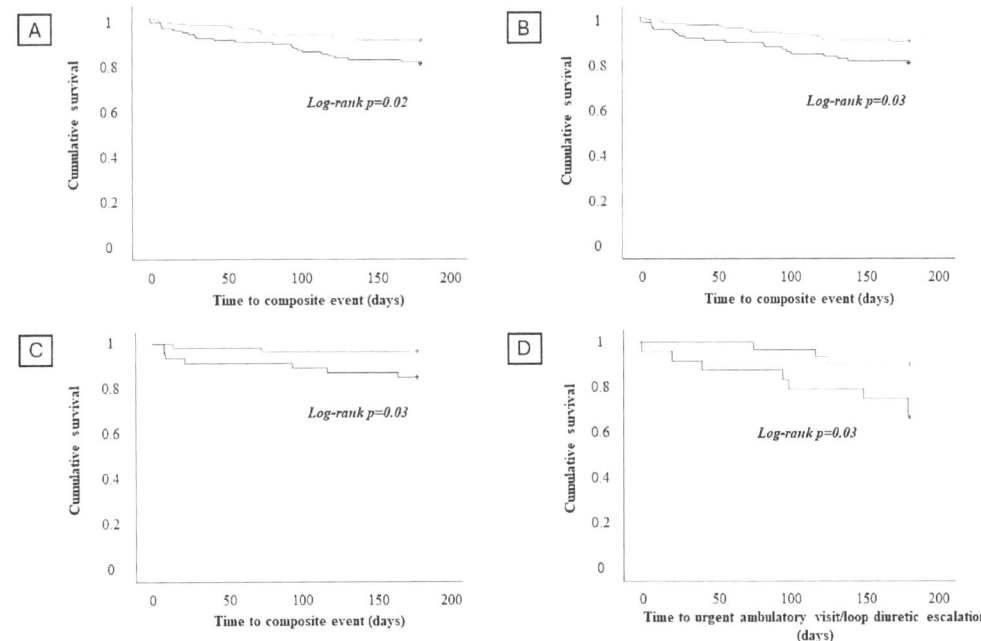

Figure 3. Survival analysis regarding the occurrence of the composite of cardiovascular (CV) death and heart failure hospitalization (HFH) in patients with an admission high-sensitivity T troponin (hs-cTnT) value below the median (blue line) and admission high-sensitivity T troponin value above the median (green line) in the overall population (**A**). Survival analysis regarding the occurrence of the composite of CV death and HFH in patients without significant in-hospital hs-cTnT increase (blue line) and with significant hs-cTnT increase (green line) in the overall population (**B**). Survival analysis regarding the occurrence of the composite of CV death and HFH in patients with an admission hs-cTnT value below the median (blue line) and admission hs-cTnT value above the median (green line) in the chronic HF subgroup (**C**). Survival analysis regarding the occurrence of worsening HF events and admission hs-cTnT values below the median (blue line) and above the median (green line) in the HFmrEF/HFpEF subgroup (**D**).

Table 4. Univariate and multivariate analysis regarding the variables considered as predictors of the composite event in the total population. High-sensitivity T troponin above the median at admission represents an independent predictor of cardiovascular death and heart failure hospitalization at 6-month follow-up in patients hospitalized with a diagnosis of heart failure.

	Univariate		
Variable	OR	95% CI	p Value
hs-cTnT above median	2.2	1.117–4.353	0.02
Age	1.01	0.986–1.044	0.33
Male sex	0.75	0.380–1.479	0.40
ACS	1.12	0.489–2.550	0.79
Arterial hypertension	0.65	0.322–1.328	0.24
Diabetes mellitus	1.64	0.838–3.201	0.15
eGFR	0.99	0.994–1.004	0.78
LVEF	0.99	0.950–1.012	0.21
Hemoglobin	0.88	0.768–1.015	0.08

Table 4. *Cont.*

	Multivariate		
Variable	OR	95% CI	p value
hs-cTnT above median	2.06	1.025–4.128	0.04
Hemoglobin	0.94	0.815–1.090	0.42

hs-cTnT—high-sensitivity cardiac troponin T; OR—odds ratio; CI—confidence interval; ACS—acute coronary syndrome; eGFR—estimated glomerular filtration rate; LVEF—left ventricular ejection fraction.

Table 5. Univariate and multivariate analysis regarding the variables considered as predictors of the composite event in the total population. High-sensitivity T troponin increase during hospitalization represents an independent predictor of cardiovascular death and heart failure hospitalization at 6-month follow-up in patients hospitalized with a diagnosis of heart failure.

	Univariate		
Variable	OR	95% CI	p Value
hs-cTnT increase	2.02	1.05–3.908	0.035
Age	1.01	0.968–10.44	0.33
Male sex	0.75	0.380–1.479	0.40
ACS	1.12	0.489–2.550	0.79
Arterial hypertension	0.65	0.322–1.328	0.24
Diabetes mellitus	1.64	0.838–3.201	0.15
eGFR	0.99	0.994–1.004	0.78
LVEF	0.98	0.950–1.012	0.21
Hemoglobin	0.88	0.768–1.015	0.08
	Multivariate		
Variable	OR	95% CI	p value
hs-cTnT increase	1.95	1.006–3.769	0.04
Hemoglobin	0.92	0.803–1.061	0.26

hs-cTnT—high-sensitivity cardiac troponin T; OR—odds ratio; CI—confidence interval; ACS—acute coronary syndrome; eGFR—estimated glomerular filtration rate; LVEF—left ventricular ejection fraction.

Table 6. Occurrence of each outcome according to high-sensitivity T troponin at hospital admission in chronic HF subgroup.

Variable	hs-cTnT below Median Value	hs-cTnT above Median Value	p Value
CV death/HFH, n (%)	2 (3.3)	7 (14.9)	0.04
CV death, n (%)	1 (1.7)	4 (8.5)	0.17
HFH, n (%)	1 (1.7)	5 (10.6)	0.08
Urgent visit/loop diuretic escalation, n (%)	8 (13.3)	12 (25.5)	0.1

CV—cardiovascular; HFH—heart failure hospitalization; hs-cTnT—high-sensitivity T troponin.

Patients with HFmrEF/HFpEF and admission hs-cTnT above the median value had a significantly higher risk of outpatient WHF (i.e., urgent ambulatory visit/loop diuretic escalation) at 6-month follow-up compared to patients with HFmrEF/HFpEF and admission hs-cTnT below the median value (8 vs. 3; 33.3% vs 10%; $p = 0.04$) (Table 8).

Table 7. Baseline features and discharge therapy of patients according to left ventricular ejection fraction.

Variable	HFrEF (N = 199)	HFmrEF/HFpEF (N = 54)	p Value
Age, years (IQR)	72 (64–80)	76 (68–81)	0.081
Male sex, n (%)	147 (73.9)	30 (55.6)	0.009
Ischemic etiology, n (%)	113 (56.8)	25 (46.3)	0.21
Arterial hypertension, n (%)	156 (78.4)	39 (72.2)	0.339
Diabetes mellitus, n (%)	59 (29.6)	13 (24.1)	0.421
Dyslipidemia, n (%)	104 (52.3)	29 (53.7)	0.851
Family history of CVD, n (%)	52 (26.1)	14 (25.9)	0.976
COPD, n (%)	51 (25.6)	16 (29.6)	0.554
Smoking habit, n (%)	75 (37.7)	21 (38.9)	0.872
Acute presentation, n (%)	120 (60.3)	26 (48.1)	0.024
Chronic presentation, n (%)	79 (39.7)	28 (51.9)	0.024
eGFR, mL/min/m^2 (IQR)	63 (44–80)	66.3 (50–84.3)	0.62
Hemoglobin, g/dL (IQR)	13 (10.9–14.3)	12.5 (11.2–14.2)	0.46
K$^+$, mmol/L (IQR)	4 (3.7–4.3)	4 (3.4–4.4)	0.55
Admission hs-cTnT, ng/mL (IQR)	0.031 (0.020–0.089)	0.031 (0.019–0.067)	0.817
Discharge hs-cTnT, ng/mL (IQR)	0.030 (0.020–0.074)	0.04 (0.02–0.079)	0.139
hs-cTnT peak, ng/mL (IQR)	0.04 (0.024–0.118)	0.044 (0.022–0.183)	0.852
hs-cTnT delta peak-admission, ng/mL (IQR)	0.001 (0–0.024)	0.003 (0–0.048)	0.375
LVEF, % (IQR)	30 (21–35)	45 (45–50)	<0.001
LVEDD, mm (IQR)	60 (54–65)	50.5 (45–56)	<0.001
IVS, mm (IQR)	11 (9–12)	11 (10–12.3)	0.077
PW, mm (IQR)	10 (9–11)	10 (9–10)	0.737
Basal RVEDD, mm (IQR)	34 (29–41)	38 (33–44)	0.1
TAPSE, mm (IQR)	18 (14–20)	19 (17–20)	0.029
ACEi, n (%)	17 (8.5)	17 (31.5)	<0.001
ARBs, n (%)	14 (7)	4 (7.4)	1
ARNI, n (%)	137 (68.8)	15 (27.8)	<0.001
BB, n (%)	189 (95)	53 (98.1)	0.466
MRAs, n (%)	165 (82.9)	29 (53.7)	<0.001
SGLT2i, n (%)	108 (54.3)	17 (31.5)	0.009
Loop diuretics, n (%)	153 (76.9)	31 (57.4)	0.004
Median NYHA, class (IQR)	3 (2–3)	3 (2–3)	1

IQR—interquartile range; CVD—cardiovascular disease; COPD—chronic obstructive pulmonary disease; eGFR—estimated glomerular filtration rate; K$^+$—potassium; hs-cTnT—high-sensitivity T troponin; HFrEF—heart failure with reduced ejection fraction; HFmrEF—heart failure with mildly reduced ejection fraction; HFpEF—heart failure with preserved ejection fraction; LVEF—left ventricular ejection fraction; LVEDD—left ventricular end diastolic diameter; IVS—interventricular septum; PW—posterior wall; RVEDD—right ventricular end diastolic diameter; TAPSE—tricuspid annular plane systolic excursion; ACEi—angiotensin-converting enzyme inhibitor; ARBs—angiotensin receptor blockers; ARNI: angiotensin receptor/neprilysin inhibitor; BB: beta blocker; MRA—mineralocorticoid receptor antagonist; SGLT2i—sodium glucose cotransporter 2 inhibitor; NYHA—New York Heart Association.

Table 8. Occurrences of each outcome in the subgroup of patients with HFpEF/HFmrEF according to hs-cTnT values at hospital admission.

Variable	hs-cTnT below Median Value	hs-cTnT above Median Value	p Value
CV death/HFH, n (%)	2 (6.7)	6 (25)	0.12
CV death, n (%)	1 (3.3)	3 (12.5)	0.31
HFH, n (%)	1 (3.3)	4 (16.7)	0.16
Urgent visit/loop diuretic escalation, n (%)	3 (10)	8 (33.3)	0.04

CV—cardiovascular; HFH—heart failure hospitalization; hs-cTnT—high-sensitivity T troponin.

Kaplan–Meier survival analysis demonstrated that patients with HFmrEF/HFpEF and an admission hs-cTnT above the median value have a significantly increased risk of experiencing an outpatient WHF event at 6-month follow-up (log rank $p = 0.03$) (Figure 3D).

4. Discussion

The identification of prognostic and predictive biomarkers is currently one of the biggest challenges for the improvement of HF management. The only validated biomarkers in HF are NPs. Beyond NPs, the most promising biomarkers are hs-cTnT and suppression of tumorigenesis-2 ligand (sST2L), and both have been shown to be independent predictors of mortality in HF [17]. However, data regarding hs-cTnT as prognostic tool in HF are discordant and often confusing, as well as scarce [18].

The results of our study highlighted the role of hs-cTnT as a valid prognostic biomarker in the total population of HF patients. More specifically, our results demonstrated that not only admission hs-cTnT values above the median, but also hs-cTnT increase during hospitalization are independent predictors of the composite of CV death and HFH at 6-month follow-up (OR: 2.06; 95% CI: 1.02–4.1; $p = 0.04$ and OR:1.95; 95%CI: 1.006–3.769; $p = 0.04$, respectively).

Previous studies revealed the possible role of troponins as predictive biomarkers of major CV events in HF patients [19–29]. Latini et al. [19] demonstrated that high levels of hs-cTnT were moderately associated with CV death in chronic HF patients, with a risk that was 5% higher when troponin levels above the median were detected. You et al. [20] identified that cardiac troponin I (cTnI) was an independent predictor of all-cause mortality in patients with acute decompensated HF. These results were confirmed in different studies including cTnI [21–23]. Del Carlo et al. [24] demonstrated a higher incidence of 1-year rehospitalization due to HF and mortality in patients with persistent troponin T levels higher than 0.02 ng/dl. Aimo et al. [25] conducted a meta-analysis analyzing a global population of 9289 in which it was confirmed that cTnT was an independent predictor of all-cause mortality and CV hospitalizations in patients with chronic HF. In a meta-analysis by Masson et al. [26] including 5284 patients, hs-cTnT levels were predictors of cardiovascular events in patients with chronic HF; however, it did not add significant prognostic discrimination. In acute decompensated HF patients, Peacock et al. [27] conducted a retrospective analysis on a population of 84872 patients hospitalized due to acute HF decompensation. A higher in-hospital mortality for patients with elevated hs-cTnT levels at admission has been observed [27]. Furthermore, Pandey et al. [28] reported that cardiac troponin elevation in patients with acute decompensated HFpEF was a predictor of adverse in-hospital and post-discharge events. In a recent meta-analysis by Evans et al. [29] including 67063 patients, hs-cTnT was associated with incident HF, improving also HF prediction.

These results, including the results of our study, are supported by a physiological explanation. It is known that the blood concentration of cardiac troponins is a consequence of myocardial cell necrosis and that every clinical condition that causes cardiomyocyte damage is also a cause of cardiac troponin blood level elevation [18,30]. In HF patients, cardiac troponin release may happen as a consequence of chronic ischemia, also in the absence of acute coronary stenosis [31]. This is due to HF-induced myocardial remodeling and subendocardial ischemia, determined by the excessive myocardial wall stress and cardiomyocyte damage [31]. Also, increased filling pressures, tachyarrhythmia or bradyarrhythmia, arterial hypotension, anemia, and endothelial dysfunction may be reasons for reduced oxygen supply to cardiomyocytes [32]. The consequence is the generation of myocardial injury, with an increase in cell permeability, allowing cytosol troponin to be released into the circulation [33,34].

Also, anemia and iron deficiency are known comorbidities associated with adverse events and worse life quality in patients with HF [1]. According to the Guidelines and the World Health Organization, anemia is defined by a hemoglobin level < 12 g/dL and <13 g/dL in females and males, respectively [1]. In our population, hemoglobin represented a predictor of CV death/HFH at univariate analysis for the total population, but it did not reach statistical significance at multivariate analysis.

Most of the mentioned studies are limited to describing an association between troponins and major CV events [35], without considering subclinical events in WHF and HF subgroups. Scenarios of WHF without hospitalization, such as escalation of diuretic therapy and/or need for urgent ambulatory visits, are also important concerns in the management of HF patients. This aspect has been highlighted by the consideration that hospitalization can be compared to the "tip of the iceberg" of a complex process of disease-worsening, which occurs outside of the hospital and is often subclinical [4,5]. It has been demonstrated that outpatient escalation of diuretics therapy increases the risk of 1-year mortality by 75% [36]. WHF is a transversal condition which involves HF patients regardless of LVEF.

HFrEF is widely studied in the scientific literature, while HFmrEF and HFpEF are entities less studied, but growing evidence demonstrates that their prognoses are similar to HFrEF [37]. In our study, we found that patients with HFmrEF/HFpEF and an admission hs-cTnT above the median value had a significant higher risk of urgent ambulatory visit/loop diuretic escalation at 6 months compared to HFmrEF/HFpEF patients with hs-cTnT below the median value ($p = 0.03$). It is known that HFpEF and HFmrEF populations have substantial differences compared to HFrEF patients. HFpEF patients are usually older and have multiple comorbidities with a less frequent history of ischemic heart disease than in HFrEF [38]. Furthermore, HFpEF has a greater association with extracardiac comorbidities, as well as with the female gender [39]. Although the mortality is similar in HFpEF and HFrEF, there has been shown to be a higher incidence of hospitalization in HFpEF, which is mainly related to worsening comorbidities [40]. It has been shown that HFmrEF has more similar outcomes to HFpEF than HFrEF [41]. The population of HFmrEF, similarly to HFpEF, is composed of older people and has a higher comorbidity burden than the HFrEF population. The prognosis of HFmrEF and HFpEF is mainly influenced by the adverse events related to comorbidities, and the role of hs-cTnT in this patient population may be explained by continuous ventricular pressure overload with consequently subendocardial ischemia [33,42].

Another important result of our study was that the risk of the composite of CV death and HFH was significantly higher in patients with chronic HF and an admission hs-cTnT above the median value compared to patients with an admission hs-cTnT below the median value ($p = 0.03$). This finding emphasizes the prognostic significance of hs-cTnT levels at hospital admission in patients with HF. Chronic HF patients with elevated hs-cTnT levels are likely to have underlying cardiac damage or stress, predisposing them to a higher risk of adverse cardiovascular outcomes. The elevated hs-cTnT levels on admission serve as a marker of continuous myocardial injury [43] in chronic HF patients. Our results seem to suggest that the long-standing steady myocardial damage in chronic HF may severely impact the prognosis.

The use of biomarkers such as NPs and cardiac troponins is suitable in most hospitals and outpatient services, and their use to manage patients is feasible and standardizable. On the contrary, other biomarkers, albeit interesting, are not always available everywhere.

NPs and cardiac troponins reflect two different pathophysiological pathways in HF [44,45], whose involvement may vary according to the HF subgroup considered. Therefore, the integrated evaluation of the latter may bring relevant information which can be integrated into clinical evaluation in light of better patient management. Importantly, our results highlight the potential role of hs-cTnT quantification, in order to predict adverse events in peculiar HF subpopulations. An emerging and challenging aspect is the possibility of using these biomarkers not only to stratify patients' prognoses, but also to guide therapy with HF disease-modifying drugs in order to identify patients at higher risk of adverse events and be more aggressive with the up-titration of therapy [6,17,46,47]. This aspect has been recently evaluated for NPs, with promising results.

Our study has several limitations. The results should be confirmed on a larger population and larger subgroups of HF patients. Due to the number of patients, multivariate analysis has not been used for subgroups. Other biomarkers have not been included in the study and compared to hs-cTnT in terms of prognostic predictivity. The trend of hs-cTnT has not been evaluated during the follow-up.

5. Conclusions

The assessment of biomarkers in HF represents a crucial aspect of patient management. Our results suggest that in-hospital hs-cTnT levels may predict the composite of CV death/HFH in patients with HF. In particular, in the subgroup of chronic HF patients, hs-cTnT may predict the composite of CV death/HFH, while in HFmrEF/HFpEF subgroup, hs-cTnT may predict out of hospital WHF events. Our results emphasize the importance of the serial assessment of hs-cTnT at admission and during hospitalization to assess the prognosis in HF patients.

Author Contributions: Conceptualization, A.D., P.S., S.P. and F.F.; data curation, A.D., P.S., S.P., M.V.M., A.D.P., R.G., V.M., A.L.F., C.C., S.M.-I., L.T., L.V., S.L.M. and G.D.P.; formal analysis, A.D., P.S., S.P. and M.V.M.; methodology, A.D., P.S., S.P. and M.V.M.; supervision, C.L., G.S., M.M., R.B., F.F. and C.D.V.; validation, C.L., G.S., M.M., R.B., F.F. and C.D.V.; visualization, C.L., G.S., M.M., R.B., F.F. and C.D.V.; writing—original draft, A.D., P.S., S.P., M.V.M., A.D.P., R.G., V.M., A.L.F., C.C., S.M.-I., L.T., L.V., S.L.M. and G.D.P.; writing—review and editing, A.D., P.S., S.P., M.V.M., C.L., G.S., M.M., R.B., F.F. and C.D.V. All authors have read and agreed to the published version of the manuscript.

Funding: This work did not receive external funding.

Institutional Review Board Statement: The study was conducted according to the guidelines of the Declaration of Helsinki and approved by the Ethics Committee of Policlinico Umberto I of Rome (protocol code 7068, approved on 8 May 2023).

Informed Consent Statement: Informed consent was obtained from all subjects involved in the study.

Data Availability Statement: Data are available upon reasonable request.

Conflicts of Interest: The authors declare no conflicts of interests.

References

1. McDonagh, T.A.; Metra, M.; Adamo, M.; Gardner, R.S.; Baumbach, A.; Böhm, M.; Burri, H.; Butler, J.; Čelutkienė, J.; Chioncel, O.; et al. 2021 ESC Guidelines for the diagnosis and treatment of acute and chronic heart failure. *Eur. Heart J.* **2021**, *42*, 3599–3726. [CrossRef] [PubMed]
2. Writing Committee; Maddox, T.M.; Januzzi, J.L., Jr.; Allen, L.A.; Breathett, K.; Butler, J.; Davis, L.L.; Fonarow, G.C.; Ibrahim, N.E.; Lindenfeld, J.; et al. 2021 Update to the 2017 ACC Expert Consensus Decision Pathway for Optimization of Heart Failure Treatment: Answers to 10 Pivotal Issues about Heart Failure with Reduced Ejection Fraction: A Report of the American College of Cardiology Solution Set Oversight Committee. *J. Am. Coll. Cardiol.* **2021**, *77*, 772–810. [CrossRef] [PubMed]
3. Tsao, C.W.; Lyass, A.; Enserro, D.; Larson, M.G.; Ho, J.E.; Kizer, J.R.; Gottdiener, J.S.; Psaty, B.M.; Vasan, R.S. Temporal trends in the incidence of and mortality associated with heart failure with preserved and reduced ejection fraction. *JACC Heart Fail.* **2018**, *6*, 678–685. [CrossRef] [PubMed]

4. Greene, S.J.; Bauersachs, J.; Brugts, J.J.; Ezekowitz, J.A.; Lam, C.S.P.; Lund, L.H.; Ponikowski, P.; Voors, A.A.; Zannad, F.; Zieroth, S.; et al. Worsening Heart Failure: Nomenclature, Epidemiology, and Future Directions: JACC Review Topic of the Week. *J. Am. Coll. Cardiol.* **2023**, *81*, 413–424. [CrossRef] [PubMed]
5. D'Amato, A.; Prosperi, S.; Severino, P.; Myftari, V.; Labbro Francia, A.; Cestiè, C.; Pierucci, N.; Marek-Iannucci, S.; Mariani, M.V.; Germanò, R.; et al. Current Approaches to Worsening Heart Failure: Pathophysiological and Molecular Insights. *Int. J. Mol. Sci.* **2024**, *25*, 1574. [CrossRef] [PubMed]
6. Tsutsui, H.; Albert, N.M.; Coats, A.J.S.; Anker, S.D.; Bayes-Genis, A.; Butler, J.; Chioncel, O.; Defilippi, C.R.; Drazner, M.H.; Felker, G.M.; et al. Natriuretic Peptides: Role in the Diagnosis and Management of Heart Failure: A Scientific Statement from the Heart Failure Association of the European Society of Cardiology, Heart Failure Society of America and Japanese Heart Failure Society. *J. Card. Fail.* **2023**, *29*, 787–804. [CrossRef] [PubMed]
7. Logeart, D.; Thabut, G.; Jourdain, P.; Chavelas, C.; Beyne, P.; Beauvais, F.; Bouvier, E.; Solal, A.C. Predischarge B-type natriuretic peptide assay for identifying patients at high risk of re-admission after decompensated heart failure. *J. Am. Coll. Cardiol.* **2004**, *43*, 635–641. [CrossRef] [PubMed]
8. Kociol, R.D.; Horton, J.R.; Fonarow, G.C.; Reyes, E.M.; Shaw, L.K.; O'Connor, C.M.; Felker, G.M.; Hernandez, A.F. Admission, discharge, or change in B-type natriuretic peptide and long-term outcomes: Data from Organized Program to Initiate Lifesaving Treatment in Hospitalized Patients with Heart Failure (OPTIMIZE-HF) linked to Medicare claims. *Circ. Heart Fail.* **2011**, *4*, 628–636. [CrossRef] [PubMed]
9. Ezekowitz, J.A.; Alemayehu, W.; Rathwell, S.; Grant, A.D.; Fiuzat, M.; Whellan, D.J.; Ahmad, T.; Adams, K.; Piña, I.L.; Cooper, L.S.; et al. The influence of comorbidities on achieving an N-terminal pro-b-type natriuretic peptide target: A secondary analysis of the GUIDE-IT trial. *ESC Heart Fail.* **2022**, *9*, 77–86. [CrossRef]
10. Del Carlo, C.H.; O'Connor, C.M. Cardiac troponins in congestive heart failure. *Am. Heart J.* **1999**, *138 Pt 1*, 646–653. [CrossRef]
11. Garg, P.; Morris, P.; Fazlanie, A.L.; Vijayan, S.; Dancso, B.; Dastidar, A.G.; Plein, S.; Mueller, C.; Haaf, P. Cardiac biomarkers of acute coronary syndrome: From history to high-sensitivity cardiac troponin. *Intern. Emerg. Med.* **2017**, *12*, 147–155. [CrossRef] [PubMed]
12. Chauin, A. The Main Causes and Mechanisms of Increase in Cardiac Troponin Concentrations Other than Acute Myocardial Infarction (Part 1): Physical Exertion, Inflammatory Heart Disease, Pulmonary Embolism, Renal Failure, Sepsis. *Vasc. Health Risk Manag.* **2021**, *17*, 601–617. [CrossRef]
13. Sandoval, Y.; Apple, F.S.; Mahler, S.A.; Body, R.; Collinson, P.O.; Jaffe, A.S.; International Federation of Clinical Chemistry and Laboratory Medicine Committee on the Clinical Application of Cardiac Biomarkers. High-Sensitivity Cardiac Troponin and the 2021 AHA/ACC/ASE/CHEST/SAEM/SCCT/SCMR Guidelines for the Evaluation and Diagnosis of Acute Chest Pain. *Circulation* **2022**, *146*, 569–581. [CrossRef]
14. Sato, Y.; Yamada, T.; Taniguchi, R.; Nagai, K.; Makiyama, T.; Okada, H.; Kataoka, K.; Ito, H.; Matsumori, A.; Sasayama, S.; et al. Persistently increased serum concentrations of cardiac troponin t in patients with idiopathic dilated cardiomyopathy are predictive of adverse outcomes. *Circulation* **2001**, *103*, 369–374. [CrossRef] [PubMed]
15. Setsuta, K.; Seino, Y.; Ogawa, T.; Arao, M.; Miyatake, Y.; Takano, T. Use of cytosolic and myofibril markers in the detection of ongoing myocardial damage in patients with chronic heart failure. *Am. J. Med.* **2002**, *113*, 717–722. [CrossRef] [PubMed]
16. Kociol, R.D.; Pang, P.S.; Gheorghiade, M.; Fonarow, G.C.; O'Connor, C.M.; Felker, G.M. Troponin elevation in heart failure prevalence, mechanisms, and clinical implications. *J. Am. Coll. Cardiol.* **2010**, *56*, 1071–1078. [CrossRef]
17. Castiglione, V.; Aimo, A.; Vergaro, G.; Saccaro, L.; Passino, C.; Emdin, M. Biomarkers for the diagnosis and management of heart failure. *Heart Fail. Rev.* **2022**, *27*, 625–643. [CrossRef]
18. Lazar, D.R.; Lazar, F.L.; Homorodean, C.; Cainap, C.; Focsan, M.; Cainap, S.; Olinic, D.M. High-Sensitivity Troponin: A Review on Characteristics, Assessment, and Clinical Implications. *Dis. Markers* **2022**, *2022*, 9713326. [CrossRef]
19. Latini, R.; Masson, S.; Anand, I.S.; Missov, E.; Carlson, M.; Vago, T.; Angelici, L.; Barlera, S.; Parrinello, G.; Maggioni, A.P.; et al. Prognostic value of very low plasma concentrations of troponin T in patients with stable chronic heart failure. *Circulation* **2007**, *116*, 1242–1249. [CrossRef]
20. You, J.J.; Austin, P.C.; Alter, D.A.; Ko, D.T.; Tu, J.V. Relation between cardiac troponin I and mortality in acute decompensated heart failure. *Am. Heart J.* **2007**, *153*, 462–470. [CrossRef]
21. Myhre, P.L.; O'Meara, E.; Claggett, B.L.; de Denus, S.; Jarolim, P.; Anand, I.S.; Beldhuis, I.E.; Fleg, J.L.; Lewis, E.; Pitt, B.; et al. Cardiac Troponin I and Risk of Cardiac Events in Patients with Heart Failure and Preserved Ejection Fraction. *Circ. Heart Fail.* **2018**, *11*, e005312. [CrossRef] [PubMed]
22. Yan, I.; Börschel, C.S.; Neumann, J.T.; Sprünker, N.A.; Makarova, N.; Kontto, J.; Kuulasmaa, K.; Salomaa, V.; Magnussen, C.; Iacoviello, L.; et al. High-Sensitivity Cardiac Troponin I Levels and Prediction of Heart Failure: Results from the BiomarCaRE Consortium. *JACC Heart Fail.* **2020**, *8*, 401–411. [CrossRef] [PubMed]
23. Stelzle, D.; Shah, A.S.V.; Anand, A.; Strachan, F.E.; Chapman, A.R.; Denvir, M.A.; Mills, N.L.; McAllister, D.A. High-sensitivity cardiac troponin I and risk of heart failure in patients with suspected acute coronary syndrome: A cohort study. *Eur. Heart J. Qual. Care Clin. Outcomes* **2018**, *4*, 36–42. [CrossRef] [PubMed]

24. Del Carlo, C.H.; Pereira-Barretto, A.C.; Cassaro-Strunz, C.; Latorre, M.d.R.; Ramires, J.A. Serial measure of cardiac troponin T levels for prediction of clinical events in decompensated heart failure. *J. Card. Fail.* **2004**, *10*, 43–48. [CrossRef] [PubMed]
25. Aimo, A.; Januzzi, J.L., Jr.; Vergaro, G.; Ripoli, A.; Latini, R.; Masson, S.; Magnoli, M.; Anand, I.S.; Cohn, J.N.; Tavazzi, L.; et al. Prognostic Value of High-Sensitivity Troponin T in Chronic Heart Failure: An Individual Patient Data Meta-Analysis. *Circulation* **2018**, *137*, 286–297. [CrossRef] [PubMed]
26. Masson, S.; Anand, I.; Favero, C.; Barlera, S.; Vago, T.; Bertocchi, F.; Maggioni, A.P.; Tavazzi, L.; Tognoni, G.; Cohn, J.N.; et al. Serial measurement of cardiac troponin T using a highly sensitive assay in patients with chronic heart failure: Data from 2 large randomized clinical trials. *Circulation* **2012**, *125*, 280–288. [CrossRef] [PubMed]
27. Peacock, W.F., 4th; De Marco, T.; Fonarow, G.C.; Diercks, D.; Wynne, J.; Apple, F.S.; Wu, A.H. Cardiac troponin and outcome in acute heart failure. *N. Engl. J. Med.* **2008**, *358*, 2117–2126. [CrossRef] [PubMed]
28. Pandey, A.; Golwala, H.; Sheng, S.; DeVore, A.D.; Hernandez, A.F.; Bhatt, D.L.; Heidenreich, P.A.; Yancy, C.W.; de Lemos, J.A.; Fonarow, G.C. Factors Associated with and Prognostic Implications of Cardiac Troponin Elevation in Decompensated Heart Failure with Preserved Ejection Fraction: Findings from the American Heart Association Get with the Guidelines-Heart Failure Program. *JAMA Cardiol.* **2017**, *2*, 136–145. [CrossRef] [PubMed]
29. Evans, J.D.W.; Dobbin, S.J.H.; Pettit, S.J.; Di Angelantonio, E.; Willeit, P. High-Sensitivity Cardiac Troponin and New-Onset Heart Failure: A Systematic Review and Meta-Analysis of 67,063 Patients with 4165 Incident Heart Failure Events. *JACC Heart Fail.* **2018**, *6*, 187–197. [CrossRef]
30. Westermann, D.; Neumann, J.T.; Sörensen, N.A.; Blankenberg, S. High-sensitivity assays for troponin in patients with cardiac disease. *Nat. Rev. Cardiol.* **2017**, *14*, 472–483. [CrossRef]
31. Januzzi, J.L., Jr.; Filippatos, G.; Nieminen, M.; Gheorghiade, M. Troponin elevation in patients with heart failure: On behalf of the third Universal Definition of Myocardial Infarction Global Task Force: Heart Failure Section. *Eur. Heart J.* **2012**, *33*, 2265–2271. [CrossRef]
32. Miller, W.L.; Hartman, K.A.; Burritt, M.F.; Grill, D.E.; Jaffe, A.S. Profiles of serial changes in cardiac troponin T concentrations and outcome in ambulatory patients with chronic heart failure. *J. Am. Coll. Cardiol.* **2009**, *54*, 1715–1721. [CrossRef]
33. Potluri, S.; Ventura, H.O.; Mulumudi, M.; Mehra, M.R. Cardiac troponin levels in heart failure. *Cardiol. Rev.* **2004**, *12*, 21–25. [CrossRef]
34. Meijers, W.C.; Bayes-Genis, A.; Mebazaa, A.; Bauersachs, J.; Cleland, J.G.F.; Coats, A.J.S.; Januzzi, J.L.; Maisel, A.S.; McDonald, K.; Mueller, T.; et al. Circulating heart failure biomarkers beyond natriuretic peptides: Review from the Biomarker Study Group of the Heart Failure Association (HFA), European Society of Cardiology (ESC). *Eur. J. Heart Fail.* **2021**, *23*, 1610–1632. [CrossRef] [PubMed]
35. Gherasim, L. Troponins in Heart Failure—A Perpetual Challenge. *Maedica* **2019**, *14*, 371–377. [CrossRef] [PubMed]
36. Madelaire, C.; Gustafsson, F.; Stevenson, L.W.; Kristensen, S.L.; Køber, L.; Andersen, J.; D'Souza, M.; Biering-Sørensen, T.; Andersson, C.; Torp-Pedersen, C.; et al. One-Year Mortality after Intensification of Outpatient Diuretic Therapy. *J. Am. Heart Assoc.* **2020**, *9*, e016010. [CrossRef]
37. Palazzuoli, A.; Beltrami, M. Are HFpEF and HFmrEF So Different? The Need to Understand Distinct Phenotypes. *Front. Cardiovasc. Med.* **2021**, *8*, 676658. [CrossRef]
38. Li, P.; Zhao, H.; Zhang, J.; Ning, Y.; Tu, Y.; Xu, D.; Zeng, Q. Similarities and Differences between HFmrEF and HFpEF. *Front. Cardiovasc. Med.* **2021**, *8*, 678614. [CrossRef]
39. Simmonds, S.J.; Cuijpers, I.; Heymans, S.; Jones, E.A.V. Cellular and Molecular Differences between HFpEF and HFrEF: A Step Ahead in an Improved Pathological Understanding. *Cells* **2020**, *9*, 242. [CrossRef] [PubMed]
40. Streng, K.W.; Nauta, J.F.; Hillege, H.L.; Anker, S.D.; Cleland, J.G.; Dickstein, K.; Filippatos, G.; Lang, C.C.; Metra, M.; Ng, L.L.; et al. Non-cardiac comorbidities in heart failure with reduced, mid-range and preserved ejection fraction. *Int. J. Cardiol.* **2018**, *271*, 132–139. [CrossRef]
41. Santas, E.; de la Espriella, R.; Palau, P.; Miñana, G.; Amiguet, M.; Sanchis, J.; Lupón, J.; Bayes-Genís, A.; Chorro, F.J.; Villota, J.N. Rehospitalization burden and morbidity risk in patients with heart failure with mid-range ejection fraction. *ESC Heart Fail.* **2020**, *7*, 1007–1014. [CrossRef] [PubMed]
42. Savarese, G.; Becher, P.M.; Lund, L.H.; Seferovic, P.; Rosano, G.M.C.; Coats, A.J.S. Global burden of heart failure: A comprehensive and updated review of epidemiology. *Cardiovasc. Res.* **2023**, *118*, 3272–3287. [CrossRef] [PubMed]
43. Agdashian, D.; Daniels, L.B. What Is the Clinical Utility of Cardiac Troponins in Heart Failure? Are They Modifiable beyond Their Prognostic Value? *Curr. Heart Fail. Rep.* **2023**, *20*, 33–43. [CrossRef] [PubMed]
44. Severino, P.; D'Amato, A.; Prosperi, S.; Myftari, V.; Canuti, E.S.; Labbro Francia, A.; Cestiè, C.; Maestrini, V.; Lavalle, C.; Badagliacca, R.; et al. Heart Failure Pharmacological Management: Gaps and Current Perspectives. *J. Clin. Med.* **2023**, *12*, 1020. [CrossRef] [PubMed]
45. Severino, P.; D'Amato, A.; Prosperi, S.; Dei Cas, A.; Mattioli, A.V.; Cevese, A.; Novo, G.; Prat, M.; Pedrinelli, R.; Raddino, R.; et al. Do the Current Guidelines for Heart Failure Diagnosis and Treatment Fit with Clinical Complexity? *J. Clin. Med.* **2022**, *11*, 857. [CrossRef] [PubMed]

46. Adamo, M.; Pagnesi, M.; Mebazaa, A.; Davison, B.; Edwards, C.; Tomasoni, D.; Arrigo, M.; Barros, M.; Biegus, J.; Celutkiene, J.; et al. NT-proBNP and high intensity care for acute heart failure: The STRONG-HF trial. *Eur. Heart J.* **2023**, *44*, 2947–2962. [CrossRef]
47. Severino, P.; Mancone, M.; D'Amato, A.; Mariani, M.V.; Prosperi, S.; Alunni Fegatelli, D.; Birtolo, L.I.; Angotti, D.; Milanese, A.; Cerrato, E.; et al. Heart failure 'the cancer of the heart': The prognostic role of the HLM score. *ESC Heart Fail.* **2024**, *11*, 390–399. [CrossRef]

Disclaimer/Publisher's Note: The statements, opinions and data contained in all publications are solely those of the individual author(s) and contributor(s) and not of MDPI and/or the editor(s). MDPI and/or the editor(s) disclaim responsibility for any injury to people or property resulting from any ideas, methods, instructions or products referred to in the content.

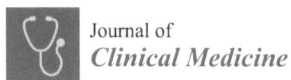

Article

Unexpected Genetic Twists in Patients with Cardiac Devices

Emilia-Violeta Goanta [1,2], Cristina Vacarescu [3,4,5,*], Georgica Tartea [2,6], Adrian Ungureanu [2], Sebastian Militaru [7], Alexandra Muraretu [2], Adelina-Andreea Faur-Grigori [4], Lucian Petrescu [3], Radu Vătășescu [8,9] and Dragos Cozma [3,4,5]

1. Doctoral School, "Victor Babes" University of Medicine and Pharmacy, 300041 Timisoara, Romania; goanta.emilia@umft.ro
2. Cardiology Department, Emergency County Hospital of Craiova, Tabaci Street, Nr. 1, 200642 Craiova, Romania; georgica.tartea@umfcv.ro (G.T.); adrian_909uai@yahoo.com (A.U.); afzanfir@gmail.com (A.M.)
3. Department of Cardiology, "Victor Babes" University of Medicine and Pharmacy, 2 Eftimie Murgu Square, 300041 Timisoara, Romania; petrescu_lucian@yahoo.com (L.P.); dragos.cozma@umft.ro (D.C.)
4. Institute of Cardiovascular Diseases Timisoara, 13A Gheorghe Adam Street, 300310 Timisoara, Romania; andreeaadelinafaur@yahoo.com
5. Research Center of the Institute of Cardiovascular Diseases Timisoara, 13A Gheorghe Adam Street, 300310 Timisoara, Romania
6. Department of Physiology, University of Medicine and Pharmacy of Craiova, 200349 Craiova, Romania
7. Department of Cardiology, Craiova University of Medicine and Pharmacy, 200349 Craiova, Romania; sebastian.militaru@umfcv.ro
8. Cardiology Department, Clinical Emergency Hospital, 014461 Bucharest, Romania; radu.vatasescu@umfcd.ro
9. Faculty of Medicine, Carol Davila University of Medicine and Pharmacy, 050474 Bucharest, Romania
* Correspondence: cristina.vacarescu@umft.ro

Abstract: Objective: To assess the frequency and types of genetic mutations in patients with arrhythmias who underwent cardiac device implantation. **Methods:** Retrospective observational study, including 38 patients with different arrhythmias and cardiac arrest as a first cardiac event. Treatment modalities encompass pacemakers, transvenous defibrillators, loop recorders, subcutaneous defibrillators, and cardiac resynchronization therapy. All patients underwent genetic testing, using commercially available panels (106–174 genes). Outcome measures include mortality, arrhythmia recurrence, and device-related complications. **Results:** Clinical parameters revealed a family history of sudden cardiac death in 19 patients (50%), who were predominantly male (58%) and had a mean age of 44.5 years and a mean left ventricle ejection fraction of 40.3%. Genetic testing identified mutations in various genes, predominantly *TMEM43* (11%). In two patients (3%) with arrhythmogenic cardiomyopathy, complete subcutaneous defibrillator extraction with de novo transvenous implantable cardioverter-defibrillator implantation was needed. The absence of multiple associations among severe gene mutations was crucial for cardiac resynchronization therapy response. Mortality in this group was around 3% in titin dilated cardiomyopathy patients. **Conclusions:** Integration of genetic testing into the decision-making process for patients with electronic devices represents a paradigm shift in personalized medicine. By identifying genetic markers associated with arrhythmia susceptibility, heart failure etiology, and cardiac resynchronization therapy response, clinicians can tailor device choices to optimize patient outcomes.

Keywords: cardiac devices; genetics; sudden cardiac death; pacemakers; defibrillators; resynchronization therapy; loop recorders

Citation: Goanta, E.-V.; Vacarescu, C.; Tartea, G.; Ungureanu, A.; Militaru, S.; Muraretu, A.; Faur-Grigori, A.-A.; Petrescu, L.; Vătășescu, R.; Cozma, D. Unexpected Genetic Twists in Patients with Cardiac Devices. *J. Clin. Med.* **2024**, *13*, 3801. https://doi.org/10.3390/jcm13133801

Academic Editors: Maurizio Taramasso and Christian Sohns

Received: 31 May 2024
Revised: 12 June 2024
Accepted: 26 June 2024
Published: 28 June 2024

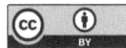

Copyright: © 2024 by the authors. Licensee MDPI, Basel, Switzerland. This article is an open access article distributed under the terms and conditions of the Creative Commons Attribution (CC BY) license (https://creativecommons.org/licenses/by/4.0/).

1. Introduction

Arrhythmias and cardiac arrest pose significant challenges in clinical management, requiring various cardiac devices and ablation procedures for treatment [1–5]. Understanding the genetics and clinical factors influencing outcomes is crucial for personalized treatment strategies [6]. Genetic testing has emerged as a valuable tool, providing insights into mutations associated with channelopathies and cardiomyopathies [6,7].

Sudden cardiac death (SCD) represents a devastating outcome, often occurring unexpectedly and leaving a profound impact on affected individuals and their families. While SCD can stem from various cardiac pathologies, channelopathies and cardiomyopathies emerge as significant contributors to this tragic event. Channelopathies encompass a group of genetic disorders characterized by abnormal ion channel function in cardiac cells, leading to arrhythmias and, in severe cases, to SCD. Similarly, cardiomyopathies entail structural abnormalities of the heart muscle, impairing its contractile function and elevating the risk of lethal arrhythmias.

It is estimated that there are about 7000 single-gene inherited disorders. Many genes responsible for hereditary cardiomyopathies, such as dilated cardiomyopathy (DCM, OMIM #604145), hypertrophic cardiomyopathy (HCM, OMIM #192600), and arrhythmogenic cardiomyopathy (ACM, OMIM #604400), as well as hereditary arrhythmias such as long QT syndromes (LQTS, OMIM #192500), Brugada syndrome (BrS, OMIM #601144), cardiac conduction defects (CCD, OMIM #115080), and catecholaminergic polymorphic ventricular tachycardia (CPVT OMIM #604772), have been identified.

Congenital LQTS is characterized by a prolonged QT interval on the baseline ECG, usually associated with T-wave abnormalities. Long QT syndrome genes can be classified into three main groups: pathogenic variants that reduce potassium outward currents, pathogenic variants that increase sodium inward currents, and pathogenic variants that increase calcium inward currents. Pathogenic variants related to potassium channels account for the vast majority of *LQTS* cases, with *KCNQ1* and *KCNH2* [8,9] being responsible for 80% of all genetically explained LQTS cases. Currently, the genes with definitive evidence include *KCNQ1*, *KCNH2*, *SCN5A*, *CALM1*, *CALM2*, and *CALM3*. The genes with moderate evidence are *CACNA1C* and *KCNE1*, and testing may be considered in patients with a high probability of diagnosis [10,11].

Brugada syndrome (BrS) is a hereditary disorder characterized by ST-segment elevation in the right precordial leads and malignant ventricular arrhythmias. This syndrome may account for approximately 18–28% of unexplained sudden cardiac arrests. Rare genetic variants in the *SCN5A* gene, leading to the loss of function of the cardiac sodium channel, are found in about 20% of the cases [12,13].

Cardiac conduction disease (CCD) is often age-dependent and is a heterogeneous progressive cardiac conduction disease (PCCD) disorder marked by impaired electrical impulse propagation in the sinoatrial node, atrioventricular (AV) node, and His–Purkinje system. On the surface ECG, sinus bradycardia, sinus pauses, prolonged P-wave duration, AV block, and different degrees of bundle branch block are typical features. The genes involved in CCD are *SCN5A* [14,15] and *TRPM4* [16].

Hypertrophic cardiomyopathy (HCM) is a relatively common hereditary disorder marked by hypertrophy of the left ventricular wall that cannot be attributed to other conditions such as hypertension or valvular heart disease. Typically, the hypertrophy is asymmetric and mainly affects the intraventricular septum. Gene panels that are generally recommended include eight sarcomere genes, including *MYH7*, *MYBPC3*, *TNNI3*, *TNNT2*, *TPM1*, *MYL2*, *MYL3*, and *ACTC1* [17]. This panel typically identifies a disease-causing variant in about 60% of familial cases [18].

Dilated cardiomyopathy (DCM) is characterized by the presence of left ventricular or biventricular dilatation and systolic dysfunction. It encompasses a wide range of genetic or acquired disorders. Approximately 100 genes have been identified as potentially related to DCM, with truncating variants in the titin gene (*TTN*) being the most common in DCM, accounting for up to 20% of cases [19]. Genetic testing panels should include the most prevalent genes such as *TTN* and *TNNT2*, as well as genes with prognostic or therapeutic implications, such as *LMNA*, *FLNC*, and *DSP*, or other genes such as *NEXN*, *ACTC1*, and *ACTN2*. The selection of genetic testing panels can be guided by the presence of specific extracardiac phenotypes, such as neuromuscular diseases (e.g., *DMD* and *EMD*), mitochondrial disease (e.g., *NDUFB3*), and congenital syndromes [20].

Arrhythmogenic cardiomyopathy (ACM) is mainly characterized by the replacement of myocardial tissue with fibrous or fibrofatty tissue, which can lead to progressive global or regional ventricular dysfunction with a high burden of ventricular arrhythmias. The recommended genetic test for ACM must include a minimal set of genes that have shown a clinical association with the disease. These genes, by frequency, include *PKP2* (20–45%), *DSP* (2–15%), *DSG2* (4–15%), *DSC2* (2–7%), *FLNC* (3%), *JUP* (1%), *TMEM43* (1%), *PLN* (1%), and *DES* (1–2%) [21]. Initial studies suggested that the *RYR2* gene is part of the genetic basis of ACM. Apart from ACM, *RYR2* mutations have been linked to CCD, DCM, and *CPVT*.

The identification of individuals at high risk of SCD due to channelopathies and cardiomyopathies poses a considerable clinical challenge. However, advances in genetic testing have revolutionized risk stratification, enabling healthcare providers to pinpoint underlying genetic mutations predisposing individuals to these.

Genetic testing in descendants of SCD victims plays a pivotal role in unraveling the basis of inherited cardiac conditions. The heritability of certain cardiac disorders, such as long QT syndrome, Brugada syndrome, and hypertrophic or arrhythmogenic cardiomyopathy, underscore the importance of identifying at-risk individuals within affected families [7,22].

The genetic make-up of individuals can influence their response to cardiac device therapy. Despite the potential benefits, incorporating genetic testing into routine clinical practice for patients with electronic cardiac devices has some challenges. Issues such as cost, accessibility, and the interpretation of genetic variants need to be addressed. Collaborative efforts between cardiologists, electrophysiologists, and genetic counsellors are essential to overcome this and integrate genetic testing into cardiac care.

2. Materials and Methods

1. Study Design: Retrospective observational study.
2. Inclusion criteria: (I) Patients diagnosed with arrhythmias as a first cardiac event (e.g., ventricular tachycardia, ventricular fibrillation, and 3rd-degree atrioventricular block) who are being treated with cardiac devices, such as pacemakers (PMKs), internal cardioverter-defibrillators (T-ICDs), subcutaneous internal cardioverter-defibrillators (S-ICDs), and undergoing genetic screening; (II) Patients with syncope of unknown cause, who are being treated with loop recorders and undergoing genetic screening; (III) Patients with cardiac resynchronization therapy (CRT) indications, heart failure (HF) belonging to New York Heart Association (NYHA) class II–IV, left ventricular ejection fraction (LVEF) $\leq$ 35%, QRS complex $\geq$ 130 ms, left bundle branch block (LBBB) pattern, and optimal pharmacological treatment 3 months prior to CRT, who are undergoing genetic testing.
3. Exclusion criteria: patients with incomplete medical records or missing genetic data.
4. Data collection:
    - 4.1 Patient demographics: age, gender, and family history of SCD.
    - 4.2 Clinical characteristics: symptoms, type of arrhythmias, and history of cardiac arrest.
    - 4.3 Cardiac imaging: (1) Echocardiographic measurements in all patients (valvular regurgitation and ejection fraction (EF)) and (2) Cardiac Magnetic Resonance Imaging (MRI) if available: ejection fraction, fibrosis, or scar.
    - 4.4 Interventions: type of cardiac device (PMK, ICD, S-ICD, CRT, or loop recorder) and type of ablation if it was performed.
    - 4.5 Genetic testing used next-generation sequencing panels. The testing focused on channelopathies and cardiomyopathies, used commercially available panels, ranged from 106–174 genes, and were chosen at the discretion of the attending physician.

Depending on availability and local collaboration protocols, certain patients had their genetic testing conducted at the Regional Center of Medical Genetics Dolj (CRGM Dolj). This was performed using the TruSightCardio panel Illumina (San Diego, CA, USA), which included 174 genes. Genomic DNA was isolated from the primary sample using commercial kits (Wizard® Genomic DNA Purification Kit, PureLink™ Genomic DNA, QIAsymphony DSP DNA). Preparation of sequencing libraries was performed according to the manufacturer's recommendations. The protocol was based on enzymatic fragmentation and selective amplification of target areas. The library obtained was sequenced on the Illumina platform with the aim of obtaining coverage of at least $50\times$ (depth) for germline variants, and at least 98% (coverage) of the targeted areas. Bioinformatics analysis was performed using a bioinformatics solution implemented locally within CRGM Dolj. Variants with convincing evidence of variant/gene–phenotype correlation according to established international databases (OMIM and Clin Var) were especially evaluated. All known modes of transmission for the presumed diseases were taken into account. Mendelian and variants with insufficient criteria for diagnosis were excluded from the report (e.g., heterozygous variants in genes known to be recessive). Bioinformatics tools such as GEMENI, (iGenomes GATK GRCh37 variants nf-core/sarek v2.7.1; Nextflow v21.04.1; BWA 0.7.17; GATK v4.1.7.0) as well as tapes/annovar, could be used for filtering and prioritization. WAS followed the AMCG variant classification, which reflected the probability that a variant is pathogenic in the following sequence: Benign, Likely Benign, Variant with Uncertain Significance (VUS—variant of unknown significance), Likely Pathogenic, and Pathogenic. Only those variants that correlate with the clinical phenotype were reported.

Some patients underwent genetic testing at the Genomic Center of the University of Medicine and Pharmacy Victor Babes Timisoara, utilizing a 174-gene sequencing panel, the TruSightCardio panel from Illumina (San Diego, CA, USA). Target enrichment was conducted with the TruSight Rapid Capture kit (Illumina). Sequence reads were aligned to the human reference genome, hg37, using the Burrows–Wheeler alignment (BWA) tool. Variants identified were annotated using ANNOVAR, as described in previous publications [23].

For some patients, NGS gene panels were utilized at Invitae laboratories (USA) to test for sequence and exon-level copy number variants, as previously described [24,25]. The prescribing physician selected one or more panels among the commercially available NGS panels at their discretion. The basic commercial panel included 106 genes, while larger panels, comprising up to 168 genes, covered a broader set of genes for the Invitae Arrhythmia and Cardiomyopathy Comprehensive Panel, Add-on Preliminary evidence Genes for Arrhythmia and Cardiomyopathy, and Add-on Sudden Unexpected Death in Epilepsy (SUDEP) Genes. Familial screening was offered to relatives of a proband with pathogenic and likely pathogenic variants. The patient and physician chose among the three laboratories based on different turnaround times and reimbursement considerations. The outcomes were device efficacy and device-related complications, arrhythmia recurrence, and mortality.

Statistical Analysis

Data are presented as mean ± standard deviation for continuous variables and as proportions for categorical variables. Continuous variables were compared between groups using an unpaired T-test (variables with normal distribution) or Chi-square test. A p-value < 0.05 was considered significant.

All the subjects included in the study gave their informed consent before inclusion. The study was conducted in accordance with the Declaration of Helsinki, and the protocol was approved by the Ethics Committee of our institute (number 46/28.09.2018).

3. Results

Thirty-eight patients, 44.5 ± 13.1 y.o. (58% males), were included. All patients received an electronic cardiac device in a tertiary center between 2018–2023. The most frequent presentation that led to the diagnosis was ventricular tachycardia in 34% of the cases, followed by cardiac arrest in 26% of the cases. Demographic, clinical, and echocardiographic parameters are found in Table 1.

Table 1. Demographic, clinical, and echocardiographic parameters. COPD—chronic obstructive pulmonary disease, SD—standard deviation, MR—mitral regurgitation, TR—tricuspid regurgitation.

Male gender, %		22 (58%)
Age, y.o., mean ± SD		44.5 ± 13.1
Main arrhythmia or symptoms leading to cardiac evaluation	Cardiac arrest	10 (26%)
	Ventricular tachycardia	34 (34%)
	Atrial fibrillation	3 (8%)
	3rd degree atrioventricular block	5 (13%)
	Heart failure symptoms	2 (5%)
	Syncope	5 (13%)
Associated pathology, n, %	Hypertension	5 (13%)
	Coronary artery disease	3 (8%)
	Diabetes Mellitus	3 (8%)
	COPD	1 (3%)
LVEF (%)		40.3 ± 14.7
Severe MR, n, %		5 (13%)
Moderate MR, n, %		13 (34%)
Mild MR, n, %		14 (37%)
Severe TR, n, %		1 (3%)
Moderate TR, n, %		8 (21%)
Mild TR, n, %		24 (63%)

Twenty patients (53%) underwent an MRI scan, and in 70% of cases, extensive fibrosis was identified during the scan. The baseline medication for all the patients is presented in Table 2.

Table 2. Cardiological medication taken by the patients included in the study; NOAC—non-vitamin K antagonist oral anticoagulant, SGLT2—sodium-glucose co-transporter 2 inhibitors, ACEI—angiotensin-converting enzyme inhibitor, ARNI—angiotensin receptor neprylisin inhibitor.

Medical Treatment	N, %
Bblockers	25 (66%)
Ivabradine	1 (3%)
Class Ic antiarrhythmic	2 (5%)
Class III antiarrhythmic	14 (37%)
NOAC	6 (16%)
Antialdosteronics	16 (42%)
SGLT2 inhibitors	9 (24%)
ARB + ARNI	13 (34%)
ACEI	6 (16%)

In accordance with the cardiac pathology being the first cardiac manifestation, patients were implanted with an electronic device, as follows: six dual-chamber PMKs, 10 single-chamber ICDs, five dual-chamber ICDs, three subcutaneous ICDs, four loop recorders, 10 CRT,3 CRT-Pacemakers (CRT-P), and seven CRT-D defibrillators (CRT-D).

Nineteen patients (50%) had a family history of SCD. All the patients were genetically tested, focusing on channelopathies and cardiomyopathies and using commercially available panels, which ranged from 106–174 genes. The results are displayed in graph no. 1. Testing identified pathogenic (P) or likely pathogenic (LP) variants in 27 patients (71%), variants of unknown significance (VUS) in seven patients (18%), and negative results in four patients (11%) (Table 3).

Table 3. Genetic testing in our group of patients.

Sex	Age (Years)	Gene	OMIM Number	Transcript	Zygosity	Classification
M	49	TMEM43	#612048	c.1073C>T (p.Ser358Leu)	heterozygous	P
M	50	TMEM43&TTN	#612048&#188840	c.1073C>T (p.Ser358Leu)&c.107635C>T (p.Gln35879*)	heterozygous	P&P
F	28	DSP	#125647	Deletion (Exons 7-10)	heterozygous	LP
M	30	TMEM43	#612048	c.1073C>T (p.Ser358Leu)	heterozygous	P
M	49	DSP	#125647	c.939C>T (Silent)	heterozygous	LP
M	48	KCNQ1	#607542	c.691C>T (p.Arg231Cys)	heterozygous	P
F	44	KCNQ1	#607542	c.604G>A (p.Asp202Asn)	heterozygous	P
M	29	DMD	#300377	Deletion (Exons 45-47)	hemizygous	P
M	24	EMD	#300384	c.187+1G>A (Splice donor)	hemizygous	P
F	50	TNNI3K	#613932	c.2302G>A (p.Glu768Lys)	heterozygous	P
M	52	RYR2	#180902	c.10631C>G (p.Pro3544Arg)	heterozygous	LP
M	50	TTN	#188840	c.93166C>T (p.Arg31056*)	heterozygous	LP
F	40	LMNA	#150330	c.604G>T (p.Glu202*)	heterozygous	P
F	47	SCN5A	#600163	c.5971C>T (p.Arg1991Trp)	heterozygous	LP
F	61	DSC2	#125645	c.397G>A (p.Ala133Thr)	heterozygous	LP
M	31	TRPM4	#606936	c.1127T>C (p.Ile376Thr)	heterozygous	P
M	63	MYBPC3	#600958	c.712C>T (p.Arg238Cys)	heterozygous	LP
F	23	CTNNA3	#607667	Deletion (Exon 10)	heterozygous	LP
M	38	SCN5A	#600163	c.2989G>A (p.Ala997Thr)	heterozygous	LP
M	46	RYR2	#180902	c.5776G>A (p.Val1926Ile)	heterozygous	LP
F	45	MYH7	#160760	c.1615A>G (p.Met539Val)	heterozygous	LP
M	47	PKP2	#602861	c.1510+1G>T	heterozygous	LP
M	38	TTN	#188840	c.69224delA	heterozygous	LP
M	55	SGCD	#601411	c.448T>G	heterozygous	VUS
F	61	TMEM43	#612048	c.1073C>T (p.Ser358Leu)	heterozygous	P
F	55	FBN1	#134797	c.718C>T	heterozygous	P
F	58	MYH7	#160760	c.1615A>G	heterozygous	LP
M	46	MYLK	#600922	c.3610C>T (p.Arg1204Trp)	heterozygous	VUS
M	53	A2ML1	#610627	c.2464G>A (p.Val822Ile)	heterozygous	VUS
M	64	SOS1	#182530	c.2165G>A (p.Arg722Lys)	heterozygous	VUS
F	26	CACNB2	#600003	c.998C>T (p.Thr333Ile)	heterozygous	VUS
F	63	AGL	#610860	c.1333A>G (p.Met445Val)	heterozygous	VUS
F	67	AGL	#610860	c.3235C>T (p.Gln1079*)	heterozygous	P
F	25	NDUFB3	#603839	c.208G>T (p.Gly70*)	heterozygous	VUS

Gene variants—pathogenic, likely pathogenic, and uncertain significance. M = male, F = female, P = pathogenic, LP = likely pathogenic, VUS = uncertain significance. c.107635C>T (p.Gln35879*) TTN: Exons 153-155 (NM_133378.4) are excluded from analysis. TTN variants are reported in the primary report based on functional effect and/or location. A complete list of variants of uncertain significance, likely benign and benign variants in TTN is available upon request. Variants are named relative to the NM_001267550.2 (meta) transcript, but only variants in the coding sequence and intronic boundaries of the clinically relevant NM_133378.4 (N2A) isoform are reported (PMID: 25589632). c.93166C>T (p.Arg31056*) TTN: Exons 45-46, 147, 149, 164, 172-201 (NM_001267550.2) are excluded from analysis. TTN variants are included in the primary report based on functional effect and/or location. A complete list of variants of uncertain significance, likely benign and benign variants in TTN is available upon request. Variants are named relative to the NM_001267550.2 (meta) transcript. c.604G>T (p.Glu202*) This sequence change creates a premature translational stop signal (p.Glu202*) in the LMNA gene. It is expected to result in an absent or disrupted protein product. Loss-of-function variants in LMNA are known to be pathogenic (PMID: 18585512, 18926329). c.3235C>T (p.Gln1079*) This sequence change creates a premature translational stop signal (p.Gln1079*) in the AGL gene. It is expected to result in an absent or disrupted protein product. This variant has been observed in individual(s) with clinical features of glycogen storage disease type III (PMID: 26885414). In at least one individual the data is consistent with the variant being in trans (on the opposite chromosome) from a pathogenic variant. ClinVar contains an entry for this variant (Variation ID: 551403). c.208G>T (p.Gly70*) This sequence change creates a premature translational stop signal (p.Gly70*) in the NDUFB3 gene. While this is not anticipated to result in nonsense mediated decay, it is expected to disrupt the last 29 amino acid(s) of the NDUFB3 protein. NDUFB11: Deletion/duplication and sequencing analysis is not offered for exon 1. COX10: Deletion/duplication and sequencing analysis is not offered for exon.

According to the recommendations of the American College of Medical Genetics and Genomics (ACMG) [26], the patients included in our study were divided into two groups. The first group included 27 patients with positive genetic tests (pathogenic and likely pathogenic), and the second group included 11 patients either with negative genetic tests or with a variant of unknown significance. We considered *TTN* and *LMNA* as a separate group (14.81% of patients). The following genes were included in the sarcomeric motor genes group: *MYBPC3, CTNNA3, MYH7, TNNI3K,* and *MYLK*. This functional gene group recorded a positive genetic test in 22.22% of patients (Figure 1A). Regarding desmosomal genes, these included *DSP, DSC2,* and *PKP2*. This functional gene group recorded a positive test in 14.81% of the patients. Another functional gene group was represented by ion channel genes, which included the following genes: *KCNQ1, RYR2, SCN5A, TRPM4,* and *CACNB2*. This gene group registered positive genetic tests in 22.22% of the patients. In addition, genes from the cytoskeleton-Z-disk gene structural group included DMD, with a positive genetic test in only one patient (3.70%). Patients with mutations in the remaining genes that were screened were categorized into an "other genes" group. These genes include *SGCD, TMEM43, FBN1, A2ML1, SOS1, AGL, NDUFB3,* and *EMD*, and were registered in 22.22% of the patients with positive genetic tests. Regarding the patients with negative genetic tests or with a variant of unknown significance (only 11 patients out of a total of 38 patients), the following genes were identified: *CACNB2* from the ion channel genes group, MYLK from the motor sarcomeric genes group, and *A2ML1, SOS1, AGL,* and *NDUFB3* from the other genes group (Figure 1B).

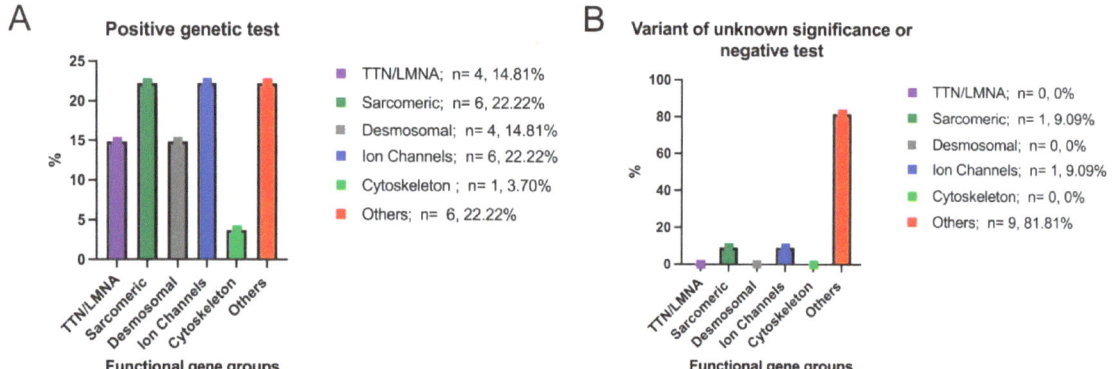

Figure 1. Distribution of positive genetic test (**A**)/variant of unknown significance or negative test (**B**) in the overall study cohort.

Seven patients (18%) had ACM, two patients (5%) had HCM, two had muscular dystrophies (one with Becker and one with Emery Dreifuss tip 1), three patients (8%) had channelopathies (two patients with LQTS type 1 and one patient with BrS syndrome), one patient (3%) had mitochondrial disease, four patients (11%) had CCD, and the rest had DCM. A more detailed image of genetic testing results is presented in Figure 2.

TMEM43 mutations (11%) were the most prevalent due to being a disease-causing variant of arrhythmogenic cardiomyopathy. In four patients (11%), genetic testing was negative, two patients had idiopathic ventricular fibrillation, one patient had ACM, and one patient had DCM. In these patients, genetic retesting will be considered using an extensive cardiology panel.

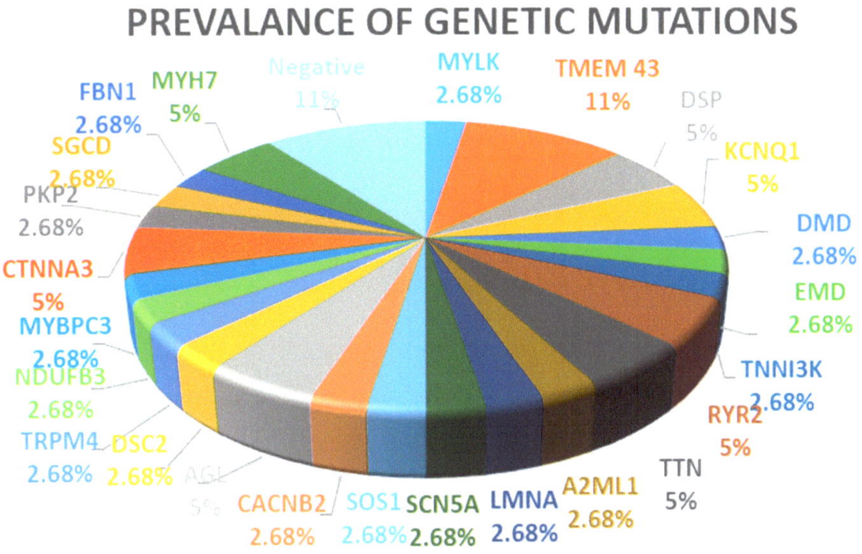

Figure 2. Prevalence of genetic mutations.

The average follow-up was 4.7 ± 1.8 years, and the longest follow-up was 6 years. During follow-up, five patients (13%) needed ventricular tachycardia ablation, two patients (5%) underwent atrial fibrillation ablation, and one patient (3%) underwent ganglion denervation.

In ten patients (26%) with DCM, CRT was performed (seven CRT-D, three CRT-P). The assessment of responses to CRT was based on the following criteria [27,28]:

- Clinical response to CRT, defined as improvement in NYHA functional class.
- Echocardiographic response (defined as >5% increase in LVEF and decreased mitral regurgitation degree).

Patients were divided into two groups: super-responders (SRs) and non-SRs (responders and hyporesponders). SR patients were defined as those with a stable ejection fraction (LVEF) $\geq$ 45%. A detailed comparison regarding SRs and non-SRs characteristics is presented in Table 4.

Comparing the SR vs. non-SR groups, we observe that the SR group has a younger average age, a 100% typical LBBB pattern, a wider QRS complex, and LV leads placed only in posterolateral or lateral positions. During a 12-month follow-up, none of the patients in the SR group experienced severe or moderate mitral regurgitation. In terms of genetic testing, there was a variation of mutations in the SR group, while the non-SR group had two patients with *VUS-AGL* and one patient with both *TTN* and *TMEM43* pathogenic mutations. No deaths were recorded in the SR group. In the non-SR group, there was one cardiac death in the patient with both *TTN* and *TMEM43* mutations due to refractory HF and electrical storm following a severe COVID infection, despite having the clinical and paraclinical criteria of a super-responder (nonischemic, younger age, typical LBBB pattern, wider QRS, and LV lead in the posterolateral position). Additionally, in the SR group, one patient with a *TNNI3K* gene mutation, who met the clinical and paraclinical criteria of a super-responder (nonischemic, younger age, typical LBBB pattern, and wider QRS) on maximal medical treatment, was initially a non-responder due to the inadequate positioning of the LV lead in the anterior wall. After proper positioning in the posterolateral wall, the patient became a super-responder, as illustrated in Figure 3.

Table 4. A comparison regarding technical aspects, echocardiography parameters, and genetic mutation in SRs versus non-SRs; LBBB—left bundle branch block, SD—standard deviation, FO—follow-up, super-responders (SRs), non-SRs (responders and hyporesponders), typical pattern—Strauss Criteria, MR—mitral regurgitation.

		SRs (N = 5, 50%)	Non-SRs (N = 5, 50%)
Age, y.o., mean ± SD		51 ± 3.3	63 ± 6.5
LV lead position n, %	Posterolateral	2 (40%)	0 (0%)
	Lateral	3 (60%)	3 (60%)
	Posterior	0 (0%)	1 (20%)
	Anterolateral	0 (0%)	1 (20%)
AV paced interval, mean ± SD		120 ± 7.5	110 ± 10
AV sensed interval, mean ± SD		100 ± 8	90 ± 6.3
LBBB	Typical pattern	5 (100%)	2 (40%)
	Atypical pattern	0 (0%)	3 (60%)
	QRS duration mean ± SD	180 ± 0	140 ± 9.8
LVEF (%)			
• Baseline		20 ± 7.1	30 ± 2.4
• 12 months FO		50 ± 3.7	35 ± 4.4
Severe MR, n, %			
• Baseline		3 (60%)	0 (0%)
• 12 months FO		0 (0%)	0 (0%)
Moderate MR, n, %			
• Baseline		2 (40%)	5 (100%)
• 12 months FO		0 (0%)	4 (80%)
Genetic testing (gene mutation)		PKP2 SGCD TNNI3K MYLK RYR2	A2ML1 AGL AGL MYBCP3 TTN&TMEM43

An upgrade to CRT-D was necessary in the non-SR group for one patient with a *VUS-AGL* mutation, a possible non-disease-causing variant. This patient had nonischemic DCM with an atypical LBBB pattern and a QRS duration of 140 ms, and was on maximal medical treatment when initially implanted with a CRT-P device. Two years after CRT implantation, due to repeated ventricular tachycardia, a CRT-D upgrade was needed, including replacement of the LV lead from the anterior position to the lateral wall. However, the patient, just like the other one with the same mutation, remained a non-responder.

Two young patients, who experienced cardiac arrest due to ventricular fibrillation as their first cardiac event, received a subcutaneous implantable cardioverter-defibrillator (S-ICD). Genetic testing later diagnosed them with arrhythmogenic cardiomyopathy, revealing one *DSP* mutation and one *TMEM43* mutation, both of which are pathogenic. During follow-up, they developed electrical storm due to multiple forms of ventricular tachycardia. Despite undergoing endoepicardial ablation procedures, they continued to experience ventricular tachycardia. Both patients experienced early battery depletion, and the patient with *DSP* mutation also showed under-sensing. Consequently, a transvenous ICD (T-ICD) was recommended with complete removal of the S-ICD system, as shown in Figure 4.

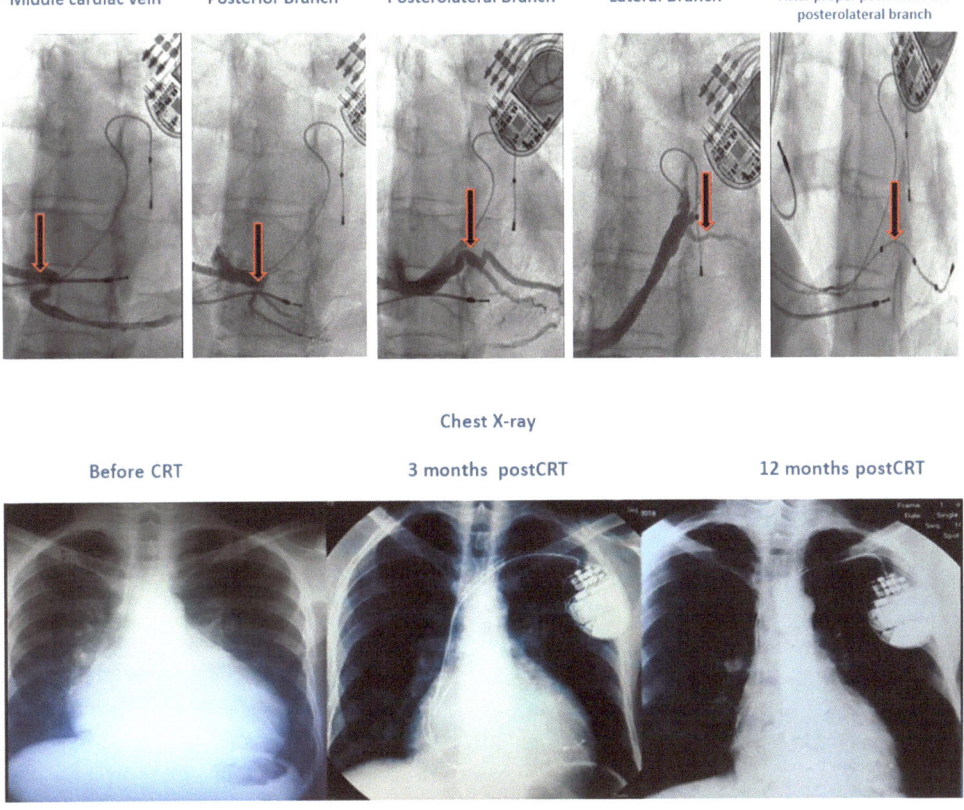

Figure 3. The evolution of a patient with a *TNNI3K* gene mutation after proper positioning of the LV lead in the posterolateral wall.

In the entire group of patients, there were two cardiac deaths, both in individuals with TTN mutations who suffered from refractory heart failure. Despite receiving maximum treatment, their condition progressed rapidly and was fulminant.

Assessing the correlation (Figure 5) between the age of the patients included in our study and the left ventricular ejection fraction (LVEF), we observed a negative correlation for all patients included in our study, meaning that the younger the patients, the higher the LVEF values, and the older the patients, the lower the LVEF values ($r = -0.5210$, $p = 0.0008$). Separating the two groups of patients, we noticed negative correlations both in patients with a positive genetic test ($r = -0.4474$, $p = 0.0193$) and in patients with a variant of unknown significance or a negative test ($r = -0.6354$, $p = 0.0357$).

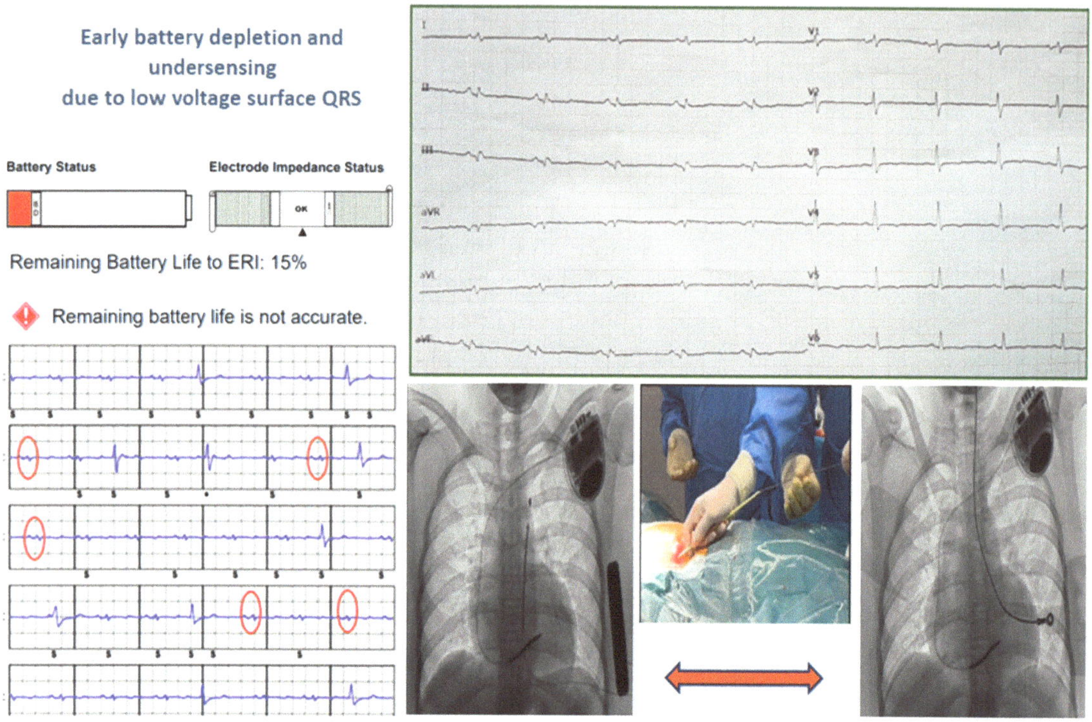

Figure 4. The cases of two young patients with S-ICD who experienced early battery depletion and under-sensing due to low voltage surface QRS. A transvenous ICD (T-ICD) was recommended with complete removal of the S-ICD system. The red circles on the ECG are highlighting QRS underdetection by the S-ICD.

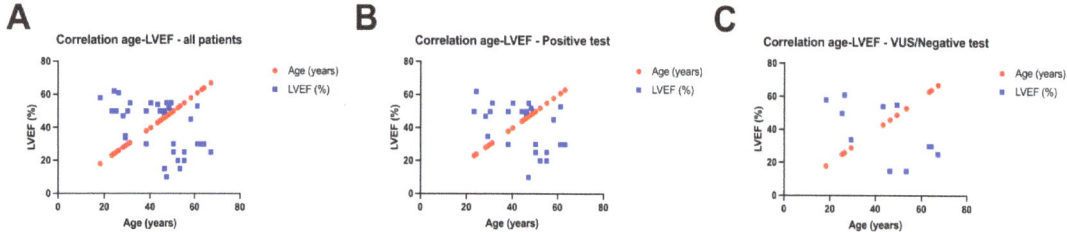

Figure 5. Correlations between left ventricular ejection fraction (LVEF) and age of all patients in the study (**A**), between LVEF and age of patients with positive genetic tests (**B**), and between LVEF and age of patients with a variant of unknown significance or a negative test (**C**).

4. Discussion

Genetic testing in patients with electronic cardiac devices holds significant promise for optimizing therapy and improving outcomes. As our understanding of the genetic basis of cardiac disorders continues to expand, integrating genetic information into the clinical decision-making process will become increasingly important. By doing so, clinicians can offer more personalized and effective treatments for patients with pacemakers, defibrillators, and resynchronization therapy devices.

Identifying a specific genetic trait can aid in patient management and guide clinical decisions. Patients with pathogenic *LMNA* variants consistently face a poor prognosis, particularly with a high risk of sudden cardiac death (SCD) due to conduction defects or ventricular arrhythmia. Preventive pacemaker (PM) or implantable cardioverter-defibrillator (ICD) therapy should be considered early for *LMNA* carriers, with ICD implantation algorithms that include pathogenic variant mechanisms (truncating vs. missense variant) due to the higher SCD risk [29,30]. Similarly, a higher risk of SCD is linked to pathogenic variants, especially truncated variants, in the *FLNC*, *DES*, *RBM20*, and *PLN* genes, warranting consideration for preventive ICD implantation in these patients [31,32]. Desmosomal pathogenic variants in individuals with dilated cardiomyopathy or biventricular arrhythmogenic cardiomyopathy are also associated with an increased risk of life-threatening ventricular arrhythmias and SCD [33].

Cardiomyopathies can be either inherited and/or acquired [34,35]. They may also be exacerbated by disease modifiers, which are conditions that can worsen or trigger cardiomyopathies (such as many cardiovascular comorbidities). Identifying an acquired cause of DCM does not rule out the presence of an underlying gene mutation; conversely, a genetic variant might require an additional acquired cause to clinically manifest [36,37].

Cardiac resynchronization therapy has emerged as a valuable treatment option for heart failure patients [38,39]. As technology advances, genetic testing plays an increasingly pivotal role in tailoring therapies to individual patients' needs. One critical decision faced by clinicians is choosing between a traditional CRT-P and a CRT-D.

After the controversial Danish trial, the ICD benefit in primary prophylaxis in patients with non-ischemic cardiomyopathy is debatable in the presence of CRT, and it seems that CRT-P is not inferior to CRT-D [28,40].

The data indicate differences within the group we studied. All patients who underwent CRT and genetic testing had non-ischemic cardiomyopathy. Among them, 70% received a CRT-D device following a cardiac arrest caused by ventricular fibrillation or ventricular tachycardia as their first cardiac event, while the remaining 30% received a CRT-P device. One patient with a *VUS-AGL* mutation, a potentially non-disease-causing variant, required an upgrade to CRT-D due to repeated ventricular tachycardia two years post-implantation, which also involved the replacement of the LV lead from the anterior position to the lateral wall. Despite these interventions, this patient, like another with the same mutation, remained a non-responder. Another patient, despite having the clinical and paraclinical criteria of a super-responder (nonischemic, younger age, typical LBBB pattern, wider QRS, and LV lead in the posterolateral position), died due to refractory HF and electrical storm, having both *TTN* and *TMEM43* mutations. It appears that patients with multiple mutations experience more severe disease and exhibit a weaker response to CRT. Furthermore, despite being a nonischemic DCM, a patient with a *TMEM43* mutation, known for its extreme arrhythmogenicity, more often has an unfavorable outcome.

In human patients, mutations in the nuclear envelope protein TMEM43 are linked to severe diseases, including ACM type 5, a devastating cardiomyopathy that leads to malignant arrhythmias and heart failure. The *TMEM43*-p.S358L mutation has been identified as the genetic cause of an aggressive form of ACM, primarily affecting males. Despite extensive in vivo studies, the pathogenic mechanisms of TMEM43-associated ACM remain poorly understood. Various research groups have developed different models using mice and zebrafish, and induced pluripotent stem cells with *TMEM43* mutations to study ACM [41–43]. However, both *TMEM43*-p.S358L knock-in and knock-out mice do not develop a cardiac phenotype under normal conditions [41], suggesting that the pathogenicity of this specific mutation requires enhancement through overexpression or additional genetic, epigenetic, or environmental factors in mice. In the study by Zink et al. [42], the first transgenic zebrafish model expressing two different potential pathogenic variants found in human patients under a heart-specific promoter was created, along with genetic mutants of *TMEM43* in zebrafish. These zebrafish lines were characterized from early embryonic stages to adulthood. The mutant p.S358L *TMEM43* was found to be unstable and partially redistributed into the cytoplasm in embryonic and adult hearts. Additionally, both *TMEM43* variants exhibited cardiac morphological defects at juvenile stages and ultrastructural changes within the myocardium, along with dysregulated gene expression in adulthood.

Conversely, a patient with a *TNNI3K* gene mutation, who met the super-responder criteria (nonischemic, younger age, typical LBBB pattern, and wider QRS) on maximal medical treatment, was initially a non-responder due to the inadequate positioning of the LV lead in the anterior wall. After proper positioning in the posterolateral wall, the patient became a super-responder.

Considering our group of patients, in order to become a super-responder, meeting the clinical and paraclinical criteria of a super-responder (nonischemic DCM, younger age, typical LBBB pattern, wider QRS complex, and appropriate LV lead position) is necessary. Additionally, the absence of multiple associations with severe gene mutations is also crucial.

Two patients diagnosed with arrhythmogenic cardiomyopathy, who experienced cardiac arrest due to ventricular fibrillation as their first cardiac event, received subcutaneous implantable cardioverter-defibrillators (S-ICDs). During follow-up, they developed electrical storm due to multiple forms of ventricular tachycardia. Both patients experienced early battery depletion, and the patient with a DSP mutation also showed under-sensing. Consequently, a transvenous ICD (T-ICD) was recommended with complete removal of the S-ICD system. The oldest lead was 6 years old. Multiple simple manual tractions were necessary to release the generator and the proximal part of the lead. For the distal part, a mechanical dilator sheath (yellow sheath, inner ID/OD 8.5/10.7Fr) was used to free the lead. The systems were completely removed without complications.

Considering this, it might be preferable to implant a T-ICD when arrhythmogenic cardiomyopathy is suspected, even if the patient experienced cardiac arrest due to ventricular fibrillation as their first cardiac event.

Studies indicate that both T-ICD and S-ICD are effective in detecting and terminating life-threatening arrhythmias in arrhythmogenic cardiomyopathy (ACM); however, the absence of antitachycardia pacing (ATP) in S-ICDs can be a limitation for patients who frequently experience ventricular tachycardia that could otherwise be managed without a shock [44,45]. Guidelines generally support the use of either device in ACM patients, emphasizing personalized treatment based on patient risk profile, lifestyle, age, and arrhythmic burden [2]. As speculated in the literature in cases of severely impaired right ventricular function, a T-ICD is better than an S-ICD [46]. In the remaining cases, an S-ICD could be taken into account, especially in younger patients or those with a higher risk of lead-related complications.

Regarding mortality, two patients died during follow-up due to refractory heart failure, both of whom had titin mutations. A significant proportion of DCM cases are linked to genetic mutations, with titin mutations being the most common type [47]. Titin is a giant protein that plays a crucial role in the elasticity and stability of cardiac sarcomeres. Studies have shown that patients with this mutation have a worse prognosis, especially a higher incidence of heart failure progression and death, but the extent of the impact can vary based on individual patient factors [48,49]. Early genetic screening and tailored therapeutic strategies are essential in managing patients with *TTN*-related DCM to improve outcomes and reduce mortality, including more aggressive heart failure management and the use of ICD to prevent sudden cardiac death.

The severity and progression of DCM exhibit significant variability among individuals, not only in sporadic cases but also within members of the same family. This variability may be explained by the fact that the clinical phenotype is influenced not only by a single causative gene variant but also by the interaction with common variants in the genome, epigenetic factors, and environmental influences. Patients with DCM who carry pathogenic variants in the *LMNA*, *RBM20*, and *DSP* genes are at higher risk for heart failure progression and may require heart transplantation [33,50].

5. Conclusions

Genetic testing has the potential to revolutionize the decision-making process in patients with cardiac electronic devices. By identifying genetic markers associated with arrhythmia susceptibility, heart failure etiology, and CRT response, clinicians can tailor therapy to individual patient needs.

Author Contributions: Concept/design: E.-V.G., D.C. and C.V.; Data collection: E.-V.G., A.-A.F.-G., A.U. and G.T.; Data analysis/interpretation: C.V., R.V., L.P., D.C. and S.M.; Drafting article: E.-V.G., A.U., G.T., and D.C.; Critical revision of article: E.-V.G., D.C., A.M. and D.C.; visualization, S.M., E.-V.G., D.C. and C.V.; supervision, E.-V.G., D.C. and R.V.; project administration, E.-V.G., D.C. and C.V. All authors have read and agreed to the published version of the manuscript.

Funding: This research received no external funding.

Institutional Review Board Statement: All the subjects included in the study gave their informed consent before inclusion. The study was conducted in accordance with the Declaration of Helsinki, and the protocol was approved by the Ethics Committee of our institute (number 46/28 September 2018).

Informed Consent Statement: Informed consent was obtained from all subjects involved in the study.

Data Availability Statement: Data available on request due to restrictions (privacy and ethical reasons).

Acknowledgments: We would like to acknowledge Victor Babes University of Medicine and Pharmacy Timisoara for their support in covering the costs of publication for this research paper.

Conflicts of Interest: The authors declare no conflicts of interest.

Abbreviations

A2ML1	Alpha 2 Macroglobulin Like 1
ACM	Arrhythmogenic Cardiomyopathy
ACMG	American College of Medical Genetics and Genomics
ACTC1	Actin Alpha Cardiac Muscle 1
ACTN2	Actinin Alpha 2
ACEI	Angiotensin-Coverting Enzyme Inhibitor
AGL	Amylo-Alpha-1, 6-Glucosidase, 4-Alpha-Glucanotransferase
ARNI	Angiotensin Receptor Neprylisin Inhibitor
ATP	Anti-Tachycardia Pacing
AV	Atrioventricular
BrS	Brugada
CACNB2	Calcium Voltage-Gated Channel Auxiliary Subunit Beta 2
CALM 1	Calmodulin 1
CALM 2	Calmodulin 2
CALM 3	Calmodulin 3
CCD	Cardiac Conduction Defects
COPD	Chronic Obstructive Pulmonary Disease
CPVT	Catecholaminergic Polymorphic Ventricular Tachycardia
CRT	Cardiac Resynchronization Therapy
CRT-D	Cardiac Resynchronization Therapy Defibrillator
CRT-P	Cardiac Resynchronization Therapy Pacemaker
CTNNA3	Catenin Alpha 3
DCM	Dilated Cardiomyopathy
DES	Desmin
DSG2	Desmoglein 2
DMD	Dystrophin
DSP	Desmoplakin
DSC2	Desmocollin 2
EF	Ejection Fraction
EMD	Emerin

FBN1	Fibrillin 1
FLNC	Filamin C
FO	Follow-Up
HCM	Hypertrophic Cardiomyopathy
HF	Heart Failure
ICD	Implantable Cardioverter Defibrillator
JUP	Junction Plakoglobin
KCNQ1	Potassium Voltage Gated Channel Subfamily Q Member 1
KCNH2	Potassium Voltage Gated Channel Subfamily H Member 2
LBBB	Left Bundle Branch Block
LP	Likely Pathogenic
LMNA	Lamin A/C
LQTs	Long QT Syndrome
LV	Left Ventricle
LVEF	Left Ventricular Ejection Fraction
MRI	Magnetic Resonance Imaging
MR	Mitral Regurgitation
MYBPC3	Myosin Binding Protein C, Cardiac
MYH7	Myosin Heavy Chain 7
MYLK	Myosin Light Chain Kinase
MYL2	Myosin Light Chain 2
MYL3	Myosin Light Chain 3
NDUFB3	NADH: Ubiquinone Oxidoreductase Subunit B3
NEXN	Nexilin F-actin binding protein
NOAC	Non-Vitamin K Antagonist Oral Anticoagulant
NYHA	New York Heart Association
P	Pathogenic
PLN	Phospholamban
PKP2	Plakophilin 2
PMK	Pacemaker
RBM20	RNA Binding Motif Protein 20
RYR2	Ryanodine Receptor 2
SCD	Sudden Cardiac Death
SCN5A	Sodium Voltage Gated Channel Alpha Subunit 5
SGCD	Sarcoglycan Delta
SGLT2	Sodium-Glucose Co-transporter 2 Inhibitors
S-ICD	Subcutaneous Implantable Cardioverter Defibrillator
SOS1	SOS Ras/Rac Guanine Nucleotide Exchange Factor 1
SR	Superresponder
SD	Standard Deviation
T-ICD	Transvenous Implantable Cardioverter Defibrillator
TMEM43	Transmembrane Protein 43
TNNI3K	TNNI3 Interacting Kinase
TNNI3	Troponin I3, Cardiac Type
TNNT2	Troponin T2, Cardiac Type
TPM1	Tropomyosin 1
TR	Tricuspid Regurgitation
TRMP4	Transient Receptor Potential Cation Channel Subfamily M Member 4
TTN	Titin
TTN-DCM	Titin Related Dilated Cardiomyopathy
VUS	Variant of Uncertain Significance

References

1. Glikson, M.; Nielsen, J.C.; Kronborg, M.B.; Michowitz, Y.; Auricchio, A.; Barbash, I.M.; Barrabe, J.A.; Boriani, G.; Braunschweig, F.; Brignole, M.; et al. 2021 ESC Guidelines on cardiac pacing and cardiac resynchronization therapy: Developed by the Task Force on cardiac pacing and cardiac resynchronization therapy of the European Society of Cardiology (ESC) With the special contribution of the European Heart Rhythm Association (EHRA). *Eur. Heart J.* **2021**, *42*, 3427–3520. [CrossRef] [PubMed]

2. Zeppenfeld, K.; Tfelt-Hansen, J.; de Riva, M.; Winkel, B.G.; Behr, E.R.; A Blom, N.; Charron, P.; Corrado, D.; Dagres, N.; de Chillou, C.; et al. 2022 ESC Guidelines for the management of patients with ventricular arrhythmias and the prevention of sudden cardiac death: Developed by the task force for the management of patients with ventricular arrhythmias and the prevention of sudden cardiac death of the European Society of Cardiology (ESC) Endorsed by the Association for European Paediatric and Congenital Cardiology (AEPC). *Eur. Heart J.* **2022**, *43*, 3997–4126. [CrossRef] [PubMed]
3. Hindricks, G.; Potpara, T.; Dagres, N.; Arbelo, E.; Bax, J.J.; Blomström-Lundqvist, C.; Boriani, G.; Castella, M.; Dan, J.-A.; Dilaveris, P.E.; et al. 2020 ESC Guidelines for the diagnosis and management of atrial fibrillation developed in collaboration with the European Association for Cardio-Thoracic Surgery (EACTS): The Task Force for the diagnosis and management of atrial fibrillation of the European Society of Cardiology (ESC) Developed with the special contribution of the European Heart Rhythm Association (EHRA) of the ESC. *Eur. Heart J.* **2021**, *42*, 373–498. [CrossRef] [PubMed]
4. Lenarczyk, R.; Zeppenfeld, K.; Tfelt-Hansen, J.; Heinzel, F.R.; Deneke, T.; Ene, E.; Meyer, C.; Wilde, A.; Arbelo, E.; Jędrzejczyk-Patej, E.; et al. Management of patients with an electrical storm or clustered ventricular arrhythmias: A clinical consensus statement of the European Heart Rhythm Association of the ESC—Endorsed by the Asia-Pacific Heart Rhythm Society, Heart Rhythm Society, and Latin-American Heart Rhythm Society. *EP Eur.* **2024**, *26*, euae049. [CrossRef]
5. Tzeis, S.; Gerstenfeld, E.P.; Kalman, J.; Saad, E.B.; Shamloo, A.S.; Andrade, J.G.; Barbhaiya, C.R.; Baykaner, T.; Boveda, S.; Calkins, H.; et al. 2024 European Heart Rhythm Association/Heart Rhythm Society/Asia Pacific Heart Rhythm Society/Latin American Heart Rhythm Society expert consensus statement on catheter and surgical ablation of atrial fibrillation. *EP Eur.* **2024**, *26*, euae043. [CrossRef]
6. Wilde, A.A.M.; Semsarian, C.; Marquez, M.F.; Shamloo, A.S.; Ackerman, M.J.; Ashley, E.A.; Sternick, E.B.; Barajas-Martinez, H.; Behr, E.R.; Bezzina, C.R.; et al. European Heart Rhythm Association (EHRA)/Heart Rhythm Society (HRS)/Asia Pacific Heart Rhythm Society (APHRS)/Latin American Heart Rhythm Society (LAHRS) Expert Consensus Statement on the state of genetic testing for cardiac diseases. *EP Eur.* **2022**, *24*, 1367. [CrossRef]
7. Arbelo, E.; Protonotarios, A.; Gimeno, J.R.; Arbustini, E.; Barriales-Villa, R.; Basso, C.; Bezzina, C.R.; Biagini, E.; A Blom, N.; A de Boer, R.; et al. 2023 ESC Guidelines for the management of cardiomyopathies: Developed by the task force on the management of cardiomyopathies of the European Society of Cardiology. *Eur. Heart J.* **2023**, *44*, 3503–3626. [CrossRef] [PubMed]
8. Adler, A.; Novelli, V.; Amin, A.S.; Abiusi, E.; Care, M.; Nannenberg, E.A.; Feilotter, H.; Amenta, S.; Mazza, D.; Bikker, H.; et al. An international, multicentered, evidence-based reappraisal of genes reported to cause congenital long QT syndrome. *Circulation* **2020**, *141*, 418–428. [CrossRef] [PubMed] [PubMed Central]
9. Shimizu, W.; Horie, M. Phenotypic manifestations of mutations in genes encoding subunits of cardiac potassium channels. *Circ. Res.* **2011**, *109*, 97–109. [CrossRef] [PubMed]
10. Crotti, L.; Odening, K.E.; Sanguinetti, M.C. Heritable arrhythmias associated with abnormal function of cardiac potassium channels. *Cardiovasc. Res.* **2020**, *116*, 1542–1556. [CrossRef] [PubMed]
11. Schwartz, P.J.; Ackerman, M.J.; Antzelevitch, C.; Bezzina, C.R.; Borggrefe, M.; Cuneo, B.F.; Wilde, A.A.M. Inherited cardiac arrhythmias. *Nat. Rev. Dis. Primers* **2020**, *6*, 58. [CrossRef] [PubMed] [PubMed Central]
12. Probst, V.; Wilde, A.A.; Barc, J.; Sacher, F.; Babuty, D.; Mabo, P.; Mansourati, J.; Le Scouarnec, S.; Kyndt, F.; Le Caignec, C.; et al. SCN5A mutations and the role of genetic background in the pathophysiology of Brugada syndrome. *Circ. Cardiovasc. Genet.* **2009**, *2*, 552–557. [CrossRef] [PubMed]
13. Bezzina, C.R.; Barc, J.; Mizusawa, Y.; Remme, C.A.; Gourraud, J.-B.; Simonet, F.; Verkerk, A.O.; Schwartz, P.J.; Crotti, L.; Dagradi, F.; et al. Common variants at SCN5A-SCN10A and HEY2 are associated with Brugada syndrome, a rare disease with high risk of sudden cardiac death. *Nat. Genet.* **2013**, *45*, 1044–1049, Erratum in *Nat. Genet.* **2013**, *45*, 1409. [CrossRef] [PubMed] [PubMed Central]
14. Neu, A.; Eiselt, M.; Paul, M.; Sauter, K.; Stallmeyer, B.; Isbrandt, D.; Schulze-Bahr, E. A homozygous SCN5A mutation in a severe, recessive type of cardiac conduction disease. *Hum. Mutat.* **2010**, *31*, E1609-21. [CrossRef] [PubMed]
15. Tan, R.B.; Gando, I.; Bu, L.; Cecchin, F.; Coetzee, W. A homozygous SCN5A mutation associated with atrial standstill and sudden death. *Pacing Clin. Electrophysiol.* **2018**, *41*, 1036–1042. [CrossRef] [PubMed]
16. Daumy, X.; Amarouch, M.-Y.; Lindenbaum, P.; Bonnaud, S.; Charpentier, E.; Bianchi, B.; Nafzger, S.; Baron, E.; Fouchard, S.; Thollet, A.; et al. Targeted resequencing identifies TRPM4 as a major gene predisposing to progressive familial heart block type I. *Int. J. Cardiol.* **2016**, *207*, 349–358. [CrossRef] [PubMed]
17. Alfares, A.A.; Kelly, M.A.; McDermott, G.; Funke, B.H.; Lebo, M.S.; Baxter, S.B.; Shen, J.; McLaughlin, H.M.; Clark, E.H.; Babb, L.J.; et al. Results of clinical genetic testing of 2,912 probands with hypertrophic cardiomyopathy: Expanded panels offer limited additional sensitivity. *Genet. Med.* **2015**, *17*, 880–888. [CrossRef] [PubMed]
18. Ho, C.Y.; Day, S.M.; Ashley, E.A.; Michels, M.; Pereira, A.C.; Jacoby, D.; Cirino, A.L.; Fox, J.C.; Lakdawala, N.K.; Ware, J.; et al. For the SHaRe Investigators. Genotype and lifetime burden of disease in hypertrophic cardiomyopathy: Insights from the Sarcomeric Human Cardiomyopathy Registry (SHaRe). *Circulation* **2018**, *138*, 1387–1398. [CrossRef] [PubMed] [PubMed Central]
19. Mazzarotto, F.; Tayal, U.; Buchan, R.J.; Midwinter, W.; Wilk, A.; Whiffin, N.; Govind, R.; Mazaika, E.; de Marvao, A.; Dawes, T.J.; et al. Reevaluating the genetic contribution of monogenic dilated cardiomyopathy. *Circulation* **2020**, *141*, 387–398. [CrossRef]
20. Haas, J.; Frese, K.S.; Peil, B.; Kloos, W.; Keller, A.; Nietsch, R.; Feng, Z.; Müller, S.; Kayvanpour, E.; Vogel, B.; et al. Atlas of the clinical genetics of human dilated cardiomyopathy. *Eur. Heart J.* **2015**, *36*, 1123–1135. [CrossRef] [PubMed]

21. Gerull, B.; Brodehl, A. Insights into Genetics and Pathophysiology of Arrhythmogenic Cardiomyopathy. *Curr. Heart Fail Rep.* **2021**, *18*, 378–390. [CrossRef] [PubMed] [PubMed Central]
22. Ackerman, M.J.; Priori, S.G.; Willems, S.; Berul, C.; Brugada, R.; Calkins, H.; Camm, A.J.; Ellinor, P.T.; Gollob, M.; Hamilton, R.; et al. HRS/EHRA expert consensus statement on the state of genetic testing for the channelopathies and cardiomyopathies this document was developed as a partnership between the Heart Rhythm Society (HRS) and the European Heart Rhythm Association (EHRA). *Heart Rhythm* **2011**, *8*, 1308–1339. [CrossRef]
23. Chirita-Emandi, A.; Andreescu, N.; Zimbru, C.G.; Tutac, P.; Arghirescu, S.; Serban, M.; Puiu, M. Challenges in reporting pathogenic/potentially pathogenic variants in 94 cancer predisposing genes—In pediatric patients screened with NGS panels. *Sci. Rep.* **2020**, *10*, 223. [CrossRef] [PubMed] [PubMed Central]
24. Lincoln, S.E.; Kobayashi, Y.; Anderson, M.J.; Yang, S.; Desmond, A.J.; Mills, M.A.; Nilsen, G.B.; Jacobs, K.B.; Monzon, F.A.; Kurian, A.W.; et al. A Systematic Comparison of Traditional and Multigene Panel Testing for Hereditary Breast and Ovarian Cancer Genes in More Than 1000 Patients. *J. Mol. Diagn.* **2015**, *17*, 533–544. [CrossRef] [PubMed]
25. Lincoln, S.E.; Truty, R.; Lin, C.-F.; Zook, J.M.; Paul, J.; Ramey, V.H.; Salit, M.; Rehm, H.L.; Nussbaum, R.L.; Lebo, M.S. A Rigorous Interlaboratory Examination of the Need to Confirm Next-Generation Sequencing–Detected Variants with an Orthogonal Method in Clinical Genetic Testing. *J. Mol. Diagn.* **2019**, *21*, 318–329. [CrossRef] [PubMed] [PubMed Central]
26. Richards, S.; Aziz, N.; Bale, S.; Bick, D.; Das, S.; Gastier-Foster, J.; Grody, W.W.; Hegde, M.; Lyon, E.; Spector, E.; et al. ACMG Laboratory Quality Assurance Committee. Standards and guidelines for the interpretation of sequence variants: A joint consensus recommendation of the American College of Medical Genetics and Genomics and the Association for Molecular Pathology. *Genet. Med.* **2015**, *17*, 405–424. [CrossRef] [PubMed] [PubMed Central]
27. Burri, H.; Prinzen, F.W.; Gasparini, M.; Leclercq, C. Left univentricular pacing for cardiac resynchronization therapy. *Europace* **2017**, *19*, 912–919. [CrossRef]
28. Køber, L.; Thune, J.J.; Nielsen, J.C.; Haarbo, J.; Videbæk, L.; Korup, E.; Jensen, G.; Hildebrandt, P.; Steffensen, F.H.; Bruun, N.E.; et al. Defibrillator Implantation in Patients with Nonischemic Systolic Heart Failure. *N. Engl. J. Med.* **2016**, *375*, 1221–1230. [CrossRef] [PubMed]
29. Thuillot, M.; Maupain, C.; Gandjbakhch, E.; Waintraub, X.; Hidden-Lucet, F.; Isnard, R.; Ader, F.; Rouanet, S.; Richard, P.; Charron, P. External validation of risk factors for malignant ventricular arrhythmias in lamin A/C mutation carriers. *Eur. J. Heart Fail* **2019**, *21*, 253–254. [CrossRef] [PubMed]
30. Peters, S.; Kumar, S.; Elliott, P.; Kalman, J.M.; Fatkin, D. Arrhythmic genotypes in familial dilated cardiomyopathy: Implications for genetic testing and clinical management. *Heart Lung Circ.* **2019**, *28*, 31–38. [CrossRef] [PubMed]
31. Ortiz-Genga, M.F.; Cuenca, S.; Ferro, M.D.; Zorio, E.; Salgado-Aranda, R.; Climent, V.; Padrón-Barthe, L.; Duro-Aguado, I.; Jiménez-Jáimez, J.; Hidalgo-Olivares, V.M.; et al. Truncating FLNC mutations are associated with high-risk dilated and arrhythmogenic cardiomyopathies. *J. Am. Coll. Cardiol.* **2016**, *68*, 2440–2451. [CrossRef] [PubMed]
32. Wahbi, K.; Béhin, A.; Charron, P.; Dunand, M.; Richard, P.; Meune, C.; Vicart, P.; Laforêt, P.; Stojkovic, T.; Bécane, H.M.; et al. High cardiovascular morbidity and mortality in myofibrillar myopathies due to DES gene mutations: A 10-year longitudinal study. *Neuromuscul. Disord.* **2012**, *22*, 211–218. [CrossRef] [PubMed]
33. Gigli, M.; Merlo, M.; Graw, S.L.; Barbati, G.; Rowland, T.J.; Slavov, D.B.; Stolfo, D.; Haywood, M.E.; Ferro, M.D.; Altinier, A.; et al. Genetic risk of arrhythmic phenotypes in patients with dilated cardiomyopathy. *J. Am. Coll. Cardiol.* **2019**, *74*, 1480–1490. [CrossRef] [PubMed] [PubMed Central]
34. Arbustini, E.; Narula, N.; Dec, G.W.; Reddy, K.S.; Greenberg, B.; Kushwaha, S.; Marwick, T.; Pinney, S.; Bellazzi, R.; Favalli, V.; et al. The MOGE(S) classification for a phenotype-genotype nomenclature of cardiomyopathy: Endorsed by the World Heart Federation. *J. Am. Coll. Cardiol.* **2013**, *62*, 2046–2072. [CrossRef]
35. Pinto, Y.M.; Elliott, P.M.; Arbustini, E.; Adler, Y.; Anastasakis, A.; Böhm, M.; Duboc, D.; Gimeno, J.; De Groote, P.; Imazio, M.; et al. MProposal for a revised definition of dilated cardiomyopathy, hypokinetic non-dilated cardiomyopathy, and its implications for clinical practice: A position statement of the ESC working group on myocardial and pericardial diseases. *Eur. Heart J.* **2016**, *37*, 1850–1858. [CrossRef]
36. Bondue, A.; Arbustini, E.; Bianco, A.; Ciccarelli, M.; Dawson, D.; De Rosa, M.; Hamdani, N.; Hilfiker-Kleiner, D.; Meder, B.; Leite-Moreira, A.F.; et al. Complex roads from genotype to phenotype in dilated cardiomyopathy: Scientific update from the Working Group of Myocardial Function of the European Society of Cardiology. *Cardiovasc. Res.* **2018**, *114*, 1287–1303. [CrossRef]
37. Hazebroek, M.; Kemna, M.; Schalla, S.; Wijk, S.S.-V.; Gerretsen, S.; Dennert, R.; Merken, J.; Kuznetsova, T.; Staessen, J.; Rocca, H.B.-L.; et al. Prevalence and prognostic relevance of cardiac involvement in ANCA-associated vasculitis: Eosinophilic granulomatosis with polyangiitis and granulomatosis with polyangiitis. *Int. J. Cardiol.* **2015**, *199*, 170–179. [CrossRef]
38. McDonagh, T.A.; Metra, M.; Adamo, M.; Gardner, R.S.; Baumbach, A.; Böhm, M.; Burri, H.; Butler, J.; Čelutkienė, J.; Chioncel, O.; et al. 2021 ESC Guidelines for the diagnosis and treatment of acute and chronic heart failure: Developed by the Task Force for the diagnosis and treatment of acute and chronic heart failure of the European Society of Cardiology (ESC) With the special contribution of the Heart Failure Association (HFA) of the ESC. *Eur. Heart J.* **2021**, *42*, 4901. [CrossRef]

39. McDonagh, T.A.; Metra, M.; Adamo, M.; Gardner, R.S.; Baumbach, A.; Bohm, M.; Burri, H.; Butler, J.; Celutkiene, J.; Chioncel, O.; et al. 2023 Focused Update of the 2021 ESC Guidelines for the diagnosis and treatment of acute and chronic heart failure: Developed by the task force for the diagnosis and treatment of acute and chronic heart failure of the European Society of Cardiology (ESC) With the special contribution of the Heart Failure Association (HFA) of the ESC. *Eur. Heart J.* **2024**, *45*, 53. [CrossRef]
40. Beggs, S.A.S.; Jhund, P.S.; Jackson, C.E.; McMurray, J.J.V.; Gardner, R.S. Non-ischaemic cardiomyopathy, sudden death and implantable defibrillators: A review and meta-analysis. *Heart* **2018**, *104*, 144–150. [CrossRef]
41. Stroud, M.J.; Fang, X.; Zhang, J.; Guimarães-Camboa, N.; Veevers, J.; Dalton, N.D.; Gu, Y.; Bradford, W.H.; Peterson, K.L.; Evans, S.M.; et al. Luma is not essential for murine cardiac development and function. *Cardiovasc. Res.* **2018**, *114*, 378–388. [CrossRef] [PubMed] [PubMed Central]
42. Zink, M.; Seewald, A.; Rohrbach, M.; Brodehl, A.; Liedtke, D.; Williams, T.; Childs, S.J.; Gerull, B. Decreased survival and cardiac performance of mutant TMEM43 in transgenic zebrafish. *Circulation* **2018**, *138* (Suppl. 1), A15878. [CrossRef] [PubMed] [PubMed Central]
43. Ratnavadivel, S.; de Toledo, M.S.; Rasmussen, T.B.; Šarić, T.; Gummert, J.; Zenke, M.; Milting, H. Human pluripotent stem cell line (HDZi001-A) derived from a patient carrying the ARVC-5 associated mutation TMEM43-p S358L. *Stem Cell Res.* **2020**, *48*, 101957. [CrossRef] [PubMed]
44. Healey, J.S.; Krahn, A.D.; Bashir, J.; Amit, G.; McIntyre, W.F.; Tsang, B.; Joza, J.; Exner, D.V.; Birnie, D.H.; Sadek, M.; et al. Perioperative Safety andarly Patient and Device Outcomes Among Subcutaneous Versus Transvenous Implantable Cardioverter Defibrillator Implantations: A Randomized, Multicenter Trial. *Ann. Intern. Med.* **2022**, *175*, 1658–1665. [CrossRef]
45. Wang, W.; Gasperetti, A.; Sears, S.F.; Tichnell, C.; Murray, B.; Tandri, H.; James, C.A.; Calkins, H. Subcutaneous and Transvenous Defibrillators in Arrhythmogenic Right Ventricular Cardiomyopathy: A Comparison of Clinical and Quality-of-Life Outcomes. *JACC Clin. Electrophysiol.* **2023**, *9*, 394–402. [CrossRef]
46. Honarbakhsh, S.; Protonotarios, A.; Monkhouse, C.; Hunter, R.J.; Elliott, P.M.; Lambiase, P.D. Right ventricular function is a predictor for sustained ventricular tachycardia requiring anti-tachycardic pacing in arrhythmogenic ventricular cardiomyopathy: Insight into transvenous vs. subcutaneous implantable cardioverter defibrillator insertion. *Europace* **2023**, *25*, euad073. [CrossRef]
47. McNally, E.M.; Mestroni, L. Dilated cardiomyopathy: Genetic determinants and mechanisms. *Circ. Res.* **2017**, *121*, 731–748. [CrossRef]
48. Herman, D.S.; Lam, L.; Taylor, M.R.; Wang, L.; Teekakirikul, P.; Christodoulou, D.; Conner, L.; DePalma, S.R.; McDonough, B.; Sparks, E.; et al. Truncations of titin causing dilated cardiomyopathy. *N. Engl. J. Med.* **2012**, *366*, 619–628. [CrossRef]
49. Chauveau, C.; Rowell, J.; Ferreiro, A. A rising titan: TTN review and mutation update. *Hum. Mutat.* **2014**, *35*, 1046–1059. [CrossRef]
50. Kayvanpour, E.; Sedaghat-Hamedani, F.; Amr, A.; Lai, A.; Haas, J.; Holzer, D.B.; Frese, K.S.; Keller, A.; Jensen, K.; Katus, H.A.; et al. Genotype-phenotype associations in dilated cardiomyopathy: Meta-analysis on more than 8000 individuals. *Clin. Res. Cardiol.* **2017**, *106*, 127–139. [CrossRef]

Disclaimer/Publisher's Note: The statements, opinions and data contained in all publications are solely those of the individual author(s) and contributor(s) and not of MDPI and/or the editor(s). MDPI and/or the editor(s) disclaim responsibility for any injury to people or property resulting from any ideas, methods, instructions or products referred to in the content.

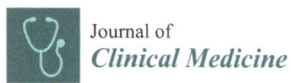

Review

A Comparative Analysis of Apical Rocking and Septal Flash: Two Views of the Same Systole?

Alexandra-Iulia Lazăr-Höcher [1,2], Dragoș Cozma [2,3,4,*], Liviu Cirin [1], Andreea Cozgarea [1,5], Adelina-Andreea Faur-Grigori [2], Rafael Catană [3], Dănuț George Tudose [6], Georgică Târtea [7], Simina Crișan [2,3,4], Dan Gaiță [2,3,4], Constantin-Tudor Luca [2,3,4] and Cristina Văcărescu [2,3,4]

1. Doctoral School, "Victor Babes" University of Medicine and Pharmacy, 300041 Timisoara, Romania; alexandra.hocher@umft.ro (A.-I.L.-H.); liviu.cirin@umft.ro (L.C.); andreea.cozgarea@umft.ro (A.C.)
2. Institute of Cardiovascular Diseases Timisoara, 13A Gheorghe Adam Street, 300310 Timisoara, Romania; andreeaadelinafaur@yahoo.com (A.-A.F.-G.); simina.crisan@umft.ro (S.C.); dan.gaita@umft.ro (D.G.); constantin.luca@umft.ro (C.-T.L.); cristina.vacarescu@umft.ro (C.V.)
3. Department of Cardiology, "Victor Babes" University of Medicine and Pharmacy, 2 Eftimie Murgu Square, 300041 Timisoara, Romania; catanarafael02@gmail.com
4. Research Center of the Institute of Cardiovascular Diseases Timisoara, 13A Gheorghe Adam Street, 300310 Timisoara, Romania
5. County Clinical Emergency Hospital of Sibiu, 550245 Sibiu, Romania
6. Institute of Cardiovascular Diseases C.C. Iliescu, Fundeni Clinical Institute, 258 Fundeni Street, 022328 Bucharest, Romania; georgedtudose@gmail.com
7. Department of Physiology, University of Medicine and Pharmacy of Craiova, 200349 Craiova, Romania; georgica.tartea@umfcv.ro
* Correspondence: dragos.cozma@umft.ro

Abstract: Heart failure (HF) is a complex medical condition characterized by both electrical and mechanical dyssynchrony. Both dyssynchrony mechanisms are intricately linked together, but the current guidelines for cardiac resynchronization therapy (CRT) rely only on the electrical dyssynchrony criteria, such as the QRS complex duration. This possible inconsistency may result in undertreating eligible individuals who could benefit from CRT due to their mechanical dyssynchrony, even if they fail to fulfill the electrical criteria. The main objective of this literature review is to provide a comprehensive analysis of the practical value of echocardiography for the assessment of left ventricular (LV) dyssynchrony using parameters such as septal flash and apical rocking, which have proven their relevance in patient selection for CRT. The secondary objectives aim to offer an overview of the relationship between septal flash and apical rocking, to emphasize the primary drawbacks and benefits of using echocardiography for evaluation of septal flash and apical rocking, and to offer insights into potential clinical applications and future research directions in this area. Conclusion: there is an opportunity to render resynchronization therapy more effective for every individual; septal flash and apical rocking could be a very useful and straightforward echocardiography resource.

Keywords: cardiac resynchronization; left ventricular dyssynchrony; septal flash; apical rocking; echocardiography

1. Introduction

Heart failure (HF) is a clinical syndrome resulting from structural and functional impairment of ventricular filling or ejection of blood. The global incidence and prevalence rates of HF have reached epidemic proportions, affecting nearly 23 million people, and in the general European population the prevalence of symptomatic HF ranges between 0.4 and 0.6%, being similar to the prevalence in the United States [1]. The prevalence of HF rises exponentially with age, being ≥10% among people aged >70 years [2].

Within the population of patients with chronic HF, intraventricular conduction abnormalities play a substantial role in elevating the risk of morbidity and mortality. These abnormalities can lead to impaired systolic function, reduced left ventricular contractility, prolonged mitral regurgitation, and abnormal septal wall motion, affecting approximately one-third of patients with heart failure and reduced ejection fraction (HFrEF) [3–9]. It is noteworthy that the prevalence of secondary mitral regurgitation (SMR) in heart failure patients reaches 50% for ischemic and 65% for nonischemic cardiomyopathy, while mild to moderate secondary mitral regurgitation occurs in 49% of patients with HF and severe secondary mitral regurgitation occurs in 24% of patients [10,11]. The presence and severity of SMR alone reveal substantial connections with both all-cause mortality and heart failure hospitalizations [11].

Cardiac resynchronization therapy (CRT) is a well-established treatment for heart failure patients with a severely reduced ejection fraction (LVEF < 35%) and a QRS duration exceeding 130 ms who remain symptomatic despite optimized medical therapy [12]. Extensive data from large-scale randomized studies consistently show that, in patients with a wide left bundle branch block (LBBB) conduction pattern and severe left ventricular (LV) systolic dysfunction, cardiac resynchronization therapy (CRT) leads to significant improvements in hard outcomes such as reduced mortality [13] and heart failure hospitalization rates [14], as well as improvement of exercise capacity, symptoms, and quality of life [15]. In addition, cardiac resynchronization therapy (CRT) can reduce secondary mitral regurgitation by enhancing the closing forces driven by ventricular resynchronization as well as by diminishing the tethering forces on the mitral apparatus [16].

In the last three decades, extensive research efforts have focused on identifying imaging-based parameters that can uncover the electromechanical factors influencing the effectiveness of cardiac resynchronization therapy (CRT) [17]. Echocardiographic assessment of ventricular or mechanical dyssynchrony before CRT, irrespective of left ventricular ejection fraction (LVEF) or QRS duration [18–20] may enhance patient selection and identify patients who may benefit from CRT [9,21]. These assessments, including apical rocking and septal flash, have shown promise in predicting favorable outcomes in CRT patients, offering an accurate and rapid bedside investigation to guide treatment decisions [22–29].

During echocardiography examination, the most frequently observed abnormal wall motions are represented by septal flash, septal rebound stretch, and apical rocking. While both "septal flash" (early inward bulge of the septum) and "septal rebound stretch" (outward extension after initial shortening) are linked to the left bundle branch block (LBBB), their underlying condition is different. The origin of septal flash is in the early activation of the right heart chamber pushing on the unopposed septum, whereas rebound stretch is caused by late activation of the left ventricle after early septal contraction [30,31]. The prevalence of septal flash in LBBB patients exhibits a wide range, typically between 45% and 63%, with variations attributed to the specific population under study and the strictness of the criteria used to define LBBB [28,32].

Septal flash (originally termed "septal beak" in 1974 by Dillon et al.), when observed through M mode echocardiography in patients with left bundle branch block (LBBB) [33], serves as a prominent marker of intraventricular dyssynchrony.

The term "septal flash" gained specificity in 2008 when Parsai et al. linked it to an indicator of asynchrony resulting from electrical abnormalities [22], defining it as an anomalous, rapid leftward motion of the interventricular septum during the isovolumetric ventricular contraction phase, which occurs before the opening of the aortic valve [34,35]. This phenomenon is primarily driven by an electrical disorder, as the left bundle branch block leads to the left ventricle's electrical activation via the right bundle branch, causing a depolarization process from right to left. This results in delayed contraction in the posterolateral walls due to slower propagation velocity through the myocardial fibers with distinct electrical properties compared to the specialized Purkinje system [30]. The septal strain pattern in the left bundle branch block (LBBB) is notable for its distinct features, which involve pre-ejection shortening followed by abrupt septal stretch during ejection [36,37].

The presence of a significant septal flash is frequently associated with a U-shaped activation pattern on electrical mapping and predicts a more favorable response to CRT intervention compared to patients with no or limited septal flash [28,38].

Moreover, in the context of left bundle branch block (LBBB), the septum, comprising approximately one-third of the left ventricle's mass, loses its contractile effectiveness, leading to a dyssynchronous contraction that impairs the heart's pumping function and results in the entire ejection fraction workload being carried by the posterior and lateral walls [39,40]. In cases of LBBB with a posterior lateral scar or myocardial ischemia, septal flash is notably absent, as these conditions do not exert the necessary forces to stretch the septum, potentially leading to a "pseudonormal" appearance initially, which can ultimately induce left ventricular remodeling [5]. This remodeling often manifests as hypertrophy of the left ventricular lateral wall and thinning of the septum [34], potentially driven by altered activation and stretch patterns in opposite LV walls that induce molecular and cellular changes [4], redistribute myocardial blood flow and oxygen uptake [41], and result in differences in septal-to-lateral wall thickness [42,43].

An apical four–chamber view M–mode of the LV (Figure 1) is shown from a patient with typical LBBB, demonstrating septal flash (red arrows) and the dyssynchrony of contractility between the interventricular septum and posterolateral wall (red circle). The septum has an initial short inward motion before the ejection phase, which is followed by the stretching of the left ventricular lateral wall.

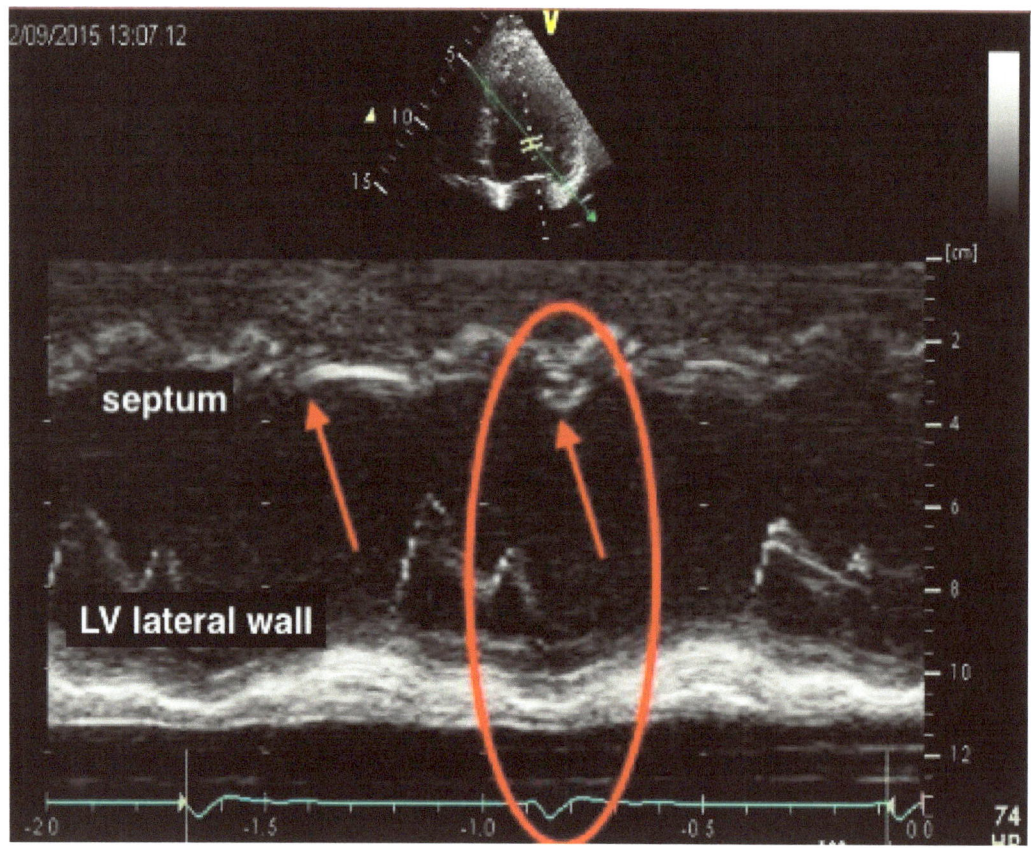

Figure 1. Septal flash on M-mode imaging.

Jansen et al. initially identified apical shuffle in 2007 as an unusual systolic septal-to-lateral movement of the left ventricle, yet they did not explore the underlying physiological mechanisms that cause this phenomenon, despite its predictive power for left ventricular reverse remodeling (sensitivity 90% and specificity 70%) [44]. Nowadays, the "apical shuffle" is known as apical rocking, and it is defined as abnormal lateral rocking of the ventricular apex caused by an intraventricular functional dyssynchrony. This dyssynchrony can be attributed to intraventricular conduction delays (e.g., LBBB), regional damage (e.g., myocardial scar), or a combination interplay of both [25,42,45,46].

Recently, the pathophysiological mechanism of apical rocking, characterized by brief early septal motion at the apex and a predominant lateral motion during ejection, has been elucidated in two distinct publications [26,47]. This phenomenon is characterized by a distinct right-to-left motion of the apical myocardium in the left ventricle (LV), occurring perpendicular to the LV's long axis [47,48]. The mechanism of apical rocking involves a contraction that causes the septum to temporarily move inward, pulling the apex closer towards it. Following that, the septum stretches as the apex is pulled laterally by the delayed activation of the lateral wall during the ejection phase [49]. This gradual process allows the ventricle to build up the necessary force to eventually open the aortic valve and efficiently pump blood out. The extent of "apical rocking" in dilated cardiomyopathy directly relates to the size of the left ventricle (left ventricular end-diastolic volume), and the QRS duration does not influence the magnitude of the movement [50].

Even though each of these easily recognizable and accessible parameters indicates an atypical myocardial motion associated with the left bundle branch block (LBBB), our comprehension of the precise physiological mechanisms that underlie septal flash and apical rocking is restricted, regardless of their efficacy in the patient selection process for CRT. This literature review aims to provide a comprehensive analysis of the practical value of echocardiography for the assessment of left ventricular (LV) dyssynchrony using parameters such as septal flash and apical rocking, which have proven their relevance in patient selection for CRT, the relationship between septal flash and apical rocking, emphasize the primary drawbacks and benefits of using echocardiography for evaluation of septal flash and apical rocking, and offer insights into potential clinical applications and future research directions in this area.

It is illustrated by the early septal contraction before aortic valve opening (AVO) associated with the pre-stretch and apical movement of the posterolateral wall towards the septum. At the end of the systolic phase, the apex undergoes rightward rotation due to the lateral wall contraction in addition to the septal stretching. The dashed line shows the longitudinal axis of the left ventricle (Figure 2).

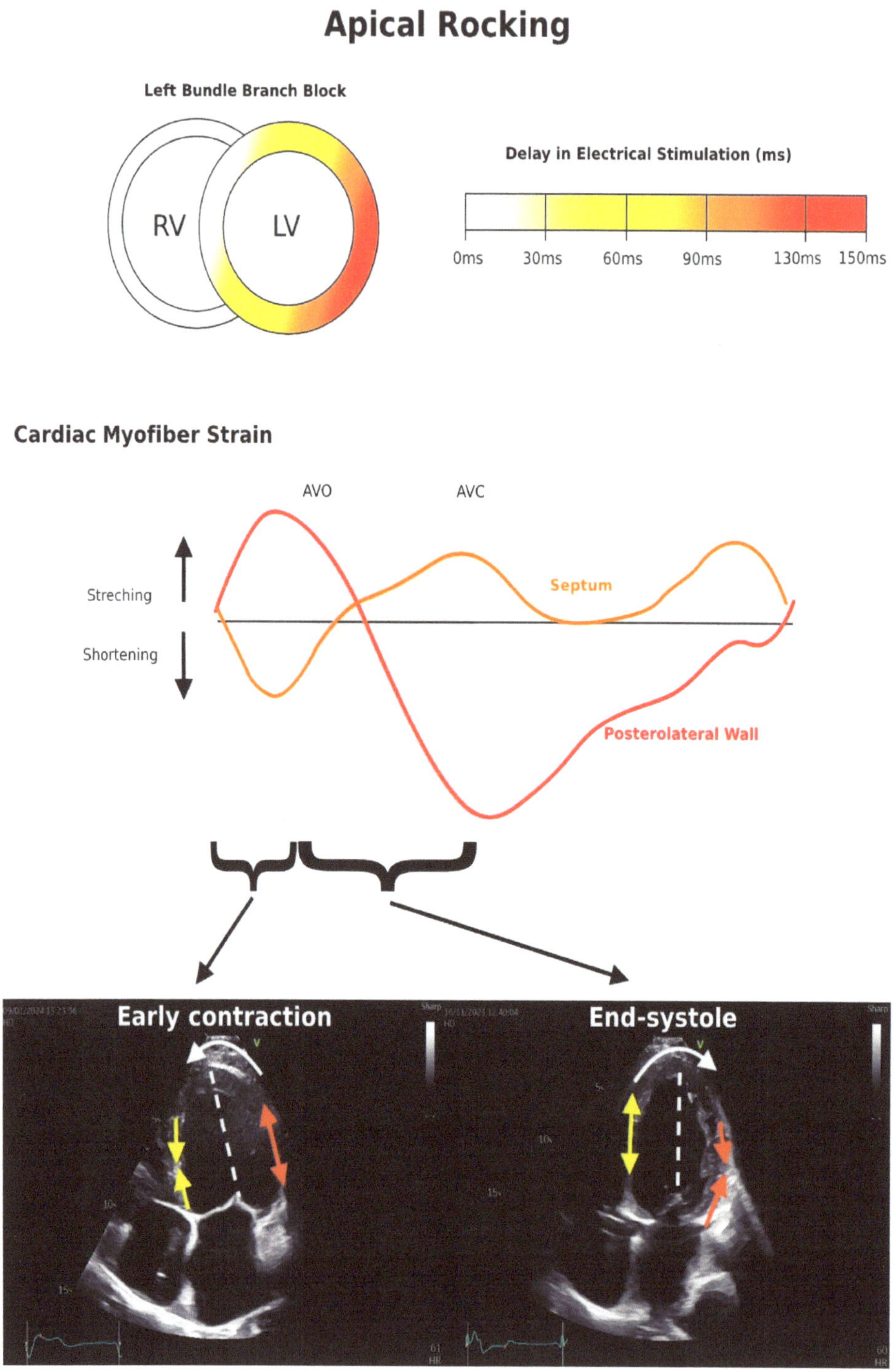

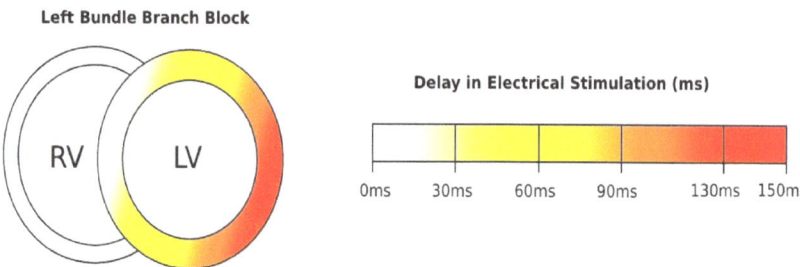

Figure 2. Computer Simulations of Cardiac Myofiber Strain in LBBB patients and two-dimensional echocardiography of apical four-chamber view illustrating the apical rocking phenomenon.

2. Materials and Methods

The selection of studies for this review followed the PRISMA (Preferred Reporting Items for Systematic Reviews and Meta-Analyses) guidelines. This review was conducted by reviewing bibliographic searches on databases such as the PubMed database, Google Scholar, and Scopus. Both manual searches and the use of MeSH terms on PubMed were employed to identify articles on septal flash and apical rocking published within no date restriction. The selection of the most relevant articles involved assessing their titles, the information provided in their abstracts, and a brief overview of the complete manuscript. The eligibility criteria was based on studies that evaluated septal flash and/or apical rocking. There was no restriction based on how septal flash and/or apical rocking was defined, with all imaging modalities being included. Articles not written in English, publications with only abstracts available, and duplicate entries were excluded from consideration.

In October 2023, the search and selection process was carried out by two experienced cardiologists with expertise in interventional arrhythmology and echocardiography. Initially, we manually scoured articles using the specific keywords "ventricular dyssynchrony" and "septal flash" and "apical rocking". Additionally, using the MeSH term option available in PubMed, we conducted another search with the following terms: (("Cardiac Resynchronization Therapy" [Mesh]) AND "Echocardiography"[Mesh]).

The PRISMA diagram below illustrates the search strategy employed along with the filters that were applied (Figure 3). The diagram was made using the draw.io application (UK).

To enhance the organization and planning of the review, all chosen articles were integrated into a Microsoft Excel (version 2021) table. This table included columns for the article's title, authors, utilized imaging method, year of publication, journal, publication type, and keywords.

We deliberated on the critical data and findings, with a particular emphasis on the correlation (Table 1) and the difference (Table 2) between septal flash and apical rocking. We categorized the articles in the following manner:

1. The strong inter-relationship between septal flash and apical rocking—19 selected articles [studied included in quantitative synthesis (n = 16); studied included in qualitative synthesis (n = 3)]; some of the most relevant, of date articles regarding the same underlying pathophysiology similarities and differences.
2. The importance of echocardiography in ventricular dyssynchrony management—23 selected articles [studied included in quantitative synthesis (n = 19); studied included in qualitative synthesis (n = 4)]; some of the most relevant articles regarding the role and limitation of the echocardiographic techniques were selected and compared with one another.

Table 1. Similarities of septal flash and apical rocking.

Feature	Septal Flash	Apical Rocking
Type of abnormality	Wall motion abnormality	Wall motion abnormality
Pathophysiology	Early activation of the right ventricle exerts pressure on the septum as a consequence of left bundle branch block (LBBB) [20,30]	Early septal contraction pulls the apex inwards, while delayed lateral wall contraction pulls the apex outwards [26,28]
Associated with	The uncoordinated contraction of the left ventricle [20,22,28,30,36,51]	The uncoordinated contraction of the left ventricle [26,28]
Observed with	Echocardiography	Echocardiography

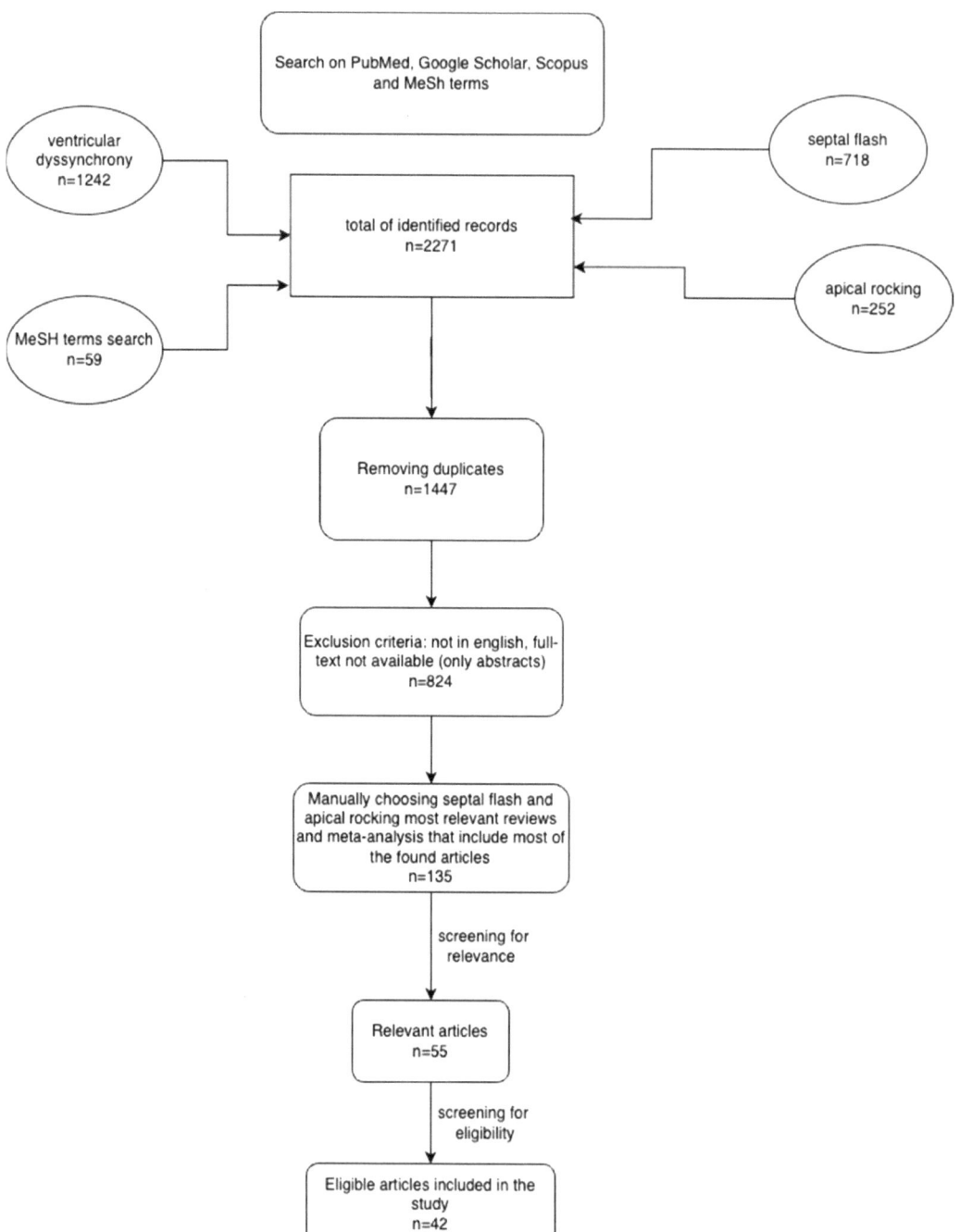

Figure 3. PRISMA chart of the article selection.

Table 2. Differences of septal flash and apical rocking.

Feature	Septal Flash	Apical Rocking
Type of abnormality	Paradoxical interventricular septum movement toward left ventricle during systole [20,30,36]	Brief early septal motion at the apex and a predominant lateral motion during ejection [26,47]
Region	Involves the interventricular septum [20,22,30,36,51]	Primarily affects the left ventricular apex [28]
Timing in the cardiac cycle	Earlier—During isovolumic contraction phase [20,30]	Later—During the ejection phase [26,28]
Clinical Significance	Associated with left bundle branch block (LBBB) and other conduction abnormalities [20,30,49]	Typically seen in patients with left ventricular dysfunction or ischemic heart disease [26]

3. Results

3.1. The Relationship between Septal Flash and Apical Rocking

Septal flash and apical rocking are related features of the typical left bundle branch block (LBBB) contraction pattern, indicating a shared underlying pathophysiology. They often coexist in the same patients, although their extent may vary.

Stankovic et al. determined that the left bundle branch block (LBBB) causes early septal contraction, seen as "septal flash", occurring before the aortic valve opens [28]. This is a quick inward and outward motion of the septum. During this septal flash, the left ventricular (LV) apex moves toward the septum, initiating the first part of the apical rocking motion. Subsequently, a delayed and more pronounced posterolateral contraction leads to stretching of the septum and movement of the LV apex in the opposite direction, completing the second phase of the apical rocking, as can be observed by experienced observers in an echocardiographic four-chamber view of a heart with dyssynchrony [22,26,30,49]. The main distinction between them lies in the timing of the cardiac cycle. Septal flash takes place during the shorter isovolumic ventricular contraction phase, whereas apical rocking occurs during ejection, which has a longer duration. The presence of septal flash and apical rocking corresponds with research that uses quantitative assessments of systolic stretch by strain imaging [37].

However, it is worth noting that they can occasionally be observed together or separately, with variations in their intensity [28]. There are some several conditions that can contribute to the diminished intensity or even the complete dispersal of these phenomena, summarizing that [30,36,51]: the passive phase of the septal flash can be impaired by contractility dysfunction or high filling pressures of the right ventricle; the active phase of the septal flash can be diminished by a delayed conduction through the right bundle branch or the presence of a septal scar; a scarred posterolateral wall will reduce the ability of the septum to stretch during the second phase of apical rocking; slow RBB conduction that is disguised inside the LBBB, resulting in slow RV contraction and septal activation (this would suggest that SF might occur only when RBB conduction is intact); a septal fascicle could bypass the slow transseptal conduction; difficulties in the alignment of the ultrasound fascicle beam with the latero-lateral movement of the septal flash or a low frame rate can impair the visualization of the septal flash [52]; the site of the left bundle branch block is important because, the more proximal the block is, the more typical septal flash is [30,36,51,53,54].

Alternatively, isolated mechanical asynchrony can imitate the genuine septal flash induced by electrical conduction irregularities. Moreover, elevated right ventricular pressures or a scarred septum can trigger a right-to-left systolic motion that may resemble septal flash. In these instances, the critical distinguishing characteristic is that the systolic motion persists longer than in the case of a genuine septal flash [20].

3.2. Echocardiography

Given its widespread availability, feasibility, and capacity to assess regional myocardial function with excellent temporal and spatial resolution, echocardiography emerges as an ideal imaging tool for the selection of patients suitable for cardiac resynchronization therapy (CRT) [49].

Early investigations into left ventricular mechanical dyssynchrony using echocardiography primarily concentrated on quantifying the delay in the contraction of opposing ventricular walls. In a small-scale study involving 24 heart failure patients, Pitzalis et al. identified that a septal-to-posterior motion delay (SPWMD) of ≥ 130 milliseconds could serve as a predictor of left ventricular reverse remodeling in patients without a history of anterior or septal infarction [55,56]. Later investigations explored the use of tissue Doppler imaging and speckle-tracking echocardiography to assess LV dyssynchrony. These techniques were employed to measure opposing wall delays or analyze variations in peak systolic velocities among different myocardial regions [13,18,57].

Another technique proposed to assess left ventricular dyssynchrony involves analyzing the unique contraction pattern associated with LBBB and comparing the contractility of opposing walls to identify septal flash (SF) [22] and/or apical rocking (ApR) [25].

Given that there is no universally preferred method for assessing these parameters, various techniques have been suggested. Septal flash is conventionally evaluated using M-mode in the parasternal long-axis view, as well as 2D and tissue Doppler imaging in either the short or long parasternal long-axis view [22,58]. The M-mode echocardiography can be applied from the parasternal views to ascertain the radial function of the interventricular septum, and the evaluation of the longitudinal displacement of the interventricular septum can be determined from the apical views using TDI-derived speckle tracking [7,59]. However, relying on longitudinal strain for assessing the accurate pattern of septal radial movement is not precise [38]. Assessing radial strain is a more intricate task, while parameters derived from longitudinal strain, such as septal rebound stretch and systolic stretch index [60,61], are more readily available, reproducible, and commonly employed in the selection of CRT patients. Marechaux et al. described three echocardiographic patterns of septal flash by applying the longitudinal strain speckle tracking specifically, as follows: pattern 1—a double-peaked systolic shortening; pattern 2—an early pre-ejection shortening peak followed by a prominent systolic stretch; pattern 3—a pseudo-normal shortening with a late systolic shortening peak, no or minimal pre-ejection septal lengthening, and less pronounced end-systolic stretch. This study concluded that the first two patterns of septal flash were strongly linked to a positive response to CRT, while the third pattern was more likely to lead to a negative response. The third pattern was also associated with a high level of scarring in the heart muscle and a more advanced stage of heart failure [62].

Voight et al. devised an algorithm for quantifying apical rocking through the measurement of apical transverse motion (ATM), which combines the longitudinal myocardial data from the interventricular septum and the lateral wall of the left ventricle. Their findings indicated that apical transverse motion serves as a valuable parameter for enhancing the identification of patients who stand to benefit from CRT therapy [25].

Nevertheless, echocardiography has significant limitations (Table 3). This approach relies on complex and time-consuming algorithms for assessing different cardiac cycles, and myocardial peak velocities can be greatly affected by factors like the filling condition and the passive motion of the analyzed wall segment. Furthermore, the expertise of the echocardiographer is essential for the accurate diagnosis of septal flash and apical rocking in candidates for cardiac resynchronization therapy (CRT). In a small, single-center study, Mada et al. demonstrated that semi-automatic detection of these particular contraction patterns using speckle tracking echocardiography was superior to inexperienced echo-readers for recognizing SF/ApR [63].

Table 3. Advantages, disadvantages, strengths, and limitations of echocardiography in the assessment of septal flash and apical rocking.

Parameter	Septal Flash	Apical Rocking
Advantages	A variety of echocardiographic techniques, including M-mode, 2D, and tissue Doppler imaging [18,55,60,62] Various septal flash echocardiographic patterns have been identified, some of which are strongly associated with a favorable response to CRT [38]	Enhances identification of patients who may benefit from CRT [25] Quantified through apical transverse motion (ATM) [25]
Disadvantages	Myocardial peak velocities can be influenced by a multitude of variables, such as passive motion and filling condition [7] Expertise of echocardiographer is essential [63]	Assessment complexity and reliance on expertise of the operator [63]
Strengths	Potential predictive value for CRT response [7,22] Different septal flash patterns were identified [38,62]	An additional parameter is provided to improve the process of selecting patients for CRT Quantifiable through specific echocardiographic measurements [25]
Limitations	Operator dependency and complexity of interpretation [56,63] Semi-automatic detection may not completely replace expertise of an experienced Echocardiographer [63] Specific septal flash patterns might not be common to all Patients [38,62] Features such as the severity of heart failure and a history of myocardial fibrosis may impact the analysis	Relies on expertise of echocardiographer for accurate evaluation [63] Algorithmic quantification may still be influenced by various factors affecting myocardial motion such as temporal and regional function Inhomogeneities [25]

4. Discussion

Echocardiography plays a pivotal role in the selection of patients undergoing cardiac resynchronization therapy (CRT) due to its broad spectrum of possibilities. Septal flash and apical rocking are practical indicators in predicting the response to cardiac resynchronization therapy (CRT), resulting in improved clinical outcomes for patients.

Cardiac resynchronization therapy (CRT) plays an essential role in treating heart failure patients with prolonged QRS duration and low LVEF [12]. International guidelines make a Class IA recommendation for CRT device implantation in symptomatic patients in sinus rhythm with an LV ejection fraction (LVEF) of $\leq 35\%$, LBBB and QRS duration (QRSd) of ≥ 150 ms, despite optimal medical therapy and a Class IIaB for symptomatic patients with heart failure in sinus rhythm with an LV ejection fraction (LVEF) of $\leq 35\%$, LBBB and QRS duration (QRSd) 130–149 ms, despite optimal medical therapy for the reduction in mortality and morbidity [12]. Despite the coexistence of electrical and mechanical dyssynchrony, the CRT guideline recommendations rely on electrical dyssynchrony criteria, due to the amount of research data using QRS duration as an enrollment criterion and findings from studies like the Predictors of Response to CRT (PROSPECT) study [13].

However, certain research data proved that septal flash is a relevant echocardiographic finding in over half of heart failure (HF) patients receiving cardiac resynchronization therapy (CRT), and it serves as a valuable predictor of favorable left ventricular reverse remodeling following CRT implantation, as evidenced by Doltra et al., who reported an 80.2%

echocardiographic response rate with reductions in LV end-systolic volumes and LVEF, along with CRT-induced correction of septal flash in 93% of patients [64]. Gabrielli et al. determined septal flash as the only independent predictor of significant left ventricular reverse remodeling [29], Gąsior et al. observed that septal flash at baseline correlated with notable enhancements in LVEF, LV end-systolic volumes, and diastolic volumes [65], and Parsai et al. reported that 88% of cases displayed the resolution of septal flash after CRT implantation, along with improvements in LV volumes, although no significant overall LVEF improvement was noted [22]. In a comprehensive, multi-center observational study known as PREDICT-CRT, a quantitative measurement of apical rocking was compared with visual assessment and showed similar accuracy in predicting the response to CRT. In addition, Stankovic et al. demonstrated that a certain pattern of LV mechanical dyssynchrony, characterized by apical rocking and septal flash, is associated with enhanced long-term survival after cardiac resynchronization therapy (CRT) [28]. Another study conducted by Parsai et al. proved that low-dose dobutamine stress echocardiography (DSE) represents a valuable approach for revealing septal flash in individuals with a viable septum, irrespective of the cause of their heart failure [23]. Low-dose DSE unveils or amplifies the extent of dyssynchronous motion induced by left bundle branch block (LBBB) and helps in the identification of patients who may experience reverse remodeling following cardiac resynchronization therapy (CRT). CRT responders exhibit a characteristic early septal contraction that pulls the apex toward the septum, aligning with other studies demonstrating this phenomenon as a brief bounce in the septum, known as septal flash [22]. The prominence of septal flash is an indicator of the inefficient work performed by the dyssynchronous left ventricle, and its disappearance following pacing is associated with the reversal of left ventricular remodeling, whereas its persistence after pacing is a sign of non-responsiveness to therapy [23]. Furthermore, Stankovic et al. concluded that the presence of septal flash and apical rocking has shown its predictive value for CRT response in individuals with chronic right ventricular pacing who require an upgrade to cardiac resynchronization therapy (CRT) [66].

Although small cohort retrospective studies have shown positive outcomes related to the utility of echo-derived parameters in predicting CRT response, the extensive PROSPECT trial did not succeed in confirming their effectiveness for identifying appropriate CRT candidates [67]. These inconclusive outcomes are ascribed to the variability in the reproducibility of echo-derived dyssynchrony parameter analysis [21], as well as the inadequacy of opposite wall delay as the sole assessment tool, which fails to fully elucidate the complex pathophysiology underlying CRT response.

Even though randomized controlled trials (RCTs) have demonstrated significant benefits of cardiac resynchronization therapy (CRT) in HFrEF patients (Table 4), a subset exhibits non-response characterized by persistent symptoms, recurrent hospitalizations for heart failure, and lack of left ventricular reverse remodeling. Non-responsiveness to CRT can be attributed to a broad range of causes, including poor lead placement in the left ventricle, suboptimal atrioventricular (AV) and ventricular-ventricular (VV) timing, left ventricular scar, and progression of heart failure [68]. The excessive focus on the idea of "non-response" to cardiac resynchronization therapy (CRT) has led to a significant lack of use of the device, leading to up to two-thirds of indicated patients failing to obtain the implant [69]. The most recent attempt in the data area focuses on identifying patients who respond to the CRT with a particularly beneficial (super) response patients because of their significantly lower cumulative risk of heart failure, mortality, and need for defibrillator therapy for ventricular tachycardia or ventricular fibrillation. Based upon the results of previous research, studies have identified the following two potential predictors of a "super-response" to treatment: left bundle branch block (LBBB) and a smaller size of the left atrium [70,71]. The MADIT-CRT trial identified female gender, absence of prior myocardial infarction, QRS duration $\geq$ 150 ms, LBBB, BMI < 30 kg/m^2, and reduced left atrial volume index as predictors of super-responsiveness to cardiac resynchronization therapy [72].

Table 4. Summary of the main cited studies providing an overview of the relationship between septal flash and apical rocking in the field of CRT.

Authors/Journal-Year/Ref	Population Study	Endpoints	Imaging Parameters	Results
C. Parsai et al., Eur. Heart J., 2009 [22]	161 pts 66 ± 10 years LVEF 24 ± 6% QRS width >120 ms	Reverse remodeling was defined as a reduction in LVESV ≥10% Clinical response was defined as a reduction in NYHA Class ≥1	SF	Presence of SF Se 64%, Sp 55%, PPV 81%, NPV 33% for the prediction of LV response remodeling
C. Parsai et al., Eur. Heart J., 2008 [23]	52 pts 69 ± 2 years LVEF 24 ± 7% QRS width >120 ms	Reduction in LVESV ≥10% Clinical response was defined as a reduction in NYHA Class ≥1, increase in 6 min walk test (>10%), and fall in BNP (≥30%)	SF	Presence of ApR and SF Se 84% and 79% and Sp 79% and Sp 74%, and accuracy of 82% and 77% for the prediction of LV response remodeling ApR [HR] 0.40, 95% confidence interval [CI] 0.30–0.53, $p < 0.0001$ and SF (HR 0.45 [CI 0.34–0.61], $p < 0.001$ is associated with lower all-cause mortality after CRT
M. Szulik et al., Eur. J. Echocardiogr., 2010 [26]	69 pts 63 ± 10 years	Reduction in LVESV > 15%	ApR	Presence of ApR resulted in an average Se = 89%, Sp = 75%, and accuracy for prediction of CRT response of 83%;
I. Stankovic et al., Eur. Heart J., 2014 [27]	58 pts 63 ± 10 years LVEF 26 ± 6% QRS width > 175 ± 25 ms	An increase >5% of LVEF during stress-echocardiography	ApR	AUC 0.88, 95% CI 0.77–0.99, $p < 0.001$ for the prediction of CRT response
I. Stankovic et al., Eur. Heart J.—Cardiovasc. Imaging, 2016 [28]	1060 pts 64 ± 11 years LVEF 27 ± 7% QRS width >170 ± 29 ms	Reduction in left LVESV ≥15% during the first year FU	SF ApR	Presence of ApR and SF Se 84% and 79%, Sp 79% and Sp 74%, and accuracy of 82% and 77% for the prediction of LV response remodeling ApR [HR] 0.40, 95% confidence interval [CI] 0.30–0.53, $p < 0.0001$ and SF (HR 0.45 [CI 0.34–0.61], $p < 0.001$ is associated with lower all-cause mortality after CRT
L. Gabrielli et al., Europace, 2014 [29]	94 pts 69 ± 8 years QRS width >166 ± 35 ms	Reduction in LVESV >15%	SF	Baseline SF predicts CRT response (OR 5.24; 95% CI 1.95–14.11)
Z. Gąsior et al., Arch. Med. Sci., 2016 [65]	133 pts 63 ± 10 years LVEF 25 ± 6% QRS width >165 ± 25 ms	Evaluation of SF implication Evaluation of myocardial contractile reserve for 12 months follow up	SF	SF presence before CRT implantation is related to significant improvement in LV systolic and diastolic volumes and LVEF ($p < 0.05$)
A. Ghani et al., Neth. Heart J., 2016 [48]	297 pts median age 68.7 years median LVEF 24 ± 8% median QRS width 160 ms	Determination of the independent association of LV ApR and CRT super-response	ApR	Super-responders had an absolute mean LVEF increase of 27% (22.05 ± 5.7 at baseline and 49.0% ± 7.5 at follow up) ApR was more common in super-responders (76%, $p < 0.001$)
A. Doltra et al., JACC Cardiovasc. Imaging, 2014 [67]	200 pts 67.37 ± 9.17 years LVEF 24 ± 6% QRS width >169.29 ± 30.38 ms	Reduction in LVESV ≥15%	SF	Baseline SF predicts CRT response in 93% of the population

Abbreviations: ApR—apical rocking, AUC—area under the curve, BNP—brain natriuretic peptide, CI—confidence interval, CRT—cardiac resynchronization therapy, FU—follow-up, LV—left ventricle, HR—hazard ration, LVEF—left ventricle ejection fraction, LVESV—left ventricle end-systolic volume, NPV—negative predictive value, NYHA—New York Heart Association functional class, OR—odds ration, PPV—positive predictive value, Se—sensibility, Sp—specificity, SF—septal flash.

Based on the fact that these two parameters are distinctive characteristics of left bundle branch block (LBBB) contraction patterns, which indicate the presence of an asynchronous left ventricular (LV) contraction, the goal of cardiac resynchronization therapy (CRT) is to correct the dyssynchrony by coordinating the contraction of the ventricles. In consequence, a coordinated contraction will enhance the function of the left ventricle and will decrease the burden of the symptoms of heart failure. In addition, the relationship between septal flash and apical rocking and favorable outcomes in patients undergoing cardiac resynchronization therapy (CRT) may be related to their link with left ventricular reverse remodeling [29,67]. The literature data have shown that there is a link between the resolution of septal flash and the reduction in apical rocking post cardiac resynchronization therapy (CRT) implantation with an increase in left ventricular (LV) function, defined as decreased end-systolic volumes [22] and increased ejection fraction percentage [65]. In patients undergoing cardiac resynchronization therapy (CRT), the presence of septal flash and apical rocking may therefore function as indicators of CRT response and subsequent left ventricle (LV) reversal remodeling, resulting in enhanced clinical outcomes [28].

However, the particular mechanisms beneath the efficacy of cardiac resynchronization treatment (CRT) for individuals with heart failure and widened QRS remain unclear, emphasizing the need for a more comprehensive assessment of their pathophysiology because dyssynchrony might be probably the most important factor, but not the only factor, influencing the success of CRT in an individual patient [49]. This increased comprehension could lead to a more accurate and focused evaluation of patients for CRT, possibly outlining the wide range of responses noticed, from significant LV reverse remodeling in "CRT super-responders" [72] to more modest effects or even deterioration of LV function [73–75]. Alternative CRT pacing, such as fusion pacing CRT or LV only pacing, was associated with a high rate of super-responders [76,77]. Fusion pacing CRT is defined as optimised LV only pacing (with or without a back-up RV lead) creating electrical and mechanical fusion with the intrinsec QRS. Avoiding RV pacing may substantially increase the structural response rate by shortening LV activation time [78]. Moreover, different "degrees" of LV only fusion, according to AV node variability and heart rate, seem to play an important role in the LV remodelling process, and post-implantation optimization by targeting electrical dyssynchrony can improve CRT response in non-responder patients [79,80]. In consequence, understanding all components of cardiac dyssynchrony is essential not only in patient selection, but also in choosing the best CRT pacing modality.

Comparing our results with those of previous studies reveals consistencies and discrepancies both in terms of results and clinical implications. Our findings mainly align with previous research in highlighting the importance of echocardiography in assessing cardiac function and identifying potential candidates for cardiac resynchronization therapy (CRT), but we also highlight the ongoing challenge of assessing septal flash and apical rocking despite their formerly established significance in improving patient selection. Compared to previous research that may have indicated specific criteria for parameters like septal flash and apical rocking [20,26,30], our results contribute to the consensus that no single echocardiographic approach has gained broad support in current clinical guidelines.

Furthermore, our review emphasizes the tendency to underestimate the strong correlation between septal flash and apical rocking. Although they often coexist in patients with left bundle branch block (LBBB) and left ventricle (LV) dyssynchrony, the inadequate application of both in the approach of these patients is neglected, and there is not enough data on the combined effectiveness of these parameters. Along with that, adopting an integrated strategy towards heart failure patients undergoing cardiac resynchronization therapy (CRT) increases the potential to significantly influence the prognosis of the group of patients now referred to as non-responders.

This review contributes to the existing literature data by providing a comprehensive assessment of septal flash and apical rocking, their close relationship, and their potential relevance. Even more, by addressing gaps in the understanding of echocardiographic analysis, our research summarizes the current evidence on septal flash and apical rocking, emphasizing that echocardiography is the most accessible, readily available imaging modality that can improve patient selection.

This review has certain limitations due to the lack of studies examining septal flash and apical rocking. Our work is restricted by the absence of established criteria for measuring septal flash and apical rocking, leading to inconsistencies during echocardiography. More research is needed to fill in the lack of data in this area. Specifically, studies should focus on quality of life measurements, cardiac event rates (such as recurrent hospitalization with heart failure), and mortality rates to thoroughly evaluate the association of septal flash and apical rocking and their potential impact on mortality.

5. Future Direction

The future perspectives of the clinical application of apical rocking and septal flash for patients undergoing cardiac resynchronization therapy (CRT) display potential in enhancing tailored therapeutic approaches and optimizing outcomes for patients. Additionally, septal flash and apical rocking may be useful parameters for tracing the evolution of CRT response [28]. Through regular assessment of these echocardiographic parameters following implantation, clinicians can continue to monitor changes in ventricular dyssynchrony and assess the effectiveness of the therapy. By applying this dynamic monitoring strategy, non-responders can be detected earlier, which allows for prompt adjustments to be implemented to optimize patient outcomes. Further research into the possible integration of apical rocking and septal flash into risk stratification models for heart failure patients may be appropriate as our understanding of their prognostic significance advances. By using clinical and demographic data with these echocardiographic parameters, it may be possible to improve risk prediction tools for the aim of selecting patients who are most prone to adverse outcomes and providing guidance for targeted interventions, such as cardiac resynchronization therapy (CRT) [18,20,26,48]. The clinical application of apical rocking and septal flash in CRT patients should benefit from validation in real-world clinical practice settings. Prospective studies should focus on patient-centered-outcome research to evaluate the effects of apical rocking and septal flash on quality of life, functional status, and healthcare use in patients who have undergone cardiac resynchronization therapy (CRT).

6. Conclusions

In conclusion, this review provides a comprehensive analysis of the practical effectiveness of septal flash and apical rocking which are valuable echocardiographic parameters to assess the left ventricle (LV) dyssynchrony and to guide the patient selection for cardiac resynchronization therapy (CRT). Even if both parameters are predictive and assist in enhancing potential cardiac resynchronization therapy (CRT) responders, their dyssynchrony causes, assessment methods, and clinical implications differ. However, their combined evaluation improves the assessment of left ventricle (LV) dyssynchrony and the cardiac resynchronization therapy (CRT) optimization for better outcomes.

Author Contributions: Conceptualization, A.-I.L.-H., C.V., D.G.T. and D.C.; methodology, A.-I.L.-H., C.V. and D.C.; software, A.-I.L.-H., L.C., A.-A.F.-G. and R.C.; validation, A.-I.L.-H., C.V.; formal analysis, A.-I.L.-H., C.V., D.G.T. and A.C.; investigation, A.-I.L.-H. and C.V.; resources, A.-I.L.-H., L.C. and G.T.; data curation, A.-I.L.-H., A.C. and R.C.; writing—original draft preparation, A.-I.L.-H. and A.-A.F.-G.; writing—review and editing A.-I.L.-H., C.V. and D.C.; visualization, S.C., C.V., G.T. and C.-T.L.; supervision, S.C., C.V. and C.-T.L.; project administration, A.-I.L.-H., C.V., D.C. and D.G.; funding acquisition, D.G., A.-I.L.-H. and C.V. All authors have read and agreed to the published version of the manuscript.

Funding: This research received no external funding. Internal Funding: We would like to acknowledge VICTOR BABES UNIVERSITY OF MEDICINE AND PHARMACY TIMISOARA for their support in covering the costs of publication for this research paper.

Institutional Review Board Statement: Not applicable.

Informed Consent Statement: Not applicable.

Data Availability Statement: Data sharing is not applicable.

Conflicts of Interest: The authors declare no conflicts of interest.

References

1. Roger, V.L. Epidemiology of Heart Failure. *Circ. Res.* **2013**, *113*, 646–659. [CrossRef]
2. Mosterd, A.; Hoes, A.W. Clinical Epidemiology of Heart Failure. *Heart* **2007**, *93*, 1137–1146. [CrossRef] [PubMed]
3. Kristensen, S.L.; Castagno, D.; Shen, L.; Jhund, P.S.; Docherty, K.F.; Rørth, R.; Abraham, W.T.; Desai, A.S.; Dickstein, K.; Rouleau, J.L.; et al. Prevalence and Incidence of Intra-ventricular Conduction Delays and Outcomes in Patients with Heart Failure and Reduced Ejection Fraction: Insights from PARADIGM-HF and ATMOSPHERE. *Eur. J. Heart Fail.* **2020**, *22*, 2370–2379. [CrossRef] [PubMed]
4. Kirk, J.A.; Kass, D.A. Cellular and Molecular Aspects of Dyssynchrony and Resynchronization. *Card. Electrophysiol. Clin.* **2015**, *7*, 585–597. [CrossRef] [PubMed]
5. Eriksson, P.; Hansson, P.-O.; Eriksson, H.; Dellborg, M. Bundle-Branch Block in a General Male Population: The Study of Men Born 1913. *Circulation* **1998**, *98*, 2494–2500. [CrossRef] [PubMed]
6. Baldasseroni, S.; Opasich, C.; Gorini, M.; Lucci, D.; Marchionni, N.; Marini, M.; Campana, C.; Perini, G.; Deorsola, A.; Masotti, G.; et al. Left Bundle-Branch Block Is Associated with Increased 1-Year Sudden and Total Mortality Rate in 5517 Outpatients with Congestive Heart Failure: A Report from the Italian Network on Congestive Heart Failure. *Am. Heart J.* **2002**, *143*, 398–405. [CrossRef] [PubMed]
7. Yu, C.-M.; Chau, E.; Sanderson, J.E.; Fan, K.; Tang, M.-O.; Fung, W.-H.; Lin, H.; Kong, S.-L.; Lam, Y.-M.; Hill, M.R.S.; et al. Tissue Doppler Echocardiographic Evidence of Reverse Remodeling and Improved Synchronicity by Simultaneously Delaying Regional Contraction After Biventricular Pacing Therapy in Heart Failure. *Circulation* **2002**, *105*, 438–445. [CrossRef] [PubMed]
8. Anderson, L.J.; Miyazaki, C.; Sutherland, G.R.; Oh, J.K. Patient Selection and Echocardiographic Assessment of Dyssynchrony in Cardiac Resynchronization Therapy. *Circulation* **2008**, *117*, 2009–2023. [CrossRef] [PubMed]
9. Yu, C.-M.; Bleeker, G.B.; Fung, J.W.-H.; Schalij, M.J.; Zhang, Q.; Van Der Wall, E.E.; Chan, Y.-S.; Kong, S.-L.; Bax, J.J. Left Ventricular Reverse Remodeling but Not Clinical Improvement Predicts Long-Term Survival After Cardiac Resynchronization Therapy. *Circulation* **2005**, *112*, 1580–1586. [CrossRef] [PubMed]
10. Van Der Bijl, P.; Khidir, M.; Ajmone Marsan, N.; Delgado, V.; Leon, M.B.; Stone, G.W.; Bax, J.J. Effect of Functional Mitral Regurgitation on Outcome in Patients Receiving Cardiac Resynchronization Therapy for Heart Failure. *Am. J. Cardiol.* **2019**, *123*, 75–83. [CrossRef] [PubMed]
11. Rossi, A.; Dini, F.L.; Faggiano, P.; Agricola, E.; Cicoira, M.; Frattini, S.; Simioniuc, A.; Gullace, M.; Ghio, S.; Enriquez-Sarano, M.; et al. Independent Prognostic Value of Functional Mitral Regurgitation in Patients with Heart Failure. A Quantitative Analysis of 1256 Patients with Ischaemic and Non-Ischaemic Dilated Cardiomyopathy. *Heart* **2011**, *97*, 1675–1680. [CrossRef] [PubMed]
12. Glikson, M.; Nielsen, J.C.; Kronborg, M.B.; Michowitz, Y.; Auricchio, A.; Barbash, I.M.; Barrabés, J.A.; Boriani, G.; Braunschweig, F.; Brignole, M.; et al. 2021 ESC Guidelines on Cardiac Pacing and Cardiac Resynchronization Therapy. *Eur. Heart J.* **2021**, *42*, 3427–3520. [CrossRef] [PubMed]
13. Moss, A.J.; Hall, W.J.; Cannom, D.S.; Klein, H.; Brown, M.W.; Daubert, J.P.; Estes, N.A.M.; Foster, E.; Greenberg, H.; Higgins, S.L.; et al. Cardiac-Resynchronization Therapy for the Prevention of Heart-Failure Events. *N. Engl. J. Med.* **2009**, *361*, 1329–1338. [CrossRef] [PubMed]
14. Tang, A.S.L.; Wells, G.A.; Talajic, M.; Arnold, M.O.; Sheldon, R.; Connolly, S.; Hohnloser, S.H.; Nichol, G.; Birnie, D.H.; Sapp, J.L.; et al. Cardiac-Resynchronization Therapy for Mild-to-Moderate Heart Failure. *N. Engl. J. Med.* **2010**, *363*, 2385–2395. [CrossRef] [PubMed]
15. Ponikowski, P.; Voors, A.A.; Anker, S.D.; Bueno, H.; Cleland, J.G.F.; Coats, A.J.S.; Falk, V.; González-Juanatey, J.R.; Harjola, V.-P.; Jankowska, E.A.; et al. 2016 ESC Guidelines for the Diagnosis and Treatment of Acute and Chronic Heart Failure: The Task Force for the Diagnosis and Treatment of Acute and Chronic Heart Failure of the European Society of Cardiology (ESC)Developed with the Special Contribution of the Heart Failure Association (HFA) of the ESC. *Eur. Heart J.* **2016**, *37*, 2129–2200. [CrossRef] [PubMed]
16. Spartera, M.; Galderisi, M.; Mele, D.; Cameli, M.; D'Andrea, A.; Rossi, A.; Mondillo, S.; Novo, G.; Esposito, R.; D'Ascenzi, F.; et al. Role of Cardiac Dyssynchrony and Resynchronization Therapy in Functional Mitral Regurgitation. *Eur. Heart J.-Cardiovasc. Imaging* **2016**, *17*, 471–480. [CrossRef] [PubMed]
17. Galli, E.; Galand, V.; Le Rolle, V.; Taconne, M.; Wazzan, A.A.; Hernandez, A.; Leclercq, C.; Donal, E. The Saga of Dyssynchrony Imaging: Are We Getting to the Point. *Front. Cardiovasc. Med.* **2023**, *10*, 1111538. [CrossRef]
18. Bax, J.J.; Bleeker, G.B.; Marwick, T.H.; Molhoek, S.G.; Boersma, E.; Steendijk, P.; Van Der Wall, E.E.; Schalij, M.J. Left Ventricular Dyssynchrony Predicts Response and Prognosis after Cardiac Resynchronization Therapy. *J. Am. Coll. Cardiol.* **2004**, *44*, 1834–1840. [CrossRef] [PubMed]
19. Notabartolo, D.; Merlino, J.D.; Smith, A.L.; DeLurgio, D.B.; Vera, F.V.; Easley, K.A.; Martin, R.P.; León, A.R. Usefulness of the Peak Velocity Difference by Tissue Doppler Imaging Technique as an Effective Predictor of Response to Cardiac Resynchronization Therapy. *Am. J. Cardiol.* **2004**, *94*, 817–820. [CrossRef]
20. Calle, S.; Delens, C.; Kamoen, V.; De Pooter, J.; Timmermans, F. Septal Flash: At the Heart of Cardiac Dyssynchrony. *Trends Cardiovasc. Med.* **2020**, *30*, 115–122. [CrossRef] [PubMed]

21. Yu, C.-M.; Fung, W.-H.; Lin, H.; Zhang, Q.; Sanderson, J.E.; Lau, C.-P. Predictors of Left Ventricular Reverse Remodeling after Cardiac Resynchronization Therapy for Heart Failure Secondary to Idiopathic Dilated or Ischemic Cardiomyopathy. *Am. J. Cardiol.* **2003**, *91*, 684–688. [CrossRef] [PubMed]
22. Parsai, C.; Bijnens, B.; Sutherland, G.R.; Baltabaeva, A.; Claus, P.; Marciniak, M.; Paul, V.; Scheffer, M.; Donal, E.; Derumeaux, G.; et al. Toward Understanding Response to Cardiac Resynchronization Therapy: Left Ventricular Dyssynchrony Is Only One of Multiple Mechanisms. *Eur. Heart J.* **2009**, *30*, 940–949. [CrossRef]
23. Parsai, C.; Baltabaeva, A.; Anderson, L.; Chaparro, M.; Bijnens, B.; Sutherland, G.R. Low-Dose Dobutamine Stress Echo to Quantify the Degree of Remodelling after Cardiac Resynchronization Therapy. *Eur. Heart J.* **2008**, *30*, 950–958. [CrossRef] [PubMed]
24. Duchateau, N.; De Craene, M.; Silva, E.; Sitges, M.; Bijnens, B.H.; Frangi, A.F. Septal Flash Assessment on CRT Candidates Based on Statistical Atlases of Motion. In *Medical Image Computing and Computer-Assisted Intervention—MICCAI 2009*; Yang, G.-Z., Hawkes, D., Rueckert, D., Noble, A., Taylor, C., Eds.; Lecture Notes in Computer Science; Springer: Berlin/Heidelberg, Germany, 2009; Volume 5762, pp. 759–766, ISBN 978-3-642-04270-6.
25. Voigt, J.-U.; Schneider, T.-M.; Korder, S.; Szulik, M.; Gurel, E.; Daniel, W.G.; Rademakers, F.; Flachskampf, F.A. Apical Transverse Motion as Surrogate Parameter to Determine Regional Left Ventricular Function Inhomogeneities: A New, Integrative Approach to Left Ventricular Asynchrony Assessment. *Eur. Heart J.* **2008**, *30*, 959–968. [CrossRef] [PubMed]
26. Szulik, M.; Tillekaerts, M.; Vangeel, V.; Ganame, J.; Willems, R.; Lenarczyk, R.; Rademakers, F.; Kalarus, Z.; Kukulski, T.; Voigt, J.-U. Assessment of Apical Rocking: A New, Integrative Approach for Selection of Candidates for Cardiac Resynchronization Therapy. *Eur. J. Echocardiogr.* **2010**, *11*, 863–869. [CrossRef] [PubMed]
27. Stankovic, I.; Aarones, M.; Smith, H.-J.; Voros, G.; Kongsgaard, E.; Neskovic, A.N.; Willems, R.; Aakhus, S.; Voigt, J.-U. Dynamic Relationship of Left-Ventricular Dyssynchrony and Contractile Reserve in Patients Undergoing Cardiac Resynchronization Therapy. *Eur. Heart J.* **2014**, *35*, 48–55. [CrossRef] [PubMed]
28. Stankovic, I.; Prinz, C.; Ciarka, A.; Daraban, A.M.; Kotrc, M.; Aarones, M.; Szulik, M.; Winter, S.; Belmans, A.; Neskovic, A.N.; et al. Relationship of Visually Assessed Apical Rocking and Septal Flash to Response and Long-Term Survival Following Cardiac Resynchronization Therapy (PREDICT-CRT). *Eur. Heart J.-Cardiovasc. Imaging* **2016**, *17*, 262–269. [CrossRef] [PubMed]
29. Gabrielli, L.; Marincheva, G.; Bijnens, B.; Doltra, A.; Tolosana, J.M.; Borras, R.; Castel, M.A.; Berruezo, A.; Brugada, J.; Mont, L.; et al. Septal Flash Predicts Cardiac Resynchronization Therapy Response in Patients with Permanent Atrial Fibrillation. *Europace* **2014**, *16*, 1342–1349. [CrossRef] [PubMed]
30. Walmsley, J.; Huntjens, P.R.; Prinzen, F.W.; Delhaas, T.; Lumens, J. Septal Flash and Septal Rebound Stretch Have Different Underlying Mechanisms. *Am. J. Physiol.-Heart Circ. Physiol.* **2016**, *310*, H394–H403. [CrossRef] [PubMed]
31. De Boeck, B.W.L.; Teske, A.J.; Meine, M.; Leenders, G.E.; Cramer, M.J.; Prinzen, F.W.; Doevendans, P.A. Septal Rebound Stretch Reflects the Functional Substrate to Cardiac Resynchronization Therapy and Predicts Volumetric and Neurohormonal Response. *Eur. J. Heart Fail.* **2009**, *11*, 863–871. [CrossRef] [PubMed]
32. Corteville, B.; De Pooter, J.; De Backer, T.; El Haddad, M.; Stroobandt, R.; Timmermans, F. The Electrocardiographic Characteristics of Septal Flash in Patients with Left Bundle Branch Block. *Europace* **2016**, *19*, euv461. [CrossRef] [PubMed]
33. Dillon, J.C.; Chang, S.; Feigenbaum, H. Echocardiographic Manifestations of Left Bundle Branch Block. *Circulation* **1974**, *49*, 876–880. [CrossRef] [PubMed]
34. Vernooy, K.; Verbeek, X.A.A.M.; Peschar, M.; Crijns, H.J.G.M.; Arts, T.; Cornelussen, R.N.M.; Prinzen, F.W. Left Bundle Branch Block Induces Ventricular Remodeling and Functional Septal Hypoperfusion. *Eur. Heart J.* **2005**, *26*, 91–98. [CrossRef] [PubMed]
35. Strauss, D.G.; Selvester, R.H.; Wagner, G.S. Defining Left Bundle Branch Block in the Era of Cardiac Resynchronization Therapy. *Am. J. Cardiol.* **2011**, *107*, 927–934. [CrossRef] [PubMed]
36. Leenders, G.E.; Lumens, J.; Cramer, M.J.; De Boeck, B.W.L.; Doevendans, P.A.; Delhaas, T.; Prinzen, F.W. Septal Deformation Patterns Delineate Mechanical Dyssynchrony and Regional Differences in Contractility: Analysis of Patient Data Using a Computer Model. *Circ. Heart Fail.* **2012**, *5*, 87–96. [CrossRef] [PubMed]
37. Lumens, J.; Tayal, B.; Walmsley, J.; Delgado-Montero, A.; Huntjens, P.R.; Schwartzman, D.; Althouse, A.D.; Delhaas, T.; Prinzen, F.W.; Gorcsan, J. Differentiating Electromechanical From Non–Electrical Substrates of Mechanical Discoordination to Identify Responders to Cardiac Resynchronization Therapy. *Circ. Cardiovasc. Imaging* **2015**, *8*, e003744. [CrossRef] [PubMed]
38. Duckett, S.G.; Camara, O.; Ginks, M.R.; Bostock, J.; Chinchapatnam, P.; Sermesant, M.; Pashaei, A.; Lambiase, P.D.; Gill, J.S.; Carr-White, G.S.; et al. Relationship between Endocardial Activation Sequences Defined by High-Density Mapping to Early Septal Contraction (Septal Flash) in Patients with Left Bundle Branch Block Undergoing Cardiac Resynchronization Therapy. *Europace* **2012**, *14*, 99–106. [CrossRef] [PubMed]
39. Russell, K.; Eriksen, M.; Aaberge, L.; Wilhelmsen, N.; Skulstad, H.; Gjesdal, O.; Edvardsen, T.; Smiseth, O.A. Assessment of Wasted Myocardial Work: A Novel Method to Quantify Energy Loss Due to Uncoordinated Left Ventricular Contractions. *Am. J. Physiol.-Heart Circ. Physiol.* **2013**, *305*, H996–H1003. [CrossRef]
40. Vaillant, C.; Martins, R.P.; Donal, E.; Leclercq, C.; Thébault, C.; Behar, N.; Mabo, P.; Daubert, J.-C. Resolution of Left Bundle Branch Block–Induced Cardiomyopathy by Cardiac Resynchronization Therapy. *J. Am. Coll. Cardiol.* **2013**, *61*, 1089–1095. [CrossRef] [PubMed]
41. Delhaas, T.; Arts, T.; Prinzen, F.W.; Reneman, R.S. Regional Fibre Stress-fibre Strain Area as an Estimate of Regional Blood Flow and Oxygen Demand in the Canine Heart. *J. Physiol.* **1994**, *477*, 481–496. [CrossRef] [PubMed]

42. Prinzen, F.W.; Cheriex, E.C.; Delhaas, T.; Van Oosterhout, M.F.M.; Arts, T.; Wellens, H.J.J.; Reneman, R.S. Asymmetric Thickness of the Left Ventricular Wall Resulting from Asynchronous Electric Activation: A Study in Dogs with Ventricular Pacing and in Patients with Left Bundle Branch Block. *Am. Heart J.* **1995**, *130*, 1045–1053. [CrossRef] [PubMed]
43. Cvijic, M.; Duchenne, J.; Ünlü, S.; Michalski, B.; Aarones, M.; Winter, S.; Aakhus, S.; Fehske, W.; Stankovic, I.; Voigt, J.-U. Timing of Myocardial Shortening Determines Left Ventricular Regional Myocardial Work and Regional Remodelling in Hearts with Conduction Delays. *Eur. Heart J. Cardiovasc. Imaging* **2018**, *19*, 941–949. [CrossRef] [PubMed]
44. Jansen, A.H.M.; Van Dantzig, J.M.; Bracke, F.; Meijer, A.; Peels, K.H.; Van Den Brink, R.B.A.; Cheriex, E.C.; Delemarre, B.J.M.; Van Der Wouw, P.A.; Korsten, H.H.M.; et al. Qualitative Observation of Left Ventricular Multiphasic Septal Motion and Septal-to-Lateral Apical Shuffle Predicts Left Ventricular Reverse Remodeling after Cardiac Resynchronization Therapy. *Am. J. Cardiol.* **2007**, *99*, 966–969. [CrossRef]
45. Vernooy, K.; Verbeek, X.A.A.M.; Peschar, M.; Prinzen, F.W. Relation Between Abnormal Ventricular Impulse Conduction and Heart Failure. *J. Intervent. Cardiol.* **2003**, *16*, 557–562. [CrossRef] [PubMed]
46. Van Oosterhout, M.F.M.; Arts, T.; Bassingthwaighte, J.B.; Reneman, R.S.; Prinzen, F.W. Relation between Local Myocardial Growth and Blood Flow during Chronic Ventricular Pacing. *Cardiovasc. Res.* **2002**, *53*, 831–840. [CrossRef] [PubMed]
47. Ghani, A.; Delnoy, P.P.H.; Ottervanger, J.P.; Misier, A.R.R.; Smit, J.J.J.; Adiyaman, A.; Elvan, A. Apical Rocking Is Predictive of Response to Cardiac Resynchronization Therapy. *Int. J. Cardiovasc. Imaging* **2015**, *31*, 717–725. [CrossRef] [PubMed]
48. Ghani, A.; Delnoy, P.P.H.M.; Smit, J.J.J.; Ottervanger, J.P.; Ramdat Misier, A.R.; Adiyaman, A.; Elvan, A. Association of Apical Rocking with Super-Response to Cardiac Resynchronisation Therapy. *Neth. Heart J.* **2016**, *24*, 39–46. [CrossRef] [PubMed]
49. Voigt, J.-U. Rocking Will Tell It. *Eur. Heart J.* **2008**, *30*, 885–886. [CrossRef] [PubMed]
50. Popovic, Z.B.; Grimm, R.A.; Ahmad, A.; Agler, D.; Favia, M.; Dan, G.; Lim, P.; Casas, F.; Greenberg, N.L.; Thomas, J.D. Longitudinal Rotation: An Unrecognised Motion Pattern in Patients with Dilated Cardiomyopathy. *Heart* **2008**, *94*, e11. [CrossRef]
51. Remme, E.W.; Niederer, S.; Gjesdal, O.; Russell, K.; Hyde, E.R.; Smith, N.; Smiseth, O.A. Factors Determining the Magnitude of the Pre-Ejection Leftward Septal Motion in Left Bundle Branch Block. *Europace* **2015**, *18*, euv381. [CrossRef] [PubMed]
52. Kvitting, J.-P.E.; Wigström, L.; Strotmann, J.M.; Sutherland, G.R. How Accurate Is Visual Assessment of Synchronicity in Myocardial Motion? An In Vitro Study with Computer-Simulated Regional Delay in Myocardial Motion: Clinical Implications for Rest and Stress Echocardiography Studies. *J. Am. Soc. Echocardiogr.* **1999**, *12*, 698–705. [CrossRef] [PubMed]
53. Gjesdal, O.; Remme, E.W.; Opdahl, A.; Skulstad, H.; Russell, K.; Kongsgaard, E.; Edvardsen, T.; Smiseth, O.A. Mechanisms of Abnormal Systolic Motion of the Interventricular Septum During Left Bundle-Branch Block. *Circ. Cardiovasc. Imaging* **2011**, *4*, 264–273. [CrossRef] [PubMed]
54. Wang, C.-L.; Wu, C.-T.; Yeh, Y.-H.; Wu, L.-S.; Chan, Y.-H.; Kuo, C.-T.; Chu, P.-H.; Hsu, L.-A.; Ho, W.-J. Left Bundle-Branch Block Contraction Patterns Identified from Radial-Strain Analysis Predicts Outcomes Following Cardiac Resynchronization Therapy. *Int. J. Cardiovasc. Imaging* **2017**, *33*, 869–877. [CrossRef]
55. Pitzalis, M.V.; Iacoviello, M.; Romito, R.; Massari, F.; Rizzon, B.; Luzzi, G.; Guida, P.; Andriani, A.; Mastropasqua, F.; Rizzon, P. Cardiac Resynchronization Therapy Tailored by Echocardiographic Evaluation of Ventricular Asynchrony. *J. Am. Coll. Cardiol.* **2002**, *40*, 1615–1622. [CrossRef] [PubMed]
56. Marcus, G.M.; Rose, E.; Viloria, E.M.; Schafer, J.; De Marco, T.; Saxon, L.A.; Foster, E. Septal to Posterior Wall Motion Delay Fails to Predict Reverse Remodeling or Clinical Improvement in Patients Undergoing Cardiac Resynchronization Therapy. *J. Am. Coll. Cardiol.* **2005**, *46*, 2208–2214. [CrossRef] [PubMed]
57. Gorcsan, J.; Kanzaki, H.; Bazaz, R.; Dohi, K.; Schwartzman, D. Usefulness of Echocardiographic Tissue Synchronization Imaging to Predict Acute Response to Cardiac Resynchronization Therapy. *Am. J. Cardiol.* **2004**, *93*, 1178–1181. [CrossRef] [PubMed]
58. Van Oosterhout, M.F.M.; Prinzen, F.W.; Arts, T.; Schreuder, J.J.; Vanagt, W.Y.R.; Cleutjens, J.P.M.; Reneman, R.S. Asynchronous Electrical Activation Induces Asymmetrical Hypertrophy of the Left Ventricular Wall. *Circulation* **1998**, *98*, 588–595. [CrossRef] [PubMed]
59. Smiseth, O.A.; Russell, K.; Skulstad, H. The Role of Echocardiography in Quantification of Left Ventricular Dyssynchrony: State of the Art and Future Directions. *Eur. Heart J. Cardiovasc. Imaging* **2012**, *13*, 61–68. [CrossRef] [PubMed]
60. Leenders, G.E.; De Boeck, B.W.L.; Teske, A.J.; Meine, M.; Bogaard, M.D.; Prinzen, F.W.; Doevendans, P.A.; Cramer, M.J. Septal Rebound Stretch Is a Strong Predictor of Outcome After Cardiac Resynchronization Therapy. *J. Card. Fail.* **2012**, *18*, 404–412. [CrossRef] [PubMed]
61. Gorcsan, J.; Anderson, C.P.; Tayal, B.; Sugahara, M.; Walmsley, J.; Starling, R.C.; Lumens, J. Systolic Stretch Characterizes the Electromechanical Substrate Responsive to Cardiac Resynchronization Therapy. *JACC Cardiovasc. Imaging* **2019**, *12*, 1741–1752. [CrossRef] [PubMed]
62. Maréchaux, S.; Guiot, A.; Castel, A.L.; Guyomar, Y.; Semichon, M.; Delelis, F.; Heuls, S.; Ennezat, P.-V.; Graux, P.; Tribouilloy, C. Relationship between Two-Dimensional Speckle-Tracking Septal Strain and Response to Cardiac Resynchronization Therapy in Patients with Left Ventricular Dysfunction and Left Bundle Branch Block: A Prospective Pilot Study. *J. Am. Soc. Echocardiogr.* **2014**, *27*, 501–511. [CrossRef] [PubMed]
63. Mada, R.O.; Lysyansky, P.; Duchenne, J.; Beyer, R.; Mada, C.; Muresan, L.; Rosianu, H.; Serban, A.; Winter, S.; Fehske, W.; et al. New Automatic Tools to Identify Responders to Cardiac Resynchronization Therapy. *J. Am. Soc. Echocardiogr.* **2016**, *29*, 966–972. [CrossRef]

64. Doltra, A.; Bijnens, B.; Tolosana, J.M.; Borràs, R.; Khatib, M.; Penela, D.; De Caralt, T.M.; Castel, M.Á.; Berruezo, A.; Brugada, J.; et al. Mechanical Abnormalities Detected With Conventional Echocardiography Are Associated With Response and Midterm Survival in CRT. *JACC Cardiovasc. Imaging* **2014**, *7*, 969–979. [CrossRef]
65. Gąsior, Z.; Płońska-Gościniak, E.; Kułach, A.; Wita, K.; Mizia-Stec, K.; Szwed, H.; Kasprzak, J.; Tomaszewski, A.; Sinkiewicz, W.; Wojciechowska, C. Impact of Septal Flash and Left Ventricle Contractile Reserve on Positive Remodeling during 1 Year Cardiac Resynchronization Therapy: The Multicenter ViaCRT Study. *Arch. Med. Sci.* **2016**, *2*, 349–352. [CrossRef]
66. Stankovic, I.; Prinz, C.; Ciarka, A.; Daraban, A.M.; Mo, Y.; Aarones, M.; Szulik, M.; Winter, S.; Neskovic, A.N.; Kukulski, T.; et al. Long-Term Outcome After CRT in the Presence of Mechanical Dyssynchrony Seen with Chronic RV Pacing or Intrinsic LBBB. *JACC Cardiovasc. Imaging* **2017**, *10*, 1091–1099. [CrossRef] [PubMed]
67. Chung, E.S.; Leon, A.R.; Tavazzi, L.; Sun, J.-P.; Nihoyannopoulos, P.; Merlino, J.; Abraham, W.T.; Ghio, S.; Leclercq, C.; Bax, J.J.; et al. Results of the Predictors of Response to CRT (PROSPECT) Trial. *Circulation* **2008**, *117*, 2608–2616. [CrossRef] [PubMed]
68. Hussein, A.A.; Wilkoff, B.L. Cardiac Implantable Electronic Device Therapy in Heart Failure. *Circ. Res.* **2019**, *124*, 1584–1597. [CrossRef] [PubMed]
69. Mullens, W.; Auricchio, A.; Martens, P.; Witte, K.; Cowie, M.R.; Delgado, V.; Dickstein, K.; Linde, C.; Vernooy, K.; Leyva, F.; et al. Optimized Implementation of Cardiac Resynchronization Therapy: A Call for Action for Referral and Optimization of Care: A Joint Position Statement from the heart failure association (hfa), european heart rhythm association (ehra), and european association of cardiovascular imaging (EACVI) of the european society of cardiology. *Eur. J. Heart Fail.* **2020**, *22*, 2349–2369. [CrossRef] [PubMed]
70. Rickard, J.; Kumbhani, D.J.; Popovic, Z.; Verhaert, D.; Manne, M.; Sraow, D.; Baranowski, B.; Martin, D.O.; Lindsay, B.D.; Grimm, R.A.; et al. Characterization of Super-Response to Cardiac Resynchronization Therapy. *Heart Rhythm* **2010**, *7*, 885–889. [CrossRef] [PubMed]
71. Reant, P.; Zaroui, A.; Donal, E.; Mignot, A.; Bordachar, P.; Deplagne, A.; Solnon, A.; Ritter, P.; Daubert, J.-C.; Clementy, J.; et al. Identification and Characterization of Super-Responders After Cardiac Resynchronization Therapy. *Am. J. Cardiol.* **2010**, *105*, 1327–1335. [CrossRef] [PubMed]
72. Hsu, J.C.; Solomon, S.D.; Bourgoun, M.; McNitt, S.; Goldenberg, I.; Klein, H.; Moss, A.J.; Foster, E. Predictors of Super-Response to Cardiac Resynchronization Therapy and Associated Improvement in Clinical Outcome. *J. Am. Coll. Cardiol.* **2012**, *59*, 2366–2373. [CrossRef] [PubMed]
73. Tayal, B.; Sogaard, P.; Delgado-Montero, A.; Goda, A.; Saba, S.; Risum, N.; Gorcsan, J. Interaction of Left Ventricular Remodeling and Regional Dyssynchrony on Long-Term Prognosis after Cardiac Resynchronization Therapy. *J. Am. Soc. Echocardiogr.* **2017**, *30*, 244–250. [CrossRef] [PubMed]
74. Ruschitzka, F.; Abraham, W.T.; Singh, J.P.; Bax, J.J.; Borer, J.S.; Brugada, J.; Dickstein, K.; Ford, I.; Gorcsan, J.; Gras, D.; et al. Cardiac-Resynchronization Therapy in Heart Failure with a Narrow QRS Complex. *N. Engl. J. Med.* **2013**, *369*, 1395–1405. [CrossRef]
75. Ichibori, H.; Fukuzawa, K.; Kiuchi, K.; Matsumoto, A.; Konishi, H.; Imada, H.; Hyogo, K.; Kurose, J.; Tatsumi, K.; Tanaka, H.; et al. Predictors and Clinical Outcomes of Transient Responders to Cardiac Resynchronization Therapy. *Pacing Clin. Electrophysiol.* **2017**, *40*, 301–309. [CrossRef] [PubMed]
76. Vătășescu, R.G.; Târtea, G.C.; Iorgulescu, C.; Cojocaru, C.; Deaconu, A.; Badiul, A.; Goanță, E.-V.; Bogdan, Ș; Cozma, D. Predictors for Super-Responders in Cardiac Resynchronization Therapy. *Am. J. Ther.* **2024**, *31*, e13–e23. [CrossRef] [PubMed]
77. Goanță, E.-V.; Luca, C.-T.; Vacarescu, C.; Crișan, S.; Petrescu, L.; Vatasescu, R.; Lazăr, M.-A.; Gurgu, A.; Turi, V.-R.; Cozma, D. Nonischemic Super-Responders in Fusion CRT Pacing with Normal Atrioventricular Conduction. *Diagnostics* **2022**, *12*, 2032. [CrossRef] [PubMed]
78. Thibault, B.; Harel, F.; Ducharme, A.; White, M.; Frasure-Smith, N.; Roy, D.; Philippon, F.; Dorian, P.; Talajic, M.; Dubuc, M.; et al. Evaluation of Resynchronization Therapy for Heart Failure in Patients With a QRS Duration Greater Than 120 Ms (GREATER-EARTH) Trial: Rationale, Design, and Baseline Characteristics. *Can. J. Cardiol.* **2011**, *27*, 779–786. [CrossRef] [PubMed]
79. Vacarescu, C.; Luca, C.-T.; Feier, H.; Gaiță, D.; Crișan, S.; Negru, A.-G.; Iurciuc, S.; Goanță, E.-V.; Mornos, C.; Lazăr, M.-A.; et al. Betablockers and Ivabradine Titration According to Exercise Test in LV Only Fusion CRT Pacing. *Diagnostics* **2022**, *12*, 1096. [CrossRef] [PubMed]
80. Brown, C.D.; Burns, K.V.; Harbin, M.M.; Espinosa, E.A.; Olson, M.D.; Bank, A.J. Cardiac Resynchronization Therapy Optimization in Nonresponders and Incomplete Responders Using Electrical Dyssynchrony Mapping. *Heart Rhythm* **2022**, *19*, 1965–1973. [CrossRef] [PubMed]

Disclaimer/Publisher's Note: The statements, opinions and data contained in all publications are solely those of the individual author(s) and contributor(s) and not of MDPI and/or the editor(s). MDPI and/or the editor(s) disclaim responsibility for any injury to people or property resulting from any ideas, methods, instructions or products referred to in the content.

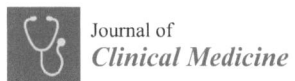

Review

Mitral Annular Plane Systolic Excursion (MAPSE): A Review of a Simple and Forgotten Parameter for Assessing Left Ventricle Function

Liviu Cirin [1,2], Simina Crișan [1,2,3,*], Constantin-Tudor Luca [1,2,3], Roxana Buzaș [4,5], Daniel Florin Lighezan [4,5], Cristina Văcărescu [1,2,3], Andreea Cozgarea [1,2,6], Cristina Tudoran [7,8,9] and Dragoș Cozma [1,2,3]

[1] Cardiology Department, "Victor Babes" University of Medicine and Pharmacy, 2 Eftimie Murgu Sq., 300041 Timisoara, Romania; cirin.liviu@umft.ro (L.C.); constantin.luca@umft.ro (C.-T.L.); cristina.vacarescu@umft.ro (C.V.); andreea.cozgarea@umft.ro (A.C.); dragos.cozma@umft.ro (D.C.)
[2] Research Center of the Institute of Cardiovascular Diseases Timisoara, 13A Gheorghe Adam Street, 300310 Timisoara, Romania
[3] Institute of Cardiovascular Diseases Timisoara, 13A Gheorghe Adam Street, 300310 Timisoara, Romania
[4] Department of Internal Medicine I, "Victor Babes" University of Medicine and Pharmacy, Eftimie Murgu Square, No. 2, 300041 Timisoara, Romania; buzas.dana@umft.ro (R.B.); dlighezan@umft.ro (D.F.L.)
[5] Center for Advanced Research in Cardiovascular Pathology and Hemostaseology, "Victor Babes" University of Medicine and Pharmacy, 300041 Timisoara, Romania
[6] County Clinical Emergency Hospital Sibiu, 550245 Sibiu, Romania
[7] Department VII, Internal Medicine II, Discipline of Cardiology, University of Medicine and Pharmacy "Victor Babes" Timisoara, E. Murgu Square, Nr. 2, 300041 Timisoara, Romania; tudoran.cristina@umft.ro
[8] County Emergency Hospital "Pius Brinzeu", L. Rebreanu, Nr. 156, 300723 Timisoara, Romania
[9] Center of Molecular Research in Nephrology and Vascular Disease, Faculty of the University of Medicine and Pharmacy "Victor Babes" Timisoara, E. Murgu Square, Nr. 2, 300041 Timisoara, Romania
* Correspondence: simina.crisan@umft.ro

Citation: Cirin, L.; Crișan, S.; Luca, C.-T.; Buzaș, R.; Lighezan, D.F.; Văcărescu, C.; Cozgarea, A.; Tudoran, C.; Cozma, D. Mitral Annular Plane Systolic Excursion (MAPSE): A Review of a Simple and Forgotten Parameter for Assessing Left Ventricle Function. *J. Clin. Med.* **2024**, *13*, 5265. https://doi.org/10.3390/jcm13175265

Academic Editor: Roberto Pedrinelli

Received: 31 July 2024
Revised: 24 August 2024
Accepted: 3 September 2024
Published: 5 September 2024

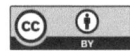

Copyright: © 2024 by the authors. Licensee MDPI, Basel, Switzerland. This article is an open access article distributed under the terms and conditions of the Creative Commons Attribution (CC BY) license (https://creativecommons.org/licenses/by/4.0/).

Abstract: Mitral annular plane systolic excursion (MAPSE) was a widely used and simple M-mode echocardiographic parameter for determining the left ventricle (LV) longitudinal systolic function. The purpose of this review is to analyze the use of MAPSE as a simple LV systolic function marker in different clinical scenarios, especially given the recent paradox of choices in ultrasound markers assessing cardiac performance. Recent data on the use of MAPSE in the assessment of LV function in different settings seem to be relatively scarce, given the wide variety of possible causes of cardiovascular pathology. There remain significant possible clinical applications of MAPSE utilization. This review included all major articles on the topic of mitral annular plane systolic excursion published and indexed in the PubMed, Google Scholar, and Scopus databases. We analyzed the potential implications of using simpler ultrasonographical tools in heart failure diagnosis, prediction, and treatment. MAPSE is a dependable, robust, and easy-to-use parameter compared to ejection fraction (EF) or global longitudinal strain (GLS) for the quick assessment of LV systolic function in various clinical settings. However, there may be a gap of evidence in certain scenarios such as conventional cardiac pacing.

Keywords: MAPSE; LVEF; echocardiography; review

1. Introduction

Mitral annular plane systolic excursion (MAPSE) is an M-mode-derived ultrasound parameter for assessing left ventricle (LV) systolic longitudinal function. It is a simple and reproducible index that correlates well with left ventricular ejection fraction (LVEF) and is a clinically established echocardiographic parameter that can be used in various stages of cardiovascular disease [1]. Even though it has long been superseded by other, more modern and complex parameters and techniques, such as tissue Doppler imaging, strain-rate imaging, or three-dimensional echocardiography, its appeal still consists in its ease of use and ready availability. The LV is conical in shape on the longitudinal section, with a central cavity surrounded by muscular walls, while, in a transverse section, it more resembles a circle. The LV wall is composed of three muscular "layers", which, based on their alignment, are a subepicardial layer, a middle layer, and a subendocardial layer. These three layers also seem to be differently oriented, thus giving birth to oblique muscle fibers in the subepicardium, circumferential in the middle layer, and longitudinal in the subendocardium [2,3]. This specific anatomical arrangement and the mechanical motion imply that, during the cardiac cycle, certain ultrasound parameters can be used for approximating LV function [4]. Several techniques and parameters have been used for the assessment of LV function by two-dimensional cardiac ultrasound. The most widely used, documented, and currently recommended by both the European Association of Cardiovascular Imaging (EACVI) and the American Society of Echocardiography (ASE) for the assessment of LVEF, is the modified Simpson's rule (biplane method of disks). Even though LVEF is a robust and reliable indicator of left ventricle systolic function, it does have its pitfalls. Due to the geometrical assumptions made by using the Simpson method, the accurate measurement of the LVEF requires good endocardial border tracing in end-systole and end-diastole and an adequate-quality image in the apical windows. These tracings eventually divide the LV cavity into a predetermined number of disks (usually 20), and since tracing of the entire LV cavity border is not achievable, some geometric assumptions need to be made.

The monoplane Simpson method requires the tracing of endocardial borders just in the apical four chambers (A4C) view, while the more precise and the preferred one, the biplane method, already requires high-quality images in two distinct views, the A4C and the apical two chamber (A2C) [5] (Figure 1).

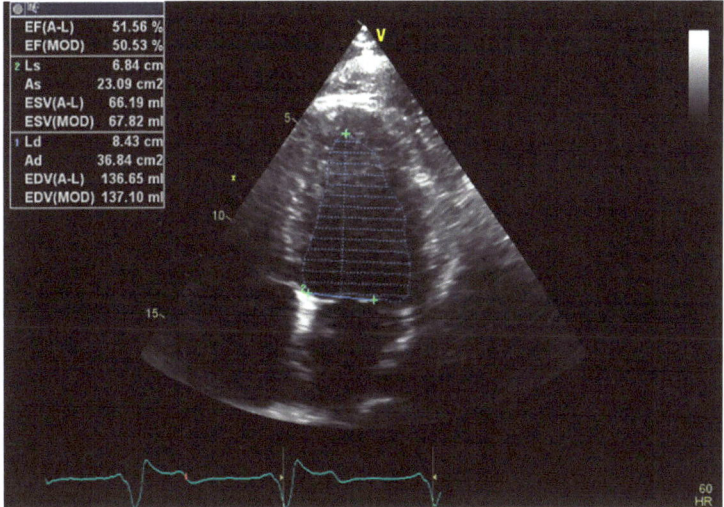

Figure 1. Example of 2D LVEF determination in the A4C view.

More modern ultrasound techniques such as two-dimensional speckle tracking echocardiography (2D-STE) with global longitudinal strain (GLS) measurement and 3D ejection fraction (3D-EF) provide excellent accuracy and, at least in the case of 3D-EF, correlate well with CMR-derived volumes and results. However, all of these techniques share the following common disadvantages: they are time consuming, operator dependent, rely on image quality, and/or require more complex and expensive ultrasound machines. On the other hand, MAPSE measurement does not require good image quality (because it is a linear measurement that is less affected by artefacts) or multiple views and is not a time-consuming technique, thus making its measurement extremely useful in case of emergency settings and poor sonographic windows [6]. There has historically been ample data published on its usefulness in evaluating the longitudinal systolic function of the LV in heart failure (HF); however, recent publications have raised the question of its validity and use as a sensitive marker of early LV dysfunction and as a prognostic tool not only for HF patients, but also in the setting of septic shock, cardio-oncology, and many others [7,8]. There appears to be a lack of validation of its use in the context of conventional, endocardial right ventricular pacing (Figure 2).

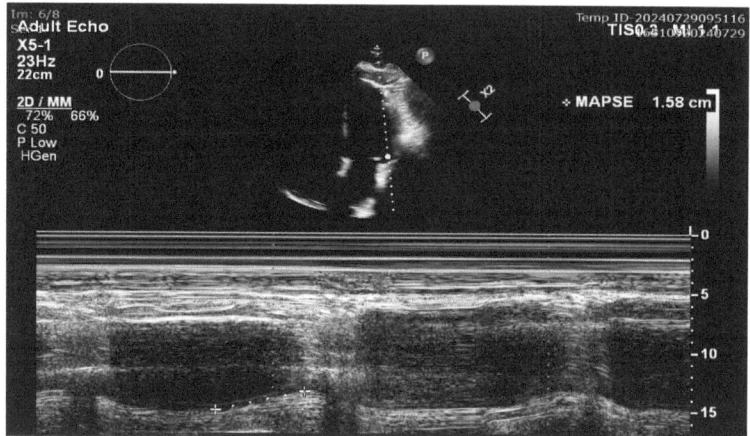

Figure 2. Lateral MAPSE measurement in the apical four chamber view.

The purpose of this article was to review the current, more recently available evidence on the use of MAPSE as a marker of cardiac function in different scenarios, as well as to offer an overview of its applications in day-to-day clinical situations.

2. Materials and Methods

We performed a literature search for different types of published studies (retrospective, prospective, and reviews) using the PubMed, Google Scholar, and Scopus databases with the keywords "MAPSE" OR "MITRAL ANNULAR PLANE SYSTOLIC EXCURSION". The selection of studies for this review followed the PRISMA (Preferred Reporting Items for Systematic Reviews and Meta-Analyses) guidelines. We performed manual searches and used MeSH (Medical Subject Headings) terms on PubMed to identify articles published on MAPSE. We excluded from selection articles not written in English, articles with subjects other than humans, articles with CMR-derived MAPSE, publications with only abstracts available, and duplicate entries. The search was performed in February 2024, with no publishing year restriction, by experienced cardiologists with expertise in echocardiography. We performed a manual initial search for articles using the specific keywords "MAPSE" and "MITRAL ANNULAR PLANE SYSTOLIC EXCURSION" in the title. In addition, using the MeSH term option available in PubMed, we conducted another search with the following terms: (("MAPSE" [Mesh])). All eligible and chosen articles were organized into a Microsoft Excel table (version 2408), which included columns for the article's title, authors, year of publication, journal, and publication type (Figure 3).

The diagram below exemplifies the methodology used by the authors for article selection and was created using Microsoft Office suite. We have found a total of 454 articles published and indexed in the search engines with the keywords of "mitral annular plane systolic excursion" and "MAPSE". Out of the total number of identified records, we discarded duplicates and articles that were not relevant or did not correspond to the inclusion criteria set at the beginning, with the final number being 25 articles (Figure 4).

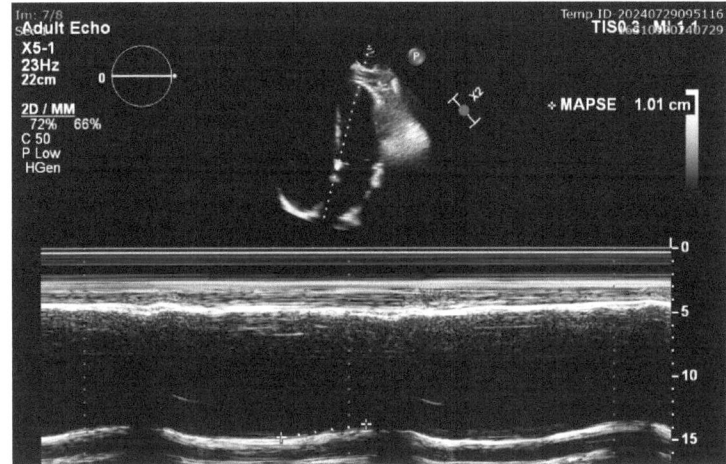

Figure 3. Example of septal MAPSE measurement in A4C view in a patient with impaired LV longitudinal function.

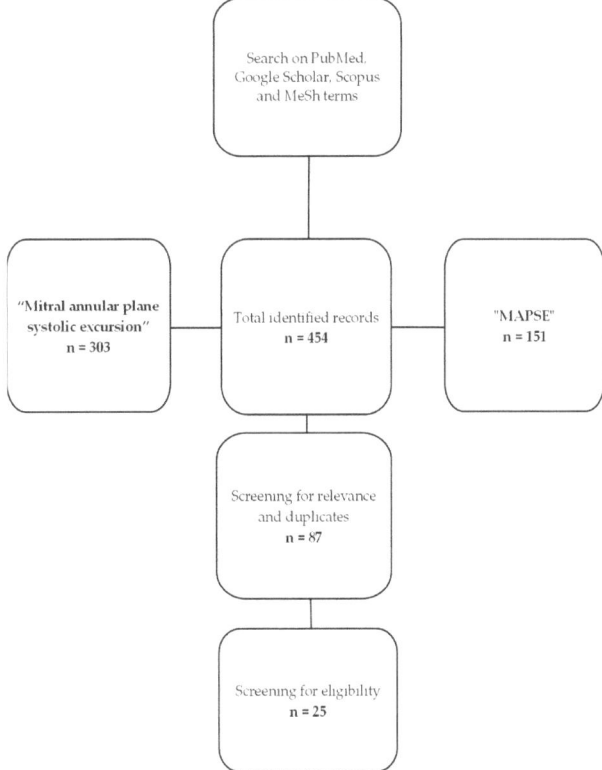

Figure 4. Flow diagram of the review process.

3. Results

We have included in the table below a selected number of relevant articles on the subject published in the last decade, having specified the title, authors, year of publication, number of patients included, and conclusions (Table 1).

Table 1. Articles published in the last decade about MAPSE. Abbreviations: Pts no, patients number; MAPSE, mitral annular plane systolic excursion; LVEF, left ventricular ejection fraction; LVT, left ventricular thrombus; TAPSE, tricuspid annular plane systolic excursion; LUSS, lung ultrasound score; APACHE II, Acute Physiology and Chronic Health Evaluation II; RA, right atrium; LV, left ventricle; MS, multiple sclerosis; ICU, intensive care unit; HFpEF, heart failure with preserved ejection fraction; LVLS, left ventricle longitudinal strain; NTpro-BNP, N-terminal prohormone of brain natriuretic peptide.

Title	Authors	Year	Pts No	Study Type	Conclusion
Cardiac dysfunction in mixed connective tissue disease: a nationwide observational study	Berger S.G. et al. [9]	2023	136	Observational	MAPSE was affected in patients with mixed connective tissue disease.
Males with abdominal aortic aneurysm have reduced left ventricular systolic and diastolic function	Åström Malm I et al. [10]	2021	307	Observational	MAPSE was reduced in subjects with abdominal aortic aneurysm.
Echocardiographic risk factors of left ventricular thrombus in patients with acute anterior myocardial infarction	Chen M et al. [11]	2021	110	Case-control	Septal MAPSE was significantly lower in the LVT group than in the control group.
Mitral Annular Plane Systolic Excursion: An Early Marker of Mortality in Severe COVID-19	Jarori U et al. [12]	2020	68	Multi-center study	MAPSE emerged as the only left heart parameter independently associated with increased mortality.
Hemodynamics in Shock Patients Assessed by Critical Care Ultrasound and Its Relationship to Outcome: A Prospective Study	Zou T et al. [13]	2020	181	Prospective	MAPSE, S′-MV, TAPSE, LUSS, APACHE II, lactate, and PaO_2/FiO_2 were independently related to 28-day mortality, with MAPSE and S′-MV responding best for left heart function.
Left Ventricular Diastolic and Systolic Functions in Patients with Hypothyroidism	Tafarshiku R et al. [14]	2020	81	Observational	In patients with hypothyroidism and a reduced waste/hip ratio, there was significant evidence for compromised LV longitudinal systolic function in the form of long-axis amplitude of motion (MAPSE) and its systolic velocity.
Intraobserver and interobserver reproducibility of M-mode and B-mode acquired mitral annular plane systolic excursion (MAPSE) and its dependency on echocardiographic image quality in children	Hensel K O et al. [6]	2018	284	Observational	Echocardiographic image quality essentially has a negligible effect on MAPSE reproducibility and measurements. MAPSE is a robust echocardiographic parameter with convincing reproducibility for the assessment of LV function in children—even in patients with substandard imaging conditions.
Value of mitral annular plane systolic excursion in the assessment of contractile reserve in patients with ischemic cardiomyopathy before cardiac revascularization	G. Magdy et al. [15]	2018	50	Retrospective	MAPSE is a rapid, simple quantitative echocardiographic method that can assess contractile reserve in patients with ischemic cardiomyopathy before cardiac revascularization.
Evaluation of sepsis induced cardiac dysfunction as a predictor of mortality	Havaldar A.A. [16]	2018	58	Prospective	Sepsis-induced cardiac dysfunction assessed by echocardiography showed that the measurement of MAPSE when combined with APACHE II was a good predictor of mortality. Among the echocardiographic parameters, MAPSE alone was a good predictor of mortality.
Impaired Cardiac Function in Patients with Multiple Sclerosis by Comparison with Normal Subjects	Mincu R.I. et al. [17]	2018	103	Prospective	Patients with MS had decreased LV systolic function compared to the control subjects, as seen by lower 2D left ventricular ejection fraction (LVEF), lower 3D LVEF, MAPSE, lower "online" longitudinal myocardial systolic velocity (S′), lower global longitudinal strain (LS), and lower 3D LS.

Table 1. Cont.

Title	Authors	Year	Pts No	Study Type	Conclusion
Left Ventricular Longitudinal Systolic Function in Septic Shock Patients with Normal Ejection Fraction: A Case-control Study	Zhang H.M. et al. [18]	2017	90	Case-control	In the heart function appraisal of septic shock patients with a normal ejection fraction, more attention should be given to longitudinal function parameters such as MAPSE.
The utilization of critical care ultrasound to assess hemody-namics and lung pathology on ICU admission and the potential for predicting outcome	Yin W et al. [19]	2017	451	Retrospective	The TAPSE, ejection fraction (EF), MAPSE, and lung ultrasound score (LUS score) were significantly related to ICU mortality.
Left ventricular longitudinal systolic dysfunction is associated with right atrial dyssynchrony in heart failure with preserved ejection fraction.	Bytyçi I et al. [20]	2016	85	Observational	In patients with HFpEF and impaired MAPSE, RA dyssynchrony increased, compared to those with normal MAPSE.
Mitral annular plane systolic excursion in the assessment of left ventricular diastolic dysfunction in obese adults	Taşolar H et al. [21]	2015	80	Prospective	MAPSE may be useful in the stratification of left ventricle diastolic dysfunction in obese adults.
M-mode apical systolic excursion: A new and simple method to evaluate global left ventricular longitudinal strain	Amado J et al. [22]	2015	31	Observational	MAPSE and especially MMASE appear to be related to global LVLS.
Effects on heart function of neoadjuvant chemotherapy and chemoradiotherapy in patients with cancer in the esophagus or gastroesophageal junction—a prospective cohort pilot study within a randomized clinical trial	Lund M et al. [23]	2015	40	Prospective multi-center	Septal MAPSE decreased significantly in the chemoradiotherapy group.
Noninvasive Risk Stratification of Patients With Transthyretin Amyloidosis	Kristen A.V. et al. [24]	2014	70	Retrospective	NT-proBNP, troponin T, MAPSE, and the LV hypertrophy index were useful as predictors of outcome. MAPSE was predictive of survival.

3.1. Heart Failure

MAPSE has a strong correlation with LVEF, which has been validated in multiple studies over time, being a valuable tool for HF screening in the mid-range and reduced phenotypes [25]. It also seems that this correlation is maintained over the whole range of HF types, with one meta-analysis discovering that MAPSE is a more sensitive and specific indicator of LV systolic function in patients with heart failure with preserved ejection fraction (HFpEF) compared to LVEF and a good predictor of mortality and risk of long-term survival in patients diagnosed with HF [26]. As far as HFpEF is concerned, an article published in 2011 by Wenzelburger et al. indicates that MAPSE correlates well with other, more complex measurements of ventricular function in this subgroup of patients at rest and during exercise, being a useful tool for HFpEF diagnosis, especially during treadmill exercise testing using a modified Bruce protocol [27]. Another study performed by Elnoamany M.F. et al. showed a significative negative correlation between MAPSE and brain natriuretic peptide (BNP) levels [28]. There also appears to be an increase in right atrial (RA) dyssynchrony (assessed as the so-called PA'-TDI interval) in HFpEF patients with reduced MAPSE values, which suggests that these patients might be at an increased risk of developing arrhythmias [20]. Left atrioventricular plane displacement (AVPD), commonly measured ultrasonographically as the MAPSE index, is related to both systolic and diastolic LV function [29].

3.2. Hypertensive Heart Disease

In hypertensive patients, especially those with concentric LV hypertrophy, there is a deterioration of longitudinal function [30]. The determination of LV longitudinal function by the measurement of left atrioventricular plane displacement using M-mode ultrasound is reliable and reproducible. Longitudinal function impairment has been demonstrated to have prognostic value and is an independent cardiovascular risk marker in these patients, as proven by data in the literature [31,32].

3.3. Ischemic Heart Disease

Several publications have reported on the correlation between MAPSE and LV systolic function in patients with ischemic heart disease. An article published in 2018 by Magdy G et al. on 50 patients with ischemic heart disease and HFrEF reports that MAPSE can be an easy tool for assessing contractile reserve before revascularization, showing a significant positive correlation with LVEF [15]. The literature also cites left atrioventricular plane displacement as a clinically useful tool in patients with stable coronary artery disease and an independent prognostic tool in these patients not influenced by previous myocardial infarction [33].

3.4. Aortic Stenosis

We do know that, in left-sided valvular heart disease, MAPSE is affected by localized wall motion abnormalities around the area of the mitral valve, by severe mitral annular calcification, and by mitral valve prosthesis [34]. In patients diagnosed with aortic valve stenosis, mitral annular plane excursion is known to be reduced, while LVEF or other LV function parameters might be within normal values. However, it does seem to be more markedly reduced in symptomatic patients compared with asymptomatic; moreover, Takeda S et al. also noticed that it may be of use as a predictor of symptom onset in this subset of patients [35].

3.5. Intensive Care Unit

MAPSE is a valuable echocardiographic tool in ICU patients too, being reported in a number of articles to reflect both systolic and diastolic function in critically ill patients, while also correlating well with myocardial injury in patients with systemic inflammatory response syndrome (SIRS) [36]. MAPSE, along with TAPSE, LVEF. and lung ultrasound score (LUS score) seem to be significantly related to ICU mortality, according to a study published by Yin W et al. in 2017 [19]. Another significant advantage regarding its use in the ICU is that MAPSE assessment does not require good image quality or an experienced operator.

3.6. Arrhythmias

Reduced MAPSE, along with LAVI (left atrial volume index), seem to play a role in predicting atrial fibrillation (AF) recurrences after catheter ablation, according to one article, and may be used as a marker in the future, with more research being required on this topic [37].

3.7. Pediatric

MAPSE variations have been described as being due to cardiac size, which implies that its use in the pediatric population should be adjusted for body size. One study concludes that it can be reliably used in children and is most significantly associated with GLS [25,38]. It also seems that MAPSE is highly reproducible in inter-observer scenarios and that image quality has minimum influence on its measurement and thus can be a robust LV evaluation tool in children [6].

3.8. Oncology

A study performed on 40 patients by Lund M et al., published in 2015, set out to evaluate the effect on LV function of chemotherapy in the case of esophagus or gastroesophageal cancer. The results found that, in a neoadjuvant chemoradiotherapy group, there was a significant decrease in LV function determined by a significant decrease in septal MAPSE (mean change -1.4 mm, with a p value of 0.02) among other ultrasound parameters [23].

3.9. COVID-19

Given the recent COVID-19 pandemic and its emerging cardiovascular implications, several authors have set out to investigate possible correlations between SARS-CoV-2 infection and cardiac dysfunction. An article published in 2020 in the Journal of the American Society of Echocardiography by Jarori U et al. suggested that MAPSE in combination with right atrial (RA) size can be used to accurately stratify the risk in patients with severe COVID-19 infection, enabling them to be more appropriately triaged and more aggressively treated early on. MAPSE, according to the same study, seems to be the only left heart parameter that was independently associated with increased mortality in this context [12].

4. Discussion

There are limitations to MAPSE use and interpretation in certain specific cases, such as after cardiac surgery, significant pericardial effusions, mitral valve disease, or localized areas of motion abnormality or fibrosis, situations in which the use of this parameter should be more carefully applied, as its result might not accurately reflect longitudinal function. As far as cardiac pacing is concerned, the data seem scarce, with no such specific situation being investigated; therefore, this is an area in which more research might be carried out as far as validating MAPSE as a tool for LV appreciation in this context. An article published by Kai H et al. in late 2012 postulates that, in patients with paradoxical septal motion (PSM), also referred to as septal bounce, such as that seen in patients with left bundle branch block or conventional RV pacing, septal MAPSE might also reflect RV abnormalities (for which we have a similar M-mode parameter that has been historically used—tricuspid annular plane systolic excursion—TAPSE). They also recommend the use of lateral MAPSE for LV longitudinal function quantification [25,39].

In recent times, with the growth of cardiac magnetic resonance (CMR) imaging, MAPSE measurement in the four-chamber cine view has become a valuable index, comparable to echocardiography. Recently published articles have suggested that CMR-derived MAPSE is a predictor of mortality in hypertensive patients and independently predicts long-term prognosis following an ST-segment elevation myocardial infarction [40,41].

The major advantages of this simple tool are its good correlation with LVEF, its simple and excellent reproducibility between users, and the fact that it is mostly independent of image quality, while its disadvantages are connected to its limitations.

The limitations of MAPSE use are related to the fact that is an M-mode parameter and thus is angle-dependent and unable to detect regional wall abnormalities. There is also a caveat in its use in the case of pericardial effusions (especially large ones that cause mobile apex) and in mitral valve disease and calcifications of the mitral ring, in which MAPSE assessment should not be performed, as its direct measurement is not accurately possible.

Gaps in Evidence and Future Perspectives

There is a lack of evidence on MAPSE usefulness in areas such as cardiac pacing and pacing-induced cardiomyopathy (PICM), where it might prove to be a useful tool for quick LV function assessment, thus justifying further research. Alatic J et al. published an article in 2022 on using MAPSE as a predictor of atrial fibrillation recurrence after pulmonary vein isolation (PVI), with the conclusion being presented in subchapter 3.6. In addition, due to the study limitations, more research is needed, as MAPSE could prove to be a diagnostic criterion in patients referred for catheter ablation of atrial fibrillation [37]. They also postulate that CMR-derived MAPSE might be used as a prognostic marker in patients with atrial fibrillation after PVI. Also, regarding CMR-derived MAPSE, there is increasing evidence of its utilization and usefulness in varying situations. A 2019 article by Romano et al. proved that its CMR-derived equivalent is a strong predictor of mortality in patients with hypertensive heart disease and that it might serve a role in identifying and stratifying the patients at a highest risk [40]. The same seems to be true in the case of acute coronary syndromes, where Mayr A et al. concluded that CMR MAPSE is a predictor of major adverse cardiovascular events (MACE) after an ST-elevation myocardial infarction, while also suggesting that more research is needed to establish a correlation between MAPSE and other markers such as left atrium parameters [41]. There is obviously room for ample research in the world of CMR-derived indices of LV longitudinal function, but we also believe that classic ultrasound M-mode-derived MAPSE still represents a field of research warranting more interest.

5. Conclusions

MAPSE seems to be a reliable and easy-to-use echocardiographic marker of LV function that not only correlates well with LVEF, but also proves to be extremely useful in the assessment of cardiac function in a wide array of clinical applications and might even have predictive value. Publications on its use in the last decade, however, seem to be insufficient, and it appears to be an underrepresented and underused LV function marker in comparison with others. There is a lack of evidence and validation regarding its use in certain specific cases such as, but not limited to, ventricular paced rhythms in patients with cardiac implantable electronic devices (CIED). It is a tried and tested ultrasound parameter that has proven to be applicable for the early detection of cardiac abnormalities, predicting the risk of heart failure and monitoring treatment response, especially in patients with poor acoustic windows.

Author Contributions: Conceptualization, L.C., C.V. and D.C.; methodology, L.C., C.V. and D.C.; software, L.C. and C.V.; validation, L.C., R.B. and C.V.; formal analysis, L.C., A.C., C.-T.L., C.V. and R.B.; investigation, L.C., A.C., R.B. and C.V.; resources, L.C., A.C., C.-T.L. and R.B.; data curation, L.C. and C.T.; writing—original draft preparation, L.C., A.C., C.V. and D.C.; writing—review and editing, L.C., A.C., S.C., C.V. and D.C.; visualization, L.C., C.V. and S.C.; supervision, R.B., D.F.L., C.V. and D.C.; project administration, L.C., C.V., D.F.L. and D.C.; funding acquisition, L.C., D.F.L. and D.C. All authors have read and agreed to the published version of the manuscript.

Funding: This research received no external funding. Internal funding: we would like to acknowledge the "Victor Babeș" University of Medicine and Pharmacy, Timișoara, for their support in covering the costs of publication for this research paper.

Informed Consent Statement: Informed consent was obtained from all subjects involved in the study.

Data Availability Statement: No new data were created or analyzed in this study. Data sharing is not applicable to this article.

Conflicts of Interest: The authors declare no conflicts of interest.

References

1. Gottdiener, J.S.; Bednarz, J.; Devereux, R.; Gardin, J.; Klein, A.; Manning, W.J.; Morehead, A.; Kitzman, D.; Oh, J.; Quinones, M.; et al. American Society of Echocardiography recommendations for use of echocardiography in clinical trials. *J. Am. Soc. Echocardiogr.* **2004**, *17*, 1086–1119. [CrossRef]
2. Savage, R.M.; Aronson, S.; Shernan, S.K. *Comprehensive Textbook of Perioperative Transesophageal Echocardiography*, 2nd ed.; Lippincott Williams and Wilkins: Philadelphia, PA, USA, 2013.
3. Smith, M.D.; MacPhail, B.; Harrison, M.R.; Lenhoff, S.J.; DeMaria, A.N. Value and limitations of transesophageal echocardiography in determination of left ventricular volumes and ejection fraction. *J. Am. Coll. Cardiol.* **1992**, *19*, 1213–1222. [CrossRef] [PubMed]
4. Chengode, S. Left ventricular global systolic function assessment by echocardiography. *Ann. Card. Anaesth.* **2016**, *19*, S26–S34. [CrossRef] [PubMed] [PubMed Central]
5. Lancellotti, P.; Cosyns, B. (Eds.) *The EACVI Echo Handbook*; ESC Publications: Oxford, UK, 2015. [CrossRef]
6. Hensel, K.O.; Roskopf, M.; Wilke, L.; Heusch, A. Intraobserver and interobserver reproducibility of M-mode and B-mode acquired mitral annular plane systolic excursion (MAPSE) and its dependency on echocardiographic image quality in children. *PLoS ONE* **2018**, *13*, e0196614. [CrossRef] [PubMed] [PubMed Central]
7. Brault, C.; Zerbib, Y.; Mercado, P.; Diouf, M.; Michaud, A.; Tribouilloy, C.; Maizel, J.; Slama, M. Mitral annular plane systolic excursion for assessing left ventricular systolic dysfunction in patients with septic shock. *BJA Open* **2023**, *7*, 100220. [CrossRef] [PubMed] [PubMed Central]
8. Habibian, M.; Lyon, A.R. Monitoring the heart during cancer therapy. *Eur. Heart J. Suppl.* **2019**, *21*, M44–M49. [CrossRef] [PubMed] [PubMed Central]
9. Berger, S.G.; Witczak, B.N.; Reiseter, S.; Schwartz, T.; Andersson, H.; Hetlevik, S.O.; Berntsen, K.S.; Sanner, H.; Lilleby, V.; Gunnarsson, R.; et al. Cardiac Dysfunction in Mixed Connective Tissue Disease: A Nationwide Observational Study. *Rheumatol. Int.* **2023**, *43*, 1055–1065. [CrossRef]
10. Åström Malm, I.; De Basso, R.; Engvall, J.; Blomstrand, P. Males with Abdominal Aortic Aneurysm Have Reduced Left Ventricular Systolic and Diastolic Function. *Clin. Physiol. Funct. Imaging* **2022**, *42*, 1–7. [CrossRef]
11. Chen, M.; Liu, D.; Weidemann, F.; Lengenfelder, B.D.; Ertl, G.; Hu, K.; Frantz, S.; Nordbeck, P. Echocardiographic Risk Factors of Left Ventricular Thrombus in Patients with Acute Anterior Myocardial Infarction. *ESC Heart Fail.* **2021**, *8*, 5248–5258. [CrossRef]
12. Jarori, U.; Maatman, T.K.; Maatman, B.; Mastouri, R.; Sawada, S.G.; Khemka, A. Mitral Annular Plane Systolic Excursion: An Early Marker of Mortality in Severe COVID-19. *J. Am. Soc. Echocardiogr.* **2020**, *33*, 1411–1413. [CrossRef]
13. Zou, T.; Yin, W.; Li, Y.; Deng, L.; Zhou, R.; Wang, X.; Chao, Y.; Zhang, L.; Kang, Y. Hemodynamics in Shock Patients Assessed by Critical Care Ultrasound and Its Relationship to Outcome: A Prospective Study. *Biomed. Res. Int.* **2020**, *2020*, 5175393. [CrossRef] [PubMed]
14. Tafarshiku, R.; Henein, M.Y.; Berisha-Muharremi, V.; Bytyçi, I.; Ibrahimi, P.; Poniku, A.; Elezi, S.; Bajraktari, G. Left Ventricular Diastolic and Systolic Functions in Patients with Hypothyroidism. *Medicina (Kaunas)* **2020**, *56*, 524. [CrossRef] [PubMed]
15. Magdy, G.; Hamdy, E.; Elzawawy, T.; Ragab, M. Value of mitral annular plane systolic excursion in the assessment of contractile reserve in patients with ischemic cardiomyopathy before cardiac revascularization. *Indian Heart J.* **2018**, *70*, 373–378. [CrossRef] [PubMed] [PubMed Central]
16. Havaldar, A.A. Evaluation of Sepsis Induced Cardiac Dysfunction as a Predictor of Mortality. *Cardiovasc. Ultrasound* **2018**, *16*, 31. [CrossRef]
17. Mincu, R.I.; Magda, S.L.; Mihaila, S.; Florescu, M.; Mihalcea, D.J.; Velcea, A.; Chiru, A.; Tiu, C.; Popescu, B.O.; Cinteza, M.; et al. Impaired Cardiac Function in Patients with Multiple Sclerosis by Comparison with Normal Subjects. *Sci. Rep.* **2018**, *8*, 3300. [CrossRef]
18. Zhang, H.-M.; Wang, X.-T.; Zhang, L.-N.; He, W.; Zhang, Q.; Liu, D.-W.; Chinese Critical Ultrasound Study Group. Left Ventricular Longitudinal Systolic Function in Septic Shock Patients with Normal Ejection Fraction: A Case-Control Study. *Chin. Med. J. (Engl.)* **2017**, *130*, 1169–1174. [CrossRef]
19. Yin, W.; Li, Y.; Zeng, X.; Qin, Y.; Wang, D.; Zou, T.; Su, L.; Kang, Y. The utilization of critical care ultrasound to assess hemodynamics and lung pathology on ICU admission and the potential for predicting outcome. *PLoS ONE* **2017**, *12*, e0182881. [CrossRef] [PubMed] [PubMed Central]
20. Bytyçi, I.; Haliti, E.; Berisha, G.; Tishukaj, A.; Shatri, F.; Bajraktari, G. Left ventricular longitudinal systolic dysfunction is associated with right atrial dyssynchrony in heart failure with preserved ejection fraction. *Rev. Port. Cardiol.* **2016**, *35*, 207–214. [CrossRef] [PubMed]
21. Taşolar, H.; Mete, T.; Çetin, M.; Altun, B.; Ballı, M.; Bayramoğlu, A.; Otlu, Y.Ö. Mitral Annular Plane Systolic Excursion in the Assessment of Left Ventricular Diastolic Dysfunction in Obese Adults. *Anatol. J. Cardiol.* **2015**, *15*, 558–564. [CrossRef]

22. Amado, J.; Islas, F.; de Isla, I.L.P.; de Diego, J.J.G.; de Agustín, A.; García-Fernandez, M.A. M-Mode Apical Systolic Excursion: A New and Simple Method to Evaluate Global Left Ventricular Longitudinal Strain. *Rev. Port. Cardiol.* **2015**, *34*, 551–554. [CrossRef]
23. Lund, M.; Alexandersson von Döbeln, G.; Nilsson, H.; Winter, R.; Lundell, L.; Tsai, J.A.; Kalman, S. Effects on heart function of neoadjuvant chemotherapy and chemoradiotherapy in patients with cancer in the esophagus or gastroesophageal junction—A prospective cohort pilot study within a randomized clinical trial. *Radiat. Oncol.* **2015**, *10*, 16. [CrossRef] [PubMed] [PubMed Central]
24. Kristen, A.V.; Scherer, K.; Buss, S.; aus dem Siepen, F.; Haufe, S.; Bauer, R.; Hinderhofer, K.; Giannitsis, E.; Hardt, S.; Haberkorn, U.; et al. Noninvasive Risk Stratification of Patients with Transthyretin Amyloidosis. *JACC Cardiovasc. Imaging* **2014**, *7*, 502–510. [CrossRef] [PubMed]
25. Hu, K.; Liu, D.; Herrmann, S.; Niemann, M.; Gaudron, P.D.; Voelker, W.; Ertl, G.; Bijnens, B.; Weidemann, F. Clinical implication of mitral annular plane systolic excursion for patients with cardiovascular disease. *Eur. Heart J. Cardiovasc. Imaging* **2013**, *14*, 205–212. [CrossRef] [PubMed]
26. Sveälv, B.G.; Olofsson, E.L.; Andersson, B. Ventricular long-axis function is of major importance for long-term survival in patients with heart failure. *Heart* **2008**, *94*, 284–289. [CrossRef] [PubMed]
27. Wenzelburger, F.W.; Tan, Y.T.; Choudhary, F.J.; Lee, E.S.; Leyva, F.; Sanderson, J.E. Mitral annular plane systolic excursion on exercise: A simple diagnostic tool for heart failure with preserved ejection fraction. *Eur. J. Heart Fail.* **2011**, *13*, 953–960. [CrossRef] [PubMed]
28. Elnoamany, M.F.; Abdelhameed, A.K. Mitral annular motion as a surrogate for left ventricular function: Correlation with brain natriuretic peptide levels. *Eur. J. Echocardiogr.* **2006**, *7*, 187–198. [CrossRef] [PubMed]
29. Willenheimer, R.; Israelsson, B.; Cline, C.; Rydberg, E.; Broms, K.; Erhardt, L. Left atrioventricular plane displacement is related to both systolic and diastolic left ventricular performance in patients with chronic heart failure. *Eur. Heart J.* **1999**, *20*, 612–618. [CrossRef] [PubMed]
30. Mizuguchi, Y.; Oishi, Y.; Miyoshi, H.; Iuchi, A.; Nagase, N.; Oki, T. Concentric left ventricular hypertrophy brings deterioration of systolic longitudinal, circumferential, and radial myocardial deformation in hypertensive patients with preserved left ventricular pump function. *J. Cardiol.* **2010**, *55*, 23–33. [CrossRef] [PubMed]
31. Ballo, P.; Barone, D.; Bocelli, A.; Motto, A.; Mondillo, S. Left Ventricular Longitudinal Systolic Dysfunction Is an Independent Marker of Cardiovascular Risk in Patients with Hypertension. *Am. J. Hypertens.* **2008**, *21*, 1047–1054. [CrossRef]
32. Ballo, P.; Quatrini, I.; Giacomin, E.; Motto, A.; Mondillo, S. Circumferential versus longitudinal systolic function in patients with hypertension: A nonlinear relation. *J. Am. Soc. Echocardiogr.* **2007**, *20*, 298–306. [CrossRef]
33. Rydberg, E.; Willenheimer, R.; Erhardt, L. Left atrioventricular plane displacement at rest is reduced in relation to severity of coronary artery disease irrespective of prior myocardial infarction. *Int. J. Cardiol.* **1999**, *69*, 201–207. [CrossRef]
34. Schick, A.L.; Kaine, J.C.; Al-Sadhan, N.A.; Lin, T.; Baird, J.; Bahit, K.; Dwyer, K.H. Focused cardiac ultrasound with mitral annular plane systolic excursion (MAPSE) detection of left ventricular dysfunction. *Am. J. Emerg. Med.* **2023**, *68*, 52–58. [CrossRef] [PubMed]
35. Takeda, S.; Rimington, H.; Smeeton, N.; Chambers, J. Long axis excursion in aortic stenosis. *Heart* **2001**, *86*, 52–56. [CrossRef] [PubMed] [PubMed Central]
36. Bergenzaun, L.; Ohlin, H.; Gudmundsson, P.; Willenheimer, R.; Chew, M.S. Mitral annular plane systolic excursion (MAPSE) in shock: A valuable echocardiographic parameter in intensive care patients. *Cardiovasc. Ultrasound* **2013**, *11*, 16. [CrossRef] [PubMed] [PubMed Central]
37. Alatic, J.; Suran, D.; Vokac, D.; Naji, F.H. Mitral Annular Plane Systolic Excursion (MAPSE) as a Predictor of Atrial Fibrillation Recurrence in Patients after Pulmonary Vein Isolation. *Cardiol. Res. Pract.* **2022**, *2022*, 2746304. [CrossRef] [PubMed] [PubMed Central]
38. Terada, T.; Mori, K.; Inoue, M.; Yasunobu, H. Mitral annular plane systolic excursion/left ventricular length (MAPSE/L) as a simple index for assessing left ventricular longitudinal function in children. *Echocardiography* **2016**, *33*, 1703–1709. [CrossRef] [PubMed]
39. Lang, R.M.; Badano, L.P.; Mor-Avi, V.; Afilalo, J.; Armstrong, A.; Ernande, L.; Flachskampf, F.A.; Foster, E.; Goldstein, S.A.; Kuznetsova, T.; et al. Recommendations for cardiac chamber quantification by echocardiography: An update from the American Society of Echocardiography and the European Association of Echocardiography. *J. Am. Soc. Echocardiogr.* **2015**, *28*, 1–39. [CrossRef] [PubMed]
40. Romano, J.; Judd, R.M.; Kim, R.J.; Kim, H.W.; Heitner, J.F.; Shah, D.J.; Devereux, R.B.; Salazar, P.; Trybula, M.; Chia, R.C.; et al. Prognostic Implications of Mitral Annular Plane Systolic Excursion in Patients with Hypertension and a Clinical Indication for Cardiac Magnetic Resonance Imaging: A Multicenter Study. *JACC Cardiovasc. Imaging* **2019**, *12*, 1769–1779. [CrossRef]
41. Mayr, A.; Pamminger, M.; Reindl, M.; Greulich, S.; Reinstadler, S.J.; Tiller, C.; Holzknecht, M.; Nalbach, T.; Plappert, D.; Kranewitter, C.; et al. Mitral annular plane systolic excursion by cardiac MR is an easy tool for optimized prognosis assessment in ST-elevation myocardial infarction. *Eur. Radiol.* **2020**, *30*, 620–629. [CrossRef] [PubMed] [PubMed Central]

Disclaimer/Publisher's Note: The statements, opinions and data contained in all publications are solely those of the individual author(s) and contributor(s) and not of MDPI and/or the editor(s). MDPI and/or the editor(s) disclaim responsibility for any injury to people or property resulting from any ideas, methods, instructions or products referred to in the content.

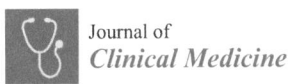

Review

Heart Rate Recovery: Up to Date in Heart Failure—A Literature Review

Andreea Cozgarea [1,2,3], Dragoș Cozma [1,2,4,*], Minodora Teodoru [3,5,*], Alexandra-Iulia Lazăr-Höcher [1,2], Liviu Cirin [2], Adelina-Andreea Faur-Grigori [1], Mihai-Andrei Lazăr [1,2,4], Simina Crișan [1,2,4], Dan Gaiță [1,2,4], Constantin-Tudor Luca [1,2,4] and Cristina Văcărescu [1,2,4]

1. Institute of Cardiovascular Diseases Timisoara, 300310 Timisoara, Romania; andreea.cozgarea@umft.ro (A.C.); alexandra.hocher@umft.ro (A.-I.L.-H.); andreeaadelinafaur@yahoo.com (A.-A.F.-G.); mihai88us@yahoo.com (M.-A.L.); simina.crisan@umft.ro (S.C.); dan.gaita@umft.ro (D.G.); constantin.luca@umft.ro (C.-T.L.); cristina.vacarescu@umft.ro (C.V.)
2. Department of Cardiology, "Victor Babeș" University of Medicine and Pharmacy, 300041 Timisoara, Romania; liviu.cirin@umft.ro
3. County Clinical Emergency Hospital of Sibiu, 550245 Sibiu, Romania
4. Research Center of the Institute of Cardiovascular Diseases Timisoara, 300310 Timisoara, Romania
5. Medical Clinical Department, Faculty of Medicine, "Lucian Blaga" University, 550024 Sibiu, Romania
* Correspondence: dragos.cozma@umft.ro (D.C.); minodora.teodoru@ulbs.ro (M.T.)

Abstract: The rising prevalence of cardiovascular disease underscores the growing significance of heart failure (HF). Pathophysiological insights into HF highlight the dysregulation of the autonomic nervous system (ANS), characterized by sympathetic overactivity and diminished vagal tone, impacting cardiovascular function. Heart rate recovery (HRR), a metric measuring the heart's ability to return to its baseline rate post-exertion, plays a crucial role in assessing cardiovascular health. Widely applied across various cardiovascular conditions including HF, coronary artery disease (CAD), and arterial hypertension (HTN), HRR quantifies the difference between peak and recovery heart rates. Given its association with elevated sympathetic tone and exercise, HRR provides valuable insights into the perspective of HF, beyond effort tolerance, reaching toward prognostic and mortality indicators. Incorporating HRR into cardiovascular evaluations enhances our understanding of autonomic regulation in HF, offering potential implications for prognostication and patient management. This review addresses the significance of HRR in HF assessment, analyzing recently conducted studies, and providing a foundation for further research and clinical application.

Keywords: heart failure; heart rate recovery; cardiac exercise stress test; autonomic nervous system

1. Introduction

Heart rate recovery (HRR) is a parameter that addresses the decrease in the heart rate following a physical exercise, reaching its resting heart rate values. It is typically measured as the difference between the maximum heart rate during effort and the heart rate at a given recovery time [1,2]. It serves as a precious tool for evaluating autonomic nervous system (ANS) imbalance and has been widely used in screening and quantifying cardiovascular risk and all-cause mortality in patients suffering from heart disease [3,4]. This process reflects the dynamic equilibrium and synchronized interaction between the reactivation of the parasympathetic nervous system and the withdrawal of the sympathetic nervous system [5].

Cardiac autonomic dysfunction is frequently linked to cardiovascular disease (CVD) and has been observed in individuals possessing such risk factors [6]. In these populations, autonomic dysfunction is predominantly characterized by diminished parasympathetic drive and increased sympathetic activity. This imbalance amplifies cardiac load, increases ventricular instability, and consequently augments the susceptibility for cardiac arrest, infarction, and sudden death. Therefore, the existence of autonomic dysfunction suggests a more deprived prognosis for individuals with cardiovascular disease and more specifically, with heart failure (HF) [7,8].

Although the recently updated guidelines from the European Society of Cardiology (ESC) explicitly classify acute and chronic HF in the realm of the left ventricular ejection fraction (LVEF), the approach fails to adequately address the diverse pathophysiological mechanisms, etiological factors, and associated comorbidities inherent to HF. Notably, patients diagnosed with HF exhibit substantial clinical similarities irrespective of their LVEF status, underscoring the inadequacy of relying solely on LVEF for complete classification and management strategies [9,10].

In conditions of impaired ventricular contraction, the sympathetic nervous system activation aims to enhance the cardiac output by accelerating the heart rate. Norepinephrine release via adrenergic pathways augments myocardial contractility and triggers activation of the renin–angiotensin–aldosterone system (RAAS), essential for maintaining adequate blood pressure and cardiac output. Chronic elevation in wall stress instigates myocardial hypertrophy and remodeling, alongside vasoconstriction, thus elevating afterload and boosting contraction while impairing myocardial relaxation. This feedback loop intensifies neurohormonal stimulation, exacerbating cardiac output compromise and perpetuating heart failure progression [11–13].

On the other hand, increased vagal tone can help protect against ischemia and arrhythmias by reducing heart rate and blood pressure. Modern therapies aim to regulate cardiac dysautonomia by increasing parasympathetic activity through interventions such as vagal nerve stimulation [14].

The purpose of this review is to provide an in-depth analysis of the existing data on HRR in heart failure patients, by identifying underlying correlations ranging from prognosis and mortality to clinical outcomes and echocardiographic evaluation. Additionally, it aims to elucidate the potential of the parameter as a diagnostic metric in detecting and/or characterizing HF patients.

2. Autonomic Influence in Exercise and the Recovery Period

Heart rate during physical exercise is influenced by both central (central command) and peripheral (metabo- and mechanoreflex) mechanisms [15]. The metaboreflex, a physiological reflex triggered during or after exercise-induced muscle ischemia, is activated by stimulation of metabo-receptors. In healthy individuals, this reflex mechanism enhances hemodynamic response, leading to increased cardiac output primarily through flow-mediated mechanisms [16]. Physical exercise causes intricate shifts between the sympathetic and parasympathetic branches of the autonomic nervous system, concluding in an augmentation of heart rate (HR) through vagal withdrawal and adrenergic discharge. This complex physiological response enhances cardiovascular parameters, including cardiac output, HR, cardiac contractility, alveolar ventilation, and venous return to the heart. As exercise intensifies, the peak of sympathetic discharge and catecholamine release induces vasoconstriction in various circulatory systems, with exceptions in muscle, coronary, and cerebral circulations [17]. Despite increased sympathetic activity during exercise, parasympathetic modulation continues to influence HR, ensuring optimal myocardial perfusion during diastolic intervals and contributing to cardioprotective effects [18].

The recovery phase after maximal exercise involves an obvious shift in autonomic tone, typified by sympathetic withdrawal and parasympathetic reactivation. Notably, parasympathetic reactivation promptly manifests within the initial minute following exercise cessation, significantly influencing HR decline. While vagal reactivation predominantly mediates the initial 30 s HR decline, the prominence of sympathetic withdrawal becomes more apparent two minutes post-exercise [6,19]. The available literature data highlight the hemodynamic changes that occur in the recovery phase, when the important HR drop may be caused by a decreased cardiac output, mediated by intrinsic regulation [20]. Autonomic influence marks both HRR and the metaboreflex. Available data reveal that HF patients exhibit an increased metaboreflex, caused by an increased sympathetic activity. This results in excessive arteriolar vasoconstriction and increased systemic vascular resistance. Consequently, ventricular contraction is compromised, leading to a reduced stroke volume. Similar changes were noted in diabetic patients or those with metabolic syndrome [21].

As opposed to heart failure, trained individuals maintain a higher cardiac output during the recovery phase, caused by the redistribution of blood to the central regions, leading to an increased preload [20]. Thus, along with the more augmented vagal activity, it explains the shifts in hemodynamics in a trained individual compared to heart failure states. While chronotropic incompetence (CI) itself serves as a marker of cardiac dysautonomia, conflictual data appeared regarding beta-blockers, that are commonly used to treat heart failure. To address this issue, a lower threshold has been introduced for patients taking beta-blockers, which defines CI as the inability to reach 62% of APMHR [22].

Exercise elicits a sophisticated autonomic response, involving sympathetic dominance and enduring parasympathetic modulation, thereby influencing the dynamics of heart rate and recovery. Considering that heart failure is a state of hypersympathetic activity, exploring the recovery phase contributes to a better understanding of the ongoing processes, allowing the evaluation of therapeutic approaches.

3. Main HRR Parameters

As early as the 1990s, the first data appeared concerning HRR, stating that a HRR < 12 beats per minute in the first minute strongly predicts overall mortality, setting a cornerstone for future studies [23]. Since then, the topic of HRR has been gaining interest among researchers, who developed various means of determining HRR, at different time intervals of the recovery period.

The following paragraph summarizes various HRRs, grouped through measurement methods.

3.1. Difference between Peak HR and HR at a Certain Moment of Recovery

- **HRR1**—HRR at 1 minute of recovery subtracted from the peak HR [24–30].
- **HRR2**—HRR at 2 min of recovery subtracted from the peak HR [25,28,29,31,32].
- **HRR150 sec**—measured as the difference between the maximum HR and the HR after 150 seconds of recovery [33].
- **HRR3**—measured as the difference between the maximum HR and the HR after three minutes of recovery [34].

3.2. A Ratio between Different Phases of the Effort

- **Heart rate recovery index**—measured as the ratio between heart rate acceleration time (AT) and heart rate deceleration time (DT) [35].

3.3. A Delay in the Maximum Heart Rate

- **Delay of peak HR**: HRR assessment 6 months after heart transplantation reflects the cardiac denervation and the loss of vagal tone, which would normally induce HR drop after exercise [32].

Given the distinct recovery phases and autonomic involvement, evaluating sympathetic nervous system activity during the post-exercise recovery phase could be crucial, given the correlation between cardiovascular issues induced by exercise and raised sympathetic activation. Moreover, while numerous population-based studies have associated HRR with mortality, there remains a gap in research regarding whether the augmentation of HRR following a therapeutic intervention serves as a predictive factor for improved survival during the subsequent follow-up period [36].

4. Clinical Applications of HRR

Ideas regarding HRR have been widely used in various clinical settings besides coronary artery disease. Heart failure, which will be thoroughly discussed further, has intricate connections with dysautonomia, implicit with the consequences of hypersympathetic states. Autonomic nervous system dysfunction is also implied in conditions such as hypertension [3], diabetes mellitus (DM) [37], metabolic syndrome and obesity [38], and obstructive sleep apnea syndrome [39].

HRR evaluation in DM plays a significant role in detecting subclinical LV dysfunction and preventing HF by evaluating diastolic functional reserve among heart failure with preserved ejection fraction (HFpEF) risk factors [40]. In a study by Vukomanovic et al., both type 2 diabetes patients and healthy individuals were enrolled to evaluate autonomic cardiac dysfunction using CPET. The results of the study revealed that patients with type 2 diabetes displayed a blunted HRR, which was associated with altered HRR, yielding significant autonomic nervous system dysfunction [41]. Moreover, another piece of research revealed the importance of dysautonomia by highlighting the associations between diastolic dysfunction and diminished functional capacity in patients with type 2 DM [42].

A recent study involving 2540 patients aimed to examine the correlations between heart rate recovery (HRR) and terminal-pro B type natriuretic peptide (NT-pro-BNP), which are both established as prognostic markers for heart failure. The study found that the NT-pro-BNP value was correlated with HRR2 and HRR3, indicating the importance of HRR in the slow recovery phase. This suggests that NT-pro-BNP is linked to the sympathetic nervous system, which is associated with heart failure processes. The study highlights the significance of cardiac dysautonomia evaluated by HRR and its connection to strong prognostic indicators of heart failure [43].

5. Methodology

The current review aims to encompass the most relevant studies conducted in the last ten years, concerning HRR in HF patients, employing two tables that hold the most relevant aspects of the studies (Tables 1 and 2).

Table 1. Heart rate recovery (HRR) studies including patients with heart failure with reduced Ejection Fraction (HFrEF).

Study (Year)	Patients Enrolled (n)	HF Population	Purpose of the Study	Exercise Test Methodology	Beta-Blocker Treatment	HRR Evaluation Method and Cut-Off	Conclusions
Andrade et al. (2022) [25]	76	HFrEF	Correlation of all-cause mortality and HRR1 and HRR2 during a 2-year follow-up	6 MWT followed by passive supine recovery.	97% of patients. Dosage N/A.	HRR1; HRR2 = HRmax-HR at 1; 2 min of recovery; Preestablished N.V. HRR1 > 12 bpm; HRR2 > 22 bpm	Decreased HRR1 and HRR2 are associated with increased mortality.
Tanaka et al. (2021) [27]	84	HFrEF with AF	Correlation of HRR and exercise capacity of HFrEF and AF patients before and after the rehabilitation program	Cycle ergometer CPET using a ramp protocol of 10 W/min until exhaustion, with an active 1 min recovery, followed by a 4 min passive recovery.	90% of patients. Dosage N/A	HRR1 = HRmax-HR at 1 min of recovery. For AF patients, HR was determined by averaging the last ten beats at each point; Cut-off N/A	Improved HRR is associated with improved exercise capacity in patients with HFrEF and AF after completing the cardiac rehabilitation program.
Cozlac et al. (2020) [35]	109	HFrEF patients following CRT implantation	Correlation of HRRI and CRT responsiveness	Cycle ergometer using the Bruce Protocol with a 25 W increase/2 min.	82.8% of the patients. Dosage N/A.	HRRI = The ratio between HR AT and DT. The cut-off for CRT response predictability was 1.51.	HRRI was significantly higher in CRT responders vs. non-responders.
Fonseca et al. (2019) [28]	116	HFrEF	Association of sarcopenia and autonomic regulation	Symptom limited cycle ergometer CPET using a ramp protocol 5–10 W/min. Active recovery for 2 min, followed by 4 min of passive recovery.	100% of sarcopenic and 94% of non-sarcopenic patients. Dosage N/A.	HRR1; HRR2 = HRmax-HR at 1; 2 min of recovery; Cut-off N/A	Sarcopenia is associated with decreased HRR1 and HRR2 in HF patients.

Table 1. Cont.

Study (Year)	Patients Enrolled (n)	HF Population	Purpose of the Study	Exercise Test Methodology	Beta-Blocker Treatment	HRR Evaluation Method and Cut-Off	Conclusions
Youn et al. (2016) [29]	107	Recovered acute decompensated HFrEF (Eligible for discharge)	Correlation between HRR and pro-inflammatory states with clinical outcomes	Treadmill CPET using a modified Bruce Protocol. Passive recovery in seated position.	Total of 33.3% in the CV-events group and 68.8% in the no-CV-events group. Dosage N/A.	HRR1; HRR2 = HRmax-HR at 1; 2 min of recovery; Cut off HRR1 < 13, HRR2 < 27	Impaired HRR is associated with an exaggerated pro-inflammatory response and independently predicts clinical outcomes.

N—Number; HF—heart failure; HFrEF—heart failure with reduced ejection fraction; AF—Atrial Fibrillation; 6 MWT—6 min walk test; HRR—heart rate recovery at a given time; HRmax—Maximum Heart Rate; HRRI—heart rate recovery index; CPET—Cardiopulmonary exercise test; Min—minute; S—Second; B.P.M.—Beats per minute; W—Watt; CRT—Cardiac Resynchronization Therapy; AT—Acceleration Time; DT—Deceleration Time; N.V.—Normal Values; N/A—Not available; CV—Cardiovascular.

The methodology used for this review implied searching on different databases, such as PubMed or Google Scholar, using relevant keywords like "heart rate recovery" and "heart failure", including Mesh terms.

The criteria for inclusion stipulated that the articles be written in English and published between 2014 and 2024, and their type should relate to patients involved in clinical studies. Furthermore, the resulting articles were manually selected considering the relevance, intending to showcase diverse clinical scenarios where HRR was employed to address heart failure.

6. HRR in Heart Failure: Bedside Studies

The resulting population heterogeneity prompted the construction of two tables to effectively organize the resulting data. Table 1 presents patients diagnosed with heart failure with reduced ejection fraction (HFrEF), offering a focused examination of this subgroup within the cohort.

In contrast, Table 2 encompasses a diverse range of study populations and comparison groups, including heart failure with preserved ejection fraction (HFpEF), heart failure with mid-range ejection fraction (HFmrEF), and comparisons between heart failure patients and healthy controls. Furthermore, two specific studies are highlighted within this framework: the study of Carneiro et al. [34], which investigated individuals at risk of developing heart failure (Stage A), and the study of Imamura et al. [32], which delves into patients recovering from advanced heart failure (Stage D), and having undergone heart transplantation.

HRR is a powerful tool for predicting morbi-mortality in various conditions and is considered a marker of cardiac dysautonomia [44].

Table 1 compresses studies conducted on HFrEF patients and reveals several HRR methods of determination, exercise protocols, and controversial aspects such as beta-blockade treatment, alongside the study objectives and results.

Our goal is to assess the various purposes for conducting exercise tests, which range from assessing the impact of reduced quality of life to establishing correlations with mortality in connection with blunted heart rate recovery. We also aim to point out the correlation between reduced heart rate recovery and pro-inflammatory states, as well as the association between exercise tests and conditions such as sarcopenia, CRT responsiveness, and the influence of cardiac rehabilitation.

Delving into HRR determination methods, the most frequently used methods are represented by HRR1 and HRR2. Cozlac et al. used another determinant, namely the heart rate recovery index (HRRI) [35]. This index evaluates both the exercise time, by assessing the heart rate acceleration time (AT), and the time of recovery, by measuring the heart rate deceleration time (DT), being defined as the ratio between AT and DT.

Although the study population is represented by HFrEF patients, and the HRR determinants are equal, cut-off values either differ between studies or have no values available for cut-off, showing a degree of inconsistency. Moreover, additional differences among the studies are evident regarding the exercise test employed, the protocols implemented, and the duration of the recovery period. These studies have employed diverse exercise protocols and test types, spanning from the six-minute walk test (6 MWT) to comprehensive cardio-pulmonary exercise tests (CPET). The recuperation period varies across studies, encompassing active recovery followed by passive recovery, solely passive recovery protocols, or instances where the recovery protocol is not specified.

Similar to a recently published study, the methodology did not exhibit a clear pattern for which exercise type and recovery protocols were used, indicating that further research and studies are necessary to validate distinct protocols for various clinical scenarios [2].

The exercise types varied from the 6 MWT to the treadmill and cycle ergometer. While maximal exercise tests like CPET are considered the benchmark for evaluating functional capacity, the 6 MWT can offer valuable insights into a patient's daily activity levels and short-term prognosis, particularly in those with heart failure and reduced ejection fraction, whether in a stable chronic condition or following an acute decompensation [45].

In contrast to the 6 MWT, both the cycle ergometer and treadmill offer a more gradual and graded exercise. The bicycle ergometer has several advantages, including a small space requirement, easy quantification of exercise, and suitability for obese patients or those with orthopedic disorders. From a safety standpoint, it is a better choice than other forms of exercise equipment, as it reduces the risk of ventricular arrhythmias and angina pectoris appearance during exercise. The reason for this is that initially, maximal exercise on a treadmill exerts more significant stress on the heart and lungs compared to bicycle ergometers. Research has shown that during exercise tests with a bicycle ergometer, untrained individuals often end the test due to fatigue in the quadriceps femoris muscles, resulting in an average 5–20% lower peak oxygen consumption (peak VO2) compared to treadmill exercise [46].

The study's population distribution is shown for example in the studies of Youn et al. or Cozlac et al. studies. The former implied symptom-limited CPET that was conducted on patients who presented with acute decompensated heart failure (ADHF), after the clinical stabilization of the patients [29]. The latter showed that an increased HRRI was associated with responder status, while a blunted HRRI was linked to non-responders in CRT patients [35].

Table 2. Heart rate recovery (HRR) studies including mixed groups of heart failure (HF) patients and healthy controls.

Study (Year)	Patients Enrolled (n)	HF Population	Purpose of the Study	Exercise Test Methodology	Beta-Blocker Treatment	HRR Evaluation Method and Cut-Off	Conclusions
Hossri et al. (2024) [24]	106	HFpEF and HFmrEF with concomitant CAD	Benefits of CPMR in HF patients with CAD	Treadmill CPET using an incremental maximal protocol, followed later by a submaximal constant load protocol at 80% of the initial test; recovery period of 6 min	87% of the patients. Dosage N/A.	HRR1 was evaluated at the first recovery min; Cut-off N/A	12 weeks of CPMR were associated with improved NYHA class, significant exercise test performance, an increased HRR, and an enhanced QOL.
Irfanullah et al. (2023) [47]	39	HFpEF, HFmrEF, HFrEF	The effects of cycle ergometer training on heart rate recovery and mindfulness in patients with NYHA Class I and II heart failure	6 MWT on a 400–700 m distance.	All patients received either beta-blockers or CCB. Dosage N/A.	HRR1; HRR2 = HRmax-HR at 1; 2 min of recovery; Cut-off N/A	HRR1 and HRR2 improved after 6 weeks of cycle-ergometer training, as well as the MAAS.
Carneiro et al. (2021) [34]	2066	Participants without HF	Incidence of HF and its type (HFpEF and HFrEF) during the follow-up period (16.8 years)	Submaximal treadmill exercise test using the Bruce protocol; recovery in a supine position.	N/A	HRR3 = HRmax-HR at 3 min of recovery; Cut-off N/A	Slower HRR3 is associated with a higher risk of developing heart failure, particularly HFrEF.
Hajdusek et al. (2017) [33]	103	78 advanced HFrEF and 25 healthy controls, assessed for device implantation or transplant eligibility	Evaluation of HRR and MCR as outcome determinants in HF, during a follow-up of ~3.4 years	Symptom limited using a bicycle CPET, with a 25 W increase/3 min.	97% of HF patients. Daily low-middle doses (12.5–50 mg Carvedilol; 2.5–200 mg Metoprolol and 2.5–10 mg Bisoprolol)	The difference between HRmax and HR at 150 s of recovery; Cut-off N/A	MCR slope correlates with distinct clinical variables compared to HRR. In heart failure patients, the MCR slope offers significant prognostic value beyond HRR.
Yayla et al. (2015) [31]	41	HFrEF and HFmrEF	Correlation between exercise training and HRR improvement, before and after entering a training program	Symptom limited bicycle CPET with 10 W/min followed by 3 min active cool-down	51.2% of patients. Dosage N/A	HRR1; HRR2 = HRmax-HR at 1; 2 min of recovery; N.V. Preestablished HRR1 > 12 bpm; HRR2 > 22 bpm	The training enhanced only HRR2, with IT showing a greater impact on the HRR2 improvement. Both HRR (1 and 2) in those with an abnormal HRR baseline have improved after exercise.

Table 2. Cont.

Study (Year)	Patients Enrolled (n)	HF Population	Purpose of the Study	Exercise Test Methodology	Beta-Blocker Treatment	HRR Evaluation Method and Cut-Off	Conclusions
Imamura et al. (2015) [32]	21	Heart transplant patients	Impact of post-heart transplantation parasympathetic reinnervation	Symptom limited Cycle-ergometer CPET using a 10 W/min incremental protocol, followed by a 5 min passive recovery in a seated position.	19% of patients. Dosage N/A.	HRR2-the difference between peak HR and HR after 2 min of recovery (measured 2 years after transplant) Delay of peak HR-the delay from the peak HR after the recovery time initiation (measured 6 months after transplant). Cut-off N/A	Parasympathetic reinnervation coincides with enhanced post-exercise recovery and heart failure-specific quality of life during the 2 years following heart transplantation.
Lindemberg et al. (2014) [26]	161. 154 completed the test	126 patients with HFrEF and 35 healthy individuals.	Correlations between HRR1 and 6 MWD	6 MWT followed by passive (seated) recovery.	70.58% of HF patients. Carvedilol mean dose 30 ± 29 mg.	HRR1 = HRmax-HR at 1 min of recovery; N.V. Preestablished HRR1 > 12 bpm	HF patients who received beta-blockers had better exercise tolerance than those without receiving beta-blocker medication, even though they had altered HRR.
Cahalin et al. (2014) [30]	240	200 patients with HFrEF and 40 patients with HFpEF	Correlations between HRR measured post 6 MWT and CPET and predictors of abnormal HRR.	6 MWT followed by a passive recovery. A symptom-limited bicycle CPET lasting 8-10 min. 1 min active cool-down period.	60% of the entire study group. Dosage N/A	HRR1 = HRmax-HR at 1 min of recovery; N.V. Preestablished HRR1 > 12 bpm	The 6 MWT and CPET were correlated concerning HRR, HR Reserve, and peak HR. Predictors of abnormal HRR were found to be Peak HR, EOV and E/e' ratio.

N—Number; HF—heart failure; HFpEF—heart failure with preserved ejection fraction; HFmrEF—heart failure with mid-range ejection fraction; HFrEF—heart failure with reduced ejection fraction; CAD—coronary artery disease; CPET—cardiopulmonary exercise test; CPMR—cardiopulmonary and metabolic rehabilitation; N/A—Not available; HRR—heart rate recovery at a given time; HRmax—maximum Heart Rate; Min—minute; N.V.—Normal Values; S—Second; B.P.M.—beats per minute; NYHA—New York Heart Association; QOL—quality of life; 6 MWT—6 min walk test; 6 MWD—6 min walk distance; CCB—calcium channel blockers; MAAS—mindful attention aware scale; W—watt; MCR—metabolic chronotropic relation; EOV—exercise oscillatory ventilation.

The presented data from the numerous studies have covered diverse study groups, comprising patients from all HF stages [48]. HRR was studied in numerous population groups, extending from HFrEF and HFmrEF to HFpEF, including cohorts of patients who were at risk of developing HF in the follow-up period, as evaluated by Carneiro et al. The study evaluated the patients enrolled in the Framingham Offspring Study to assess the association between decreased HRR and incidental HF during an average follow-up period of 16.8 years. Considering that nearly 40% of the patients were on antihypertensive treatment, 16% on lipid-lowering treatment, 12% were smokers and 9.3% were suffering from type 2 Diabetes Mellitus (T2DM), they could be considered at risk for developing HF (Stage A heart failure) [48]. Thus, it is noteworthy to mention the correlation between blunted HRR and an increased risk of developing HF, particularly HFrEF [29,34,35].

Conversely, Imamura et al. comprised the opposite spectrum of HF patients, namely those who underwent a heart transplantation, underlining the broad range of HRR applicability [32].

Research has suggested that cardiac rehabilitation programs may have a beneficial effect on HRR. Several studies have indicated that there is a significant improvement in HRR following enrolment in a rehabilitation program [24,27,34]. Not only did rehabilitation result in improved HRR, but CAD patients were shown to have attenuated exercise-induced arrhythmias and less frequent myocardial ischemia responses. Moreover, HRR appears to be correlated with other HF determinants, such as the NYHA class, the BORG scale on exertion perception, and quality of life questionaries [27].

It is common for patients with heart failure to experience mental health concerns like anxiety and depression, which can sometimes be underestimated. Research conducted by Irfanullah et al. has revealed that cardiac rehabilitation not only enhanced HRR but also has a considerable positive effect on mindfulness scale assessment. This is a crucial finding as mindfulness has been shown to promote an increase in vagal stimulation, which is advantageous for heart failure patients and may help to improve their mental and physical well-being [47].

Controversial aspects are contained in the tables, regarding the beta-blocker (BB) treatment and its influences on HRR determinations. β-blocker therapy leads to a decrease in neurohormone levels and an increase in β-receptor sensitivity, ultimately resulting in accentuated inotropy. Additionally, it has been suggested that, among other medications, β-blockers may experience reduced efficacy over time [49].

HRR was not statistically different in patients who were on BBs, compared to those who did not, as stated in several studies [2,29]. This suggests that HRR predominantly reflects vagal tone and remains a viable method for risk stratification across all patients, regardless of β-blocker therapy [2].

In the study of Hajdusek et al., a statistical difference was observed in the baseline characteristics of patients concerning beta-blockers. This was performed by comparing individuals with heart failure with reduced ejection fraction (HFrEF) who were administered beta-blockers (BBs), and healthy controls who did not have any medical reason for receiving BBs. However, HRR was found to reflect the vagal tone and was not associated with BB usage [33].

Yaylali et al. studied HF patients who were enrolled in a cardiac rehabilitation program, pointing out that significantly more patients on BBs had normal baseline HRR1 and HRR2, before starting the rehabilitation program [31].

Lindemberg et al. conducted a study with patients divided into three groups: G1 comprised HF patients treated with BB, G2 consisted of HF patients not treated with BB, and G3 included healthy patients. Even though the patients who received BB had an altered HRR, they showed better exercise tolerance, according to the study's findings [26].

Various studies that determined HRR are displayed in the tables, but the methods they used were not consistent. Most studies rely on HRR1 evaluation using a cut-off value that was put in place over 30 years ago. However, two studies used statistical methods to evaluate their HRR cut-off; Cozlac et al. referred the HRRI value to the area under the receiver operating characteristic (AuROC) [35]. Likewise, Youn et al. stood out as they use Contal and O'Quigley's method to establish a cut-off value [29]. In contrast, other studies do not have a clear cut-off value, or they depend on preexisting cut-off values.

Figure 1 shows a graphical representation of the parameters used for assessing HRR. Whereas the most used evaluation methods use the difference between peak HR and HR at a certain moment of recovery (HRR1 and HRR2), a ratio between the exercise phase and the recovery period, such as HRRI, is also displayed. The significant benefit of using HRRI is that it takes into account the entire exercise period and reports a single value that assesses both acceleration and deceleration time.

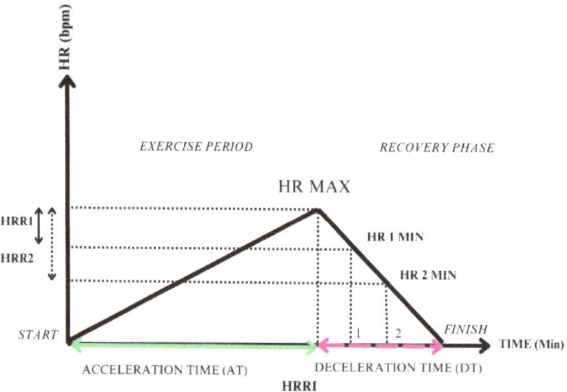

Figure 1. Graphical interpretation of heart rate recovery parameters. HRR1: HR MAX- HR1min (heart rate recovery at 1 min); HRR2: HR MAX-HR2 2 min (heart rate recovery at 2 min); HRRI: AT/DT (heart rate recovery index).

7. Echocardiographic Correlations

Echocardiography is a significant part of cardiovascular assessment. The following section contains research data that revealed associations between certain echocardiographic determinants and HRR.

LVEF is a cornerstone parameter for evaluating systolic function, yet its exclusive use is inadequate, particularly given the increasing prevalence of HFpEF. Comprehensive assessments now require additional evaluations, including diastolic function assessment, tissue Doppler imaging (TDI), and evaluation of left atrial enlargement [10]. Researchers have revealed that an examination of cardiac hemodynamic parameters, particularly through tissue Doppler echocardiography, indicates a clear correlation between left ventricular diastolic function and HRR. Patients showing decreased left ventricular filling pressures and exhibiting lower E/e' ratios demonstrate accelerated HRR and a more pronounced chronotropic response, underscoring the intricate relationship between cardiac autonomic function and adaptive responses to exercise [50]. As previously stated in the HF bedside studies, Cahalin et al. revealed that echocardiography can serve as a predictor for HRR values, involving mainly the E/e' ratio for evaluating the diastolic filling pattern [30].

Whereas conventional echocardiography has a certain contribution, diastolic assessment during stress echocardiography has shown superior results to conventional echocardiography and has been widely evaluated and incorporated in HFpEF diagnostic scores. The most evaluated parameters represent peak tricuspid regurgitation velocity jet and subsequently, pulmonary artery systolic pressure (PASP) and mitral E/E' to objectify elevated LV filling pressures [51].

The relationship between HRR and left atrial function and size is worth mentioning. Interestingly, blunted HRR has been shown to relate positively to the left atrial volume index, indicating that cardiac dysautonomia mechanisms may contribute to cardiac remodeling processes [51]. As shown in a recent study, abnormal strain rates during the reservoir, conduit, and contraction phases of the left atrium were associated with blunted HRR 120 s in patients with ST-segment elevation myocardial infarction [52].

8. Discussion

This current review discussed the topic of HRR and the main studies that involved HF patients, in which various aspects and correlations of HRR were determined. The main HRR studies that were conducted in the last decade underscore the inconsistency of HRR determinants, underlining that each method has its weaknesses and strengths.

Since the recovery phase is influenced differently by the autonomic nervous system, we consider that it is crucial to comprehend the whole-effort dynamics to better assess heart failure conditions.

Ranging from chronic inflammatory states, metabolic imbalance, and sarcopenia to cardiac outcomes, HF predictability, and mortality, we encompassed the various applicability of HRR in our presented study.

Available data suggest facilitated patient risk quantification with the help of HRR, considering that patients with blunted HRR indices exhibit increased risks of mortality, recurrent HF hospitalizations, and adverse cardiac events [25,29,44]. By identifying high-risk individuals, we presume that clinicians could adapt management strategies accordingly to HRR values.

Another key determinant of cardiac dysautonomia is reflected by heart rate variability (HRV). HRV refers to the variation in the time intervals between successive heartbeats (i.e., the R-R interval) and has been proven to have decreased values in HF [53]. While they both serve as prognostic markers [54,55], they differ in their measurement methods and the information they provide. Firstly, HRV is usually measured on standard resting electrocardiograms (ECG) or during Holter monitoring [56]. HRR on the other hand, is measured after a graded exercise and offers more complex information about both the resting HR and the recovery HR at a given time.

The mutual regulation system observed between HRV and HRR implies a potential connection between the two measures. If so, resting HRV indicators could serve as predictors of HRR before encountering stressors like exercise [57].

However, the diagnostic utility of HRR remains to be further proven, as it would be a crucial aspect to implement HRR among well-established tools, such as natriuretic peptides, in the diagnostic of heart failure.

Exercise stress tests have been helping clinicians evaluate treatment response in advanced HF states, that require CRT. A recently published article underlines the importance of ET in tailoring beta-blockers and ivabradine in CRT fusion pacing. Monitoring dynamic changes of the HR over time can help evaluate the efficacy of treatment regimens and guide adjustments as needed [58]. Therefore, our perspectives may shift towards better HRR comprehension, which may be useful in guiding medical treatment in HF patients. Therapeutic interventions aimed at improving cardiac function, such as medication adjustments, lifestyle improvements, and cardiac rehabilitation programs, may lead to enhancements in autonomic function and subsequently improved HRR.

As previously exposed, exercise training represents a cornerstone of HF management, promoting cardiovascular fitness and improving symptoms, further enhancing the quality of life of HF patients. Among improving cardiovascular fitness, exercise modulates dysautonomia, improves inflammatory states, and prevents muscle loss, which has been proven to be a consequence of the pathophysiology of heart failure [59].

Therapeutic interventions targeting autonomic modulation vary widely, starting with medical treatment, such as beta-blockers, angiotensin-converting enzyme inhibitors (ACEIs), or digoxin. More recently, studies have shown that sodium-glucose cotransporter-2 inhibitors (SGLT2-i) may improve cardiac autonomic dysfunction in type 2DM patients, as published in the SCAN Study, which may lead to new research directions toward HF patients [60]. Besides medical therapies, dysautonomia may be targeted with device-based options, such as CRT, vagal nerve stimulation (VNS), or renal denervation [61].

9. Further Perspectives

Assessing HRR in the treatment of HF patients will offer a simple approach to risk stratification, treatment monitoring, and proactive management.

HRR has been identified as a potential indicator of premature cardiac impairment, such as altered diastolic dysfunction, as demonstrated in a study involving obese adolescents. This underscores its significance as a clinically relevant outcome marker [62]. Although the available determination methods prove some degree of inconsistency with the used parameters, the field is open for novel implementations.

Future studies may show interest in establishing connections between abnormal HRR, HF, and atrial remodeling. Considering the intricate synergy between dysautonomia, electrical and mechanical remodeling, and heart failure progression, the area of research deserves to be unveiled.

Another key aspect concerns inflammation, frequently measured by high-sensitive C reactive protein (hs-CRP) [63] or the neutrophil-to-lymphocyte ratio (NLR) [64], which is known to be linked to the risk of developing cardiovascular disease, such as heart failure [65] and atrial fibrillation [66]. Further studies are necessary to evaluate the risk of quantifying atrial fibrillation in the realm of blunted HRR.

Moreover, delayed HRR has been proven to be independently associated with NLR, indicative of systemic inflammation [63]. This underscores the implications of vagal modulation in inflammation and suggests future perspectives for managing heart failure.

10. Conclusions

In summary, this study underscores the necessity of integrating heart rate recovery (HRR) into cardiovascular assessments, as it is associated with both morbidity and mortality in numerous cardiovascular conditions. The connections between HRR and the autonomic nervous system make HRR an accountable index, for both the assessment of the pathophysiologic dynamic processes and their consequences [67]. However, the domain of heart rate recovery stands as a focal point for future research endeavors, particularly in the context of heart failure, where the potential diagnostic utility of HRR remains to be fully elucidated. As mentioned before, the recently published studies encompassing HF patients lack a standardized evaluation protocol that could be easily applied throughout practices, emphasizing the importance of future research in this area of expertise.

Establishing the diagnostic power of HRR through further investigation holds significant promise, especially considering its ease of evaluation. Such advancements could revolutionize cardiovascular diagnostics, offering clinicians a simple yet potent tool for enhancing risk assessment and patient care.

Author Contributions: Conceptualization, A.C., C.V. and D.C.; methodology, A.C., M.T. and C.-T.L.; software, A.C., M.T., A.-I.L.-H. and M.-A.L.; validation, A.C., D.C., C.V. and D.G.; formal analysis, A.C., A.-I.L.-H. and M.T.; investigation, A.C., D.C., C.V. and M.-A.L.; resources, A.C., L.C., M.T. and A.-A.F.-G.; data curation, A.C., C.V., L.C. and M.T.; writing—original draft preparation, A.C., D.C., C.V. and A.-A.F.-G.; writing—review and editing, A.C., D.C., M.T., C.V. and C.-T.L.; visualization, A.C., D.C., C.V. and S.C.; supervision, A.C., D.C. and S.C.; project administration, A.C., M.T. and C.V.; funding acquisition, A.C., D.G. and D.C. All authors have read and agreed to the published version of the manuscript.

Funding: This research received no external funding. Internal funding: We would like to acknowledge VICTOR BABES UNIVERSITY OF MEDICINE AND PHARMACY TIMISOARA for their support in covering the costs of publication for this research paper.

Institutional Review Board Statement: Not applicable.

Informed Consent Statement: Not applicable.

Data Availability Statement: Data sharing is not applicable.

Conflicts of Interest: The authors declare no conflicts of interest.

References

1. Dewar, A.; Kass, L.; Stephens, R.C.M.; Tetlow, N.; Desai, T. Heart Rate Recovery Assessed by Cardiopulmonary Exercise Testing in Patients with Cardiovascular Disease: Relationship with Prognosis. *Int. J. Environ. Res. Public Health* **2023**, *20*, 4678. [CrossRef] [PubMed]
2. Yu, Y.; Liu, T.; Wu, J.; Zhu, P.; Zhang, M.; Zheng, W.; Gu, Y. Heart rate recovery in hypertensive patients: Relationship with blood pressure control. *J. Hum. Hypertens.* **2017**, *31*, 354–360. [CrossRef] [PubMed]
3. Manolis, A.A.; Manolis, T.A.; Manolis, A.S. Neurohumoral Activation in Heart Failure. *Int. J. Mol. Sci.* **2023**, *24*, 15472. [CrossRef] [PubMed]
4. Fecchio, R.Y.; Brito, L.; Leicht, A.S.; Forjaz, C.L.M.; Peçanha, T. Reproducibility of post-exercise heart rate recovery indices: A systematic review. *Auton. Neurosci.* **2019**, *221*, 102582. [CrossRef] [PubMed]
5. Qiu, S.; Cai, X.; Sun, Z.; Li, L.; Zuegel, M.; Steinacker, J.M.; Schumann, U.; Yin, J.; Jin, X.; Shan, Z.; et al. Heart Rate Recovery and Risk of Cardiovascular Events and All-Cause Mortality: A Meta-Analysis of Prospective Cohort Studies. *J. Am. Heart Assoc.* **2017**, *6*, e005505. [CrossRef] [PubMed]
6. Peçanha, T.; Silva-Júnior, N.D.; Forjaz, C.L.D.M. Heart rate recovery: Autonomic determinants, methods of assessment and association with mortality and cardiovascular diseases. *Clin. Physiol. Funct. Imaging* **2014**, *34*, 327–339. [CrossRef] [PubMed]
7. Okutucu, S.; Karakulak, U.N.; Aytemir, K.; Oto, A. Heart rate recovery: A practical clinical indicator of abnormal cardiac autonomic function. *Expert Rev. Cardiovasc. Ther.* **2011**, *9*, 1417–1430. [CrossRef] [PubMed]
8. Imai, K.; Sato, H.; Hori, M.; Kusuoka, H.; Ozaki, H.; Yokoyama, H.; Takeda, H.; Inoue, M.; Kamada, T. Vagally mediated heart rate recovery after exercise is accelerated in athletes but blunted in patients with chronic heart failure. *J. Am. Coll. Cardiol.* **1994**, *24*, 1529–1535. [CrossRef] [PubMed]
9. McDonagh, T.A.; Metra, M.; Adamo, M.; Gardner, R.S.; Baumbach, A.; Böhm, M.; Burri, H.; Butler, J.; Čelutkienė, J.; Chioncel, O.; et al. 2023 Focused Update of the 2021 ESC Guidelines for the diagnosis and treatment of acute and chronic heart failure: Developed by the task force for the diagnosis and treatment of acute and chronic heart failure of the European Society of Cardiology (ESC) With the special contribution of the Heart Failure Association (HFA) of the ESC. *Eur. Heart J.* **2023**, *44*, 3627–3639. [CrossRef]
10. Severino, P.; D'amato, A.; Prosperi, S.; Cas, A.D.; Mattioli, A.V.; Cevese, A.; Novo, G.; Prat, M.; Pedrinelli, R.; Raddino, R.; et al. Do the Current Guidelines for Heart Failure Diagnosis and Treatment Fit with Clinical Complexity? *J. Clin. Med.* **2022**, *11*, 857. [CrossRef]
11. Gronda, E.; Dusi, V.; D'elia, E.; Iacoviello, M.; Benvenuto, E.; Vanoli, E. Sympathetic activation in heart failure. *Eur. Heart J. Suppl.* **2022**, *24*, E4–E11. [CrossRef] [PubMed]
12. Borovac, J.A.; D'Amario, D.; Bozic, J.; Glavas, D. Sympathetic nervous system activation and heart failure: Current state of evidence and the pathophysiology in the light of novel biomarkers. *World J. Cardiol.* **2020**, *12*, 373–408. [CrossRef] [PubMed]
13. Zhang, D.Y.; Anderson, A.S. The Sympathetic Nervous System and Heart Failure. *Cardiol. Clin.* **2014**, *32*, 33–45. [CrossRef] [PubMed]
14. Kumar, H.U.; Nearing, B.D.; Mittal, S.; Premchand, R.K.; Libbus, I.; DiCarlo, L.A.; Amurthur, B.; KenKnight, B.H.; Anand, I.S.; Verrier, R.L. Autonomic regulation therapy in chronic heart failure with preserved/mildly reduced ejection fraction: ANTHEM-HFpEF study results. *Int. J. Cardiol.* **2023**, *381*, 37–44. [CrossRef] [PubMed]
15. Peçanha, T.; de Brito, L.C.; Fecchio, R.Y.; de Sousa, P.N.; Junior, N.D.d.S.; de Abreu, A.P.; da Silva, G.V.; Mion-Junior, D.; Forjaz, C.L.d.M. Metaboreflex activation delays heart rate recovery after aerobic exercise in never-treated hypertensive men. *J. Physiol.* **2016**, *594*, 6211–6223. [CrossRef] [PubMed]
16. Roberto, S.; Mulliri, G.; Milia, R.; Solinas, R.; Pinna, V.; Sainas, G.; Piepoli, M.F.; Crisafulli, A. Hemodynamic response to muscle reflex is abnormal in patients with heart failure with preserved ejection fraction. *J. Appl. Physiol.* **2017**, *122*, 376–385. [CrossRef] [PubMed]
17. Hellsten, Y.; Nyberg, M. Cardiovascular Adaptations to Exercise Training. In *Comprehensive Physiology*; Wiley: Hoboken, NY, USA, 2015; pp. 1–32. [CrossRef]
18. Gourine, A.V.; Ackland, G.L. Cardiac vagus and exercise. *Physiology* **2019**, *34*, 71–80. [CrossRef] [PubMed]
19. Kannankeril, P.J.; Le, F.K.; Kadish, A.H.; Goldberger, J.J. Parasympathetic Effects on Heart Rate Recovery after Exercise. *J. Investig. Med.* **2004**, *52*, 394–401. [CrossRef] [PubMed]
20. Facioli, T.P.; Philbois, S.V.; Gastaldi, A.C.; Almeida, D.S.; Maida, K.D.; Rodrigues, J.A.L.; Sanchez-Delgado, J.C.; Souza, H.C.D. Study of heart rate recovery and cardiovascular autonomic modulation in healthy participants after submaximal exercise. *Sci. Rep.* **2021**, *11*, 3620. [CrossRef]
21. Roberto, S.; Milia, R.; Doneddu, A.; Pinna, V.; Palazzolo, G.; Serra, S.; Orrù, A.; Kakhak, S.A.H.; Ghiani, G.; Mulliri, G.; et al. Hemodynamic abnormalities during muscle metaboreflex activation in patients with type 2 diabetes mellitus. *J. Appl. Physiol.* **2019**, *126*, 444–453. [CrossRef]
22. Smarz, K.; Tysarowski, M.; Zaborska, B.; Pilichowska-Paszkiet, E.; Sikora-Frac, M.; Budaj, A.; Jaxa-Chamiec, T. Chronotropic incompetence limits aerobic exercise capacity in patients taking beta-blockers: Real-life observation of consecutive patients. *Healthcare* **2021**, *9*, 212. [CrossRef] [PubMed]
23. Cole, C.R.; Foody, J.M.; Blackstone, E.H.; Lauer, M.S. Heart Rate Recovery after Submaximal Exercise Testing as a Predictor of Mortality in a Cardiovascularly Healthy Cohort. *Ann. Intern. Med.* **2000**, *132*, 552–555. [CrossRef] [PubMed]

24. Hossri, C.A.C.; Araujo, F.; Baldi, B.; Otterstetter, R.; Uemoto, V.; Carvalho, C.; Mastrocola, L.; Albuquerque, A. Association among cardiopulmonary and metabolic rehabilitation, arrhythmias, and myocardial ischemia responses of patients with HFpEF or HFmrEF. *Braz. J. Med. Biol. Res.* **2024**, *57*, e13174. [CrossRef]
25. Andrade, G.N.; Rodrigues, T.; Takada, J.; Braga, L.; Umeda, I.; Nascimento, J.; Pereira-Filho, P.; Grupi, C.; Salemi, V.; Jacob-Filho, W.; et al. Prolonged heart rate recovery time after 6-minute walk test is an independent risk factor for cardiac events in heart failure: A prospective cohort study. *Physiotherapy* **2022**, *114*, 77–84. [CrossRef] [PubMed]
26. Lindemberg, S.; Chermont, S.; Quintão, M.; Derossi, M.; Guilhon, S.; Bernardez, S.; Marchese, L.; Martins, W.; Nóbrega, A.C.L.; Mesquita, E.T. Heart Rate Recovery in the First Minute at the Six-Minute Walk Test in Patients with Heart Failure. *Arq. Bras. Cardiol.* **2014**, *102*, 279–287. [CrossRef] [PubMed]
27. Tanaka, S.; Miyamoto, T.; Mori, Y.; Harada, T.; Tasaki, H. Heart rate recovery is useful for evaluating the recovery of exercise tolerance in patients with heart failure and atrial fibrillation. *Heart Vessels* **2021**, *36*, 1551–1557. [CrossRef] [PubMed]
28. da Fonseca, G.W.P.; dos Santos, M.R.; de Souza, F.R.; da Costa, M.J.A.; von Haehling, S.; Takayama, L.; Pereira, R.M.R.; Negrão, C.E.; Anker, S.D.; Alves, M.J.d.N.N. Sympatho-Vagal Imbalance is Associated with Sarcopenia in Male Patients with Heart Failure. *Arq. Bras. Cardiol.* **2019**, *112*, 739–746. [CrossRef] [PubMed]
29. Youn, J.C.; Lee, H.S.; Choi, S.-W.; Han, S.-W.; Ryu, K.-H.; Shin, E.-C.; Kang, S.-M. Post-exercise heart rate recovery independently predicts clinical outcome in patients with acute decompensated heart failure. *PLoS ONE* **2016**, *11*, e0154534. [CrossRef] [PubMed]
30. Cahalin, L.P.; Arena, R.; Labate, V.; Bandera, F.; Guazzi, M. Predictors of abnormal heart rate recovery in patients with heart failure reduced and preserved ejection fraction. *Eur. J. Prev. Cardiol.* **2014**, *21*, 906–914. [CrossRef]
31. Yaylali, Y.T.; Fındıkoglu, G.; Yurtdas, M.; Konukcu, S.; Senol, H. The effects of baseline heart rate recovery normality and exercise training protocol on heart rate recovery in patients with heart failure. *Anatol. J. Cardiol.* **2015**, *15*, 727–734. [CrossRef]
32. Imamura, T.; Kinugawa, K.; Okada, I.; Kato, N.; Fujino, T.; Inaba, T.; Maki, H.; Hatano, M.; Kinoshita, O.; Nawata, K.; et al. Parasympathetic Reinnervation Accompanied by Improved Post-Exercise Heart Rate Recovery and Quality of Life in Heart Transplant Recipients. *Int. Heart J.* **2015**, *56*, 180–185. [CrossRef] [PubMed]
33. Hajdusek, P.; Kotrc, M.; Kautzner, J.; Melenovsky, V.; Benesova, E.; Jarolim, P.; Benes, J. Heart rate response to exercise in heart failure patients: The prognostic role of metabolic–chronotropic relation and heart rate recovery. *Int. J. Cardiol.* **2017**, *228*, 588–593. [CrossRef] [PubMed]
34. Carneiro, H.A.; Song, R.J.; Lee, J.; Schwartz, B.; Vasan, R.S.; Xanthakis, V. Association of Blood Pressure and Heart Rate Responses to Submaximal Exercise with Incident Heart Failure: The Framingham Heart Study. *J. Am. Heart Assoc.* **2021**, *10*, e019460. [CrossRef] [PubMed]
35. Cozlac, A.-R.; Petrescu, L.; Crisan, S.; Luca, C.T.; Vacarescu, C.; Streian, C.G.; Lazar, M.-A.; Gurgu, A.; Dragomir, A.; Goanta, E.V.; et al. A Novel and Simple Exercise Test Parameter to Assess Responsiveness to Cardiac Resynchronization Therapy. *Diagnostics* **2020**, *10*, 920. [CrossRef] [PubMed]
36. Peçanha, T.; Bartels, R.; Brito, L.C.; Paula-Ribeiro, M.; Oliveira, R.S.; Goldberger, J.J. Methods of assessment of the post-exercise cardiac autonomic recovery: A methodological review. *Int. J. Cardiol.* **2017**, *227*, 795–802. [CrossRef] [PubMed]
37. Sydó, N.; Sydó, T.; Merkely, B.; Carta, K.G.; Murphy, J.G.; Lopez-Jimenez, F.; Allison, T.G. Impaired Heart Rate Response to Exercise in Diabetes and Its Long-term Significance. *Mayo Clin. Proc.* **2016**, *91*, 157–165. [CrossRef] [PubMed]
38. Alihanoglu, Y.I.; Yildiz, B.S.; Kilic, I.D.; Uludag, B.; Demirci, E.E.; Zungur, M.; Evrengul, H.; Kaftan, A.H. Impaired systolic blood pressure recovery and heart rate recovery after graded exercise in patients with metabolic syndrome. *Medicine* **2015**, *94*, e428. [CrossRef] [PubMed]
39. Maeder, M.T.; Ammann, P.; Schoch, O.D.; Rickli, H.; Korte, W.; Hürny, C.; Myers, J.; Münzer, T. Determinants of postexercise heart rate recovery in patients with the obstructive sleep apnea syndrome. *Chest* **2010**, *137*, 310–317. [CrossRef] [PubMed]
40. Shim, C.Y. Stress Testing in Heart Failure with Preserved Ejection Fraction. *Heart Fail Clin.* **2021**, *17*, 435–445. [CrossRef]
41. Vukomanovic, V.; Suzic-Lazic, J.; Celic, V.; Cuspidi, C.; Grassi, G.; Galderisi, M.; Djukic, V.; Tadic, M. Is there association between left atrial function and functional capacity in patients with uncomplicated type 2 diabetes? *Int. J. Cardiovasc. Imaging* **2020**, *36*, 15–22. [CrossRef]
42. Tadic, M.; Suzic-Lazic, J.; Vukomanovic, V.; Cuspidi, C.; Ilic, S.; Celic, V. Functional capacity and left ventricular diastolic function in patients with type 2 diabetes. *Acta Diabetol.* **2021**, *58*, 107–113. [CrossRef] [PubMed]
43. Lin, Y.T.; Lin, L.Y.; Chuang, K.J. N terminal prohormone of brain natriuretic peptide is associated with improved heart rate recovery after treadmill exercise test. *Int. J. Cardiol. Cardiovasc. Risk Prev.* **2023**, *18*, 200203. [CrossRef] [PubMed]
44. van de Vegte, Y.J.; van der Harst, P.; Verweij, N. Heart rate recovery 10 seconds after cessation of exercise predicts death. *J. Am. Heart Assoc.* **2018**, *7*, e008341. [CrossRef] [PubMed]
45. Giannitsi, S.; Bougiakli, M.; Bechlioulis, A.; Kotsia, A.; Michalis, L.K.; Naka, K.K. 6-minute walking test: A useful tool in the management of heart failure patients. *Ther. Adv. Cardiovasc. Dis.* **2019**, *13*, 1–10. [CrossRef] [PubMed]
46. Ren, C.; Zhu, J.; Shen, T.; Song, Y.; Tao, L.; Xu, S.; Zhao, W.; Gao, W. Comparison Between Treadmill and Bicycle Ergometer Exercises in Terms of Safety of Cardiopulmonary Exercise Testing in Patients with Coronary Heart Disease. *Front. Cardiovasc. Med.* **2022**, *9*, 864637. [CrossRef]
47. Irfanullah, M.W.; Yaqoob, N.; Shah, S.; Tariq, I.; Chaudhary, F.; Ibrahim, U.; Huma, Z.E.; Khan, N. Effects of Cycle Ergometer Training on Heart Rate Recovery and Mind Fullness in NYHA class I, II Heart Failure Patients. *Pak. J. Med. Health Sci.* **2023**, *17*, 10–13. [CrossRef]

48. Bozkurt, B.; Coats, A.J.; Tsutsui, H.; Abdelhamid, M.; Adamopoulos, S.; Albert, N.; Anker, S.D.; Atherton, J.; Böhm, M.; Butler, J.; et al. Universal definition and classification of heart failure: A report of the Heart Failure Society of America, Heart Failure Association of the European Society of Cardiology, Japanese Heart Failure Society and Writing Committee of the Universal Definition of Heart Failure: Endorsed by the Canadian Heart Failure Society, Heart Failure Association of India, Cardiac Society of Australia and New Zealand, and Chinese Heart Failure Association. *Eur. J. Heart Fail.* **2021**, *23*, 352–380. [CrossRef]
49. Maldonado-Martín, S.; Brubaker, P.H.; Ozemek, C.; Jayo-Montoya, J.A.; Becton, J.T.; Kitzman, D.W. Impact of β-Blockers on Heart Rate and Oxygen Uptake During Exercise and Recovery in Older Patients with Heart Failure With Preserved Ejection Fraction. *J. Cardiopulm. Rehabil. Prev.* **2020**, *40*, 174. [CrossRef]
50. Skaluba, S.J.; Litwin, S.E. Doppler-derived left ventricular filling pressures and the regulation of heart rate recovery after exercise in patients with suspected coronary artery disease. *Am. J. Cardiol.* **2005**, *95*, 832–837. [CrossRef]
51. Gharacholou, S.M.; Scott, C.G.; Borlaug, B.A.; Kane, G.C.; McCully, R.B.; Oh, J.K.; Pellikka, P.A. Relationship between diastolic function and heart rate recovery after symptom-limited exercise. *J. Card. Fail.* **2012**, *18*, 34–40. [CrossRef]
52. Mashayekhi, B.; Mohseni-Badalabadi, R.; Hosseinsabet, A.; Ahmadian, T. Correlation between Heart rate recovery and Left Atrial phasic functions evaluated by 2D speckle-tracking Echocardiography after Acute Myocardial infarction. *BMC Cardiovasc. Disord.* **2023**, *23*, 164. [CrossRef] [PubMed]
53. Arshi, B.; Geurts, S.; Tilly, M.J.; Berg, M.v.D.; Kors, J.A.; Rizopoulos, D.; Ikram, M.A.; Kavousi, M. Heart rate variability is associated with left ventricular systolic, diastolic function and incident heart failure in the general population. *BMC Med.* **2022**, *20*, 91. [CrossRef] [PubMed]
54. Tsai, C.H.; Ma, H.-P.; Hung, C.-S.; Huang, S.-H.; Chuang, B.-L.; Lin, C.; Lo, M.-T.; Peng, C.-K.; Lin, Y.-H. Usefulness of heart rhythm complexity in heart failure detection and diagnosis. *Sci. Rep.* **2020**, *10*, 14916. [CrossRef]
55. Lahiri, M.K.; Kannankeril, P.J.; Goldberger, J.J. Assessment of Autonomic Function in Cardiovascular Disease. Physiological Basis and Prognostic Implications. *J. Am. Coll. Cardiol.* **2008**, *51*, 1725–1733. [CrossRef]
56. Julario, R.; Mulia, E.P.B.; Rachmi, D.A.; A'yun, M.Q.; Septianda, I.; Dewi, I.P.; Juwita, R.R.; Dharmadjati, B.B. Evaluation of heart rate variability using 24-hour Holter electrocardiography in hypertensive patients. *J. Arrhythm.* **2021**, *37*, 157–164. [CrossRef]
57. Bechke, E.; Kliszczewicz, B.; McLester, C.; Tillman, M.; Esco, M.; Lopez, R. An examination of single day vs. multi-day heart rate variability and its relationship to heart rate recovery following maximal aerobic exercise in females. *Sci. Rep.* **2020**, *10*, 14760. [CrossRef]
58. Vacarescu, C.; Luca, C.-T.; Feier, H.; Gaiță, D.; Crișan, S.; Negru, A.-G.; Iurciuc, S.; Goanță, E.-V.; Mornos, C.; Lazăr, M.-A.; et al. Betablockers and Ivabradine Titration According to Exercise Test in LV Only Fusion CRT Pacing. *Diagnostics* **2022**, *12*, 1096. [CrossRef]
59. Fiuza-Luces, C.; Santos-Lozano, A.; Joyner, M.; Carrera-Bastos, P.; Picazo, O.; Zugaza, J.L.; Izquierdo, M.; Ruilope, L.M.; Lucia, A. Exercise benefits in cardiovascular disease: Beyond attenuation of traditional risk factors. *Nat. Rev. Cardiol.* **2018**, *15*, 731–743. [CrossRef]
60. Sardu, C.; Massetti, M.M.; Rambaldi, P.; Gatta, G.; Cappabianca, S.; Sasso, F.C.; Santamaria, M.; Volpicelli, M.; Ducceschi, V.; Signoriello, G.; et al. SGLT2-inhibitors reduce the cardiac autonomic neuropathy dysfunction and vaso-vagal syncope recurrence in patients with type 2 diabetes mellitus: The SCAN study. *Metabolism* **2022**, *137*, 155243. [CrossRef] [PubMed]
61. van Bilsen, M.; Patel, H.C.; Bauersachs, J.; Böhm, M.; Borggrefe, M.; Brutsaert, D.; Coats, A.J.; de Boer, R.A.; de Keulenaer, G.W.; Filippatos, G.S.; et al. The autonomic nervous system as a therapeutic target in heart failure: A scientific position statement from the Translational Research Committee of the Heart Failure Association of the European Society of Cardiology. *Eur. J. Heart Fail.* **2017**, *19*, 1361–1378. [CrossRef]
62. Franssen, W.M.A.; Beyens, M.; Al Hatawe, T.; Frederix, I.; Verboven, K.; Dendale, P.; Eijnde, B.O.; Massa, G.; Hansen, D. Cardiac function in adolescents with obesity: Cardiometabolic risk factors and impact on physical fitness. *Int. J. Obes.* **2019**, *43*, 1400–1410. [CrossRef] [PubMed]
63. Ackland, G.L.; Minto, G.; Clark, M.; Whittle, J.; Stephens, R.C.; Owen, T.; Prabhu, P.; del Arroyo, A.G. Autonomic regulation of systemic inflammation in humans: A multi-center, blinded observational cohort study. *Brain Behav. Immun.* **2018**, *67*, 47–53. [CrossRef] [PubMed]
64. Teodoru, M.; Negrea, M.O.; Cozgarea, A.; Cozma, D.; Boicean, A. Enhancing Pulmonary Embolism Mortality Risk Stratification Using Machine Learning: The Role of the Neutrophil-to-Lymphocyte Ratio. *J. Clin. Med.* **2024**, *13*, 1191. [CrossRef] [PubMed]
65. Adamo, L.; Rocha-Resende, C.; Prabhu, S.D.; Mann, D.L. Reappraising the role of inflammation in heart failure. *Nat. Rev. Cardiol.* **2020**, *17*, 269–285. [CrossRef] [PubMed]
66. Rachieru, C.; Luca, C.T.; Văcărescu, C.; Petrescu, L.; Cirin, L.; Cozma, D. Future Perspectives to Improve CHA2 DS2 VASc Score: The Role of Left Atrium Remodelling, Inflammation and Genetics in Anticoagulation of Atrial Fibrillation. *Clin. Interv. Aging* **2023**, *18*, 1737–1748. [CrossRef]
67. da Fonseca, R.X.; da Cruz, C.J.G.; Soares, E.M.K.V.K.; Garcia, G.L.; Porto, L.G.G.; Molina, G.E. Post-exercise heart rate recovery and its speed are associated with resting-reactivity cardiovagal modulation in healthy women. *Sci. Rep.* **2024**, *14*, 5526. [CrossRef]

Disclaimer/Publisher's Note: The statements, opinions and data contained in all publications are solely those of the individual author(s) and contributor(s) and not of MDPI and/or the editor(s). MDPI and/or the editor(s) disclaim responsibility for any injury to people or property resulting from any ideas, methods, instructions or products referred to in the content.

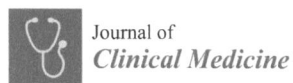 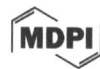

Article

Impact of Newly Diagnosed Left Bundle Branch Block on Long-Term Outcomes in Patients with STEMI

Larisa Anghel [1,2], Cristian Stătescu [1,2,*], Radu Andy Sascău [1,2,*], Bogdan-Sorin Tudurachi [1,2], Andreea Tudurachi [2], Laura-Cătălina Benchea [1,2], Cristina Prisacariu [1,2] and Rodica Radu [1,2]

[1] Internal Medicine Department, "Grigore T. Popa" University of Medicine and Pharmacy, 700503 Iași, Romania; larisa.anghel@umfiasi.ro (L.A.); bogdan-sorin.tudurachi@d.umfiasi.ro (B.-S.T.); benchea.laura-catalina@d.umfiasi.ro (L.-C.B.); cristina.prisacariu@umfiasi.ro (C.P.); rodica.radu@umfiasi.ro (R.R.)

[2] Cardiology Department, Cardiovascular Diseases Institute "Prof. Dr. George I. M. Georgescu", 700503 Iași, Romania; leonteandreea32@gmail.com

* Correspondence: cristian.statescu@umfiasi.ro (C.S.); radu.sascau@umfiasi.ro (R.A.S.); Tel.: +40-0232-211834 (C.S.)

Abstract: Background/Objectives: This study assessed the long-term prognostic implications of newly developed left bundle branch block (LBBB) in patients with ST-elevation myocardial infarction (STEMI) and a single coronary lesion, following primary percutaneous coronary intervention (PCI). **Methods:** Among 3526 patients admitted with acute myocardial infarction between January 2011 and December 2013, 42 were identified with STEMI, a single coronary lesion, and newly diagnosed LBBB. A control group of 42 randomly selected STEMI patients without LBBB was also included. All participants were prospectively evaluated with a median follow-up duration of 9.4 years. Demographic, clinical, and laboratory data were analyzed to assess the impact of LBBB on long-term outcomes. **Results:** The baseline characteristics were similar between the groups. The STEMI with new LBBB group had significantly higher rates of new myocardial infarction, revascularization, and mortality, highlighting the severe prognostic implications and elevated risk for adverse outcomes compared to STEMI without LBBB. The multivariate Cox regression analysis demonstrated that the presence of LBBB (HR: 2.15, 95% CI: 1.28–3.62, $p = 0.003$), lower LVEF (HR: 1.45, 95% CI: 1.22–1.72, $p < 0.001$), and longer pain-to-admission time (HR: 1.32, 95% CI: 1.09–1.61, $p = 0.008$) were significant independent predictors of adverse outcomes. **Conclusions:** Newly acquired LBBB in STEMI patients is associated with poorer long-term outcomes. Early identification and management of factors such as reduced LVEF and timely hospital admission, specifically in patients with new-onset LBBB, can improve prognosis.

Keywords: STEMI; new left bundle branch block; heart failure; long-term outcomes; percutaneous coronary intervention; prognostic; prospective study

Citation: Anghel, L.; Stătescu, C.; Sascău, R.A.; Tudurachi, B.-S.; Tudurachi, A.; Benchea, L.-C.; Prisacariu, C.; Radu, R. Impact of Newly Diagnosed Left Bundle Branch Block on Long-Term Outcomes in Patients with STEMI. *J. Clin. Med.* **2024**, *13*, 5479. https://doi.org/10.3390/jcm13185479

Academic Editor: Zhibing Lu

Received: 13 August 2024
Revised: 11 September 2024
Accepted: 13 September 2024
Published: 15 September 2024

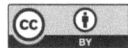

Copyright: © 2024 by the authors. Licensee MDPI, Basel, Switzerland. This article is an open access article distributed under the terms and conditions of the Creative Commons Attribution (CC BY) license (https://creativecommons.org/licenses/by/4.0/).

1. Introduction

Acute myocardial infarction with ST-segment elevation (STEMI), one of the most prevalent causes of death and morbidity worldwide, is a life-threatening disorder that requires prompt diagnosis and is frequently the early clinical manifestation of cardiovascular disease. In the assessment of individuals with STEMI, the resting 12-lead electrocardiogram (ECG) serves as the primary diagnostic tool. It is recommended that the ECG results be interpreted as promptly as possible at the first medical contact, ideally within 10 min [1]. Beyond the importance of analyzing the ischemic findings, it is necessary to assess the existence of various conduction disturbances that may occur in the setting of acute coronary syndromes. This is because alterations in the QRS duration and pattern are considered to indicate more acute ischemia and a faster progression of myocardial necrosis compared to changes in the ST-segment alone [2–4].

The American Heart Association (AHA) and European Society of Cardiology (ESC) acknowledge the challenge of diagnosing STEMI in the presence of left bundle branch block (LBBB) and determining whether the LBBB is recent or pre-existing, especially when there is no prior electrocardiogram available for comparison [1,5]. Recent studies observed that individuals with bundle branch block (BBB) who had acute myocardial infarction (AMI) had a higher prevalence of three-vessel and left main disease. Also, the occurrence of pulmonary edema, cardiogenic shock, and significant adverse cardiac events is greater in these patients [6,7]. However, other studies revealed no significant associations between the presence of new permanent LBBB or RBBB and the severity of coronary artery atherosclerosis, as measured by Gensini Score (GS) [8].

In the realm of cardiology, the onset of a new LBBB in patients with STEMI represents a pivotal diagnostic and prognostic marker. This study delves into the long-term impact of new LBBB on the incidence of heart failure among STEMI patients, a topic that has garnered attention due to its significant implications for patient outcomes and management strategies.

Our objective was to quantify the specific impact of newly developed LBBB on the long-term prognosis of patients with STEMI and a single coronary lesion who underwent primary percutaneous coronary intervention (PCI). We focused on assessing the prognostic significance of LBBB in terms of mortality risk and the development of heart failure, with the goal of aiding clinicians in optimizing treatment strategies and enhancing patient outcomes.

2. Materials and Methods

2.1. Patient Recruitment

This is a prospective observational study, conducted at a primary PCI academic hospital in Eastern Romania, the only hospital in the region with 24 h primary PCI. The study specifically focused on patients aged 18 years or older who met the criteria for STEMI, as defined by the fourth myocardial infarction classification, and a single atherosclerotic coronary lesion [1]. Patients were enrolled consecutively over the study period to minimize selection bias and ensure a representative sample. The inclusion criteria were refined to include only patients with acute STEMI who presented within 12 h of symptom onset. Considering that our hospital is the only primary PCI hospital in the region with 24 h primary PCI services, and given the significant distances between primary PCI centers in this area, we included patients who presented at more than 12 h after symptom onset, but only in the presence of ongoing symptoms suggestive of ischemia, hemodynamic instability, or life-threatening arrhythmias. This inclusion was necessary to reflect real-world clinical practice in our region, where delayed presentation is common due to geographic constraints. STEMI was defined by standard ECG criteria (ST-segment elevation in at least two contiguous leads) and elevated cardiac biomarkers. All participants underwent a prospective evaluation with a median follow-up of 9.4 years. Throughout this period, various biological parameters were assessed to examine the impact of an acute coronary event on lifestyle changes and to evaluate the predictive value of newly developed left bundle branch block (LBBB) regarding mortality and heart failure onset. Patients with type 2 myocardial infarction, defined as myocardial ischemia due to an imbalance between oxygen supply and demand without coronary artery occlusion, as well as those with a prior history of STEMI, PCI, or coronary artery bypass grafting, were excluded from the study (Figure 1).

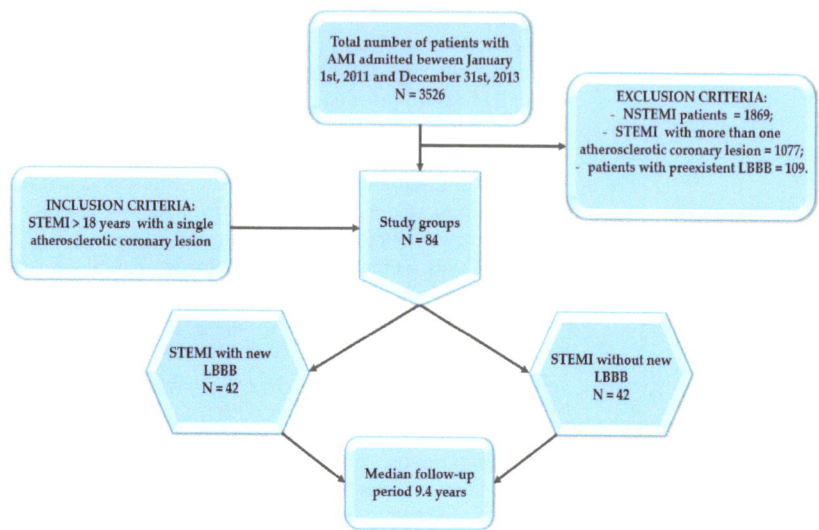

Figure 1. Study flow. AMI, acute myocardial infarction; LBBB, left bundle branch block; NSTEMI, acute myocardial infarction without ST-segment elevation; STEMI, acute myocardial infarction with ST-segment elevation.

2.2. Data Collection Method

All study participants were interviewed during their hospitalization to document their cardiovascular risk factors. Special attention was placed on accurately recording the precise onset time of chest pain related to acute myocardial infarction. A family history of premature coronary artery disease was defined as the occurrence of sudden death or coronary artery disease in first-degree male relatives under 55 years of age or in first-degree female relatives under 65 years of age.

Peripheral blood samples were collected immediately upon admission of patients to the emergency department or before the urgent coronary angiography, in order to determine the blood cell counts, biochemical analysis of lipids (total cholesterol, low-density lipoprotein cholesterol (LDLc), high-density lipoprotein cholesterol (HDLc), triglycerides), myocardial cytolysis markers (myocardial creatine kinase (CK-MB) and troponin T), glucose metabolism, aspartate aminotransferase (AST), alanine aminotransferase (ALT), and renal function analysis. The glycemic status of the patients was determined using criteria established by the European Diabetes Society: 1. normal glycemic control, defined as fasting blood glucose (FPG) levels below 5.6 mmol/L (100 mg/dL). 2. A diabetes diagnosis was made if patients had two FPG values equal to or greater than 7.0 mmol/L (126 mg/dL) (venous plasma glucose). Patients were classified as diabetic if they had a known history of diabetes, fasting blood glucose levels of 126 mg/dL or higher, or were receiving treatment with oral antidiabetic medications or insulin. These criteria were employed to assess and categorize the glycemic status of the patients in the study [9]. Hypertension was defined as blood pressure measurements equal to or exceeding 140/90 mmHg or a documented history of previous antihypertensive treatment [10]. Body mass index (BMI = weight in kg/height^2 in m^2) and smoking status were also evaluated. Obesity was defined as BMI $\geq$ 30 kg/m^2.

Electrocardiographic recognition of myocardial infarction in patients with LBBB poses challenges in the emergency department due to the masking effect of ST-segment deviations inherent in LBBB. Various diagnostic criteria have been proposed over the years to aid clinicians in making accurate diagnoses in such cases, with the Sgarbossa criteria being the most widely recognized. The original Sgarbossa criteria require at least 3 points to diagnose STEMI in the presence of LBBB, based on the following: (1) concordant ST-segment elevation of 1 mm or more in at least one lead (5 points); (2) ST-segment depression of 1 mm or more in leads V1-V3 (3 points); and (3) discordant ST-segment elevation of more than 5 mm in at least one lead (2 points). To enhance both sensitivity and specificity, achieving 91% and 90%, respectively, Smith et al. modified the Sgarbossa criteria, and replaced the absolute ST-segment elevation criterion with a relative ST/S ratio of less than 0.25 [3,4]. Patients were classified as having newly developed LBBB if the condition was documented on the initial electrocardiogram at admission, and this condition persisted at the patient's discharge, without any prior history of LBBB, as confirmed by reviewing previous ECGs when available. Patients with myocardial infarction without prior ECG data were excluded to ensure accurate classification and to include only those with definitively new-onset LBBB. This approach was employed to maintain the accuracy of the classification and the reliability of our findings regarding the impact of new LBBB on long-term outcomes in STEMI patients.

All patients underwent echocardiographic evaluation, with left ventricular ejection fraction (LVEF) measured using the biplane method of discs, based on the modified Simpson's rule [11].

All patients included in the study underwent cardiac catheterization, and coronary artery stenosis was considered to be present when there was a reduction in the lumen diameter of any of the three coronary arteries or their main branches by more than 50%. The culprit lesion was identified based on angiographic findings consistent with acute thrombus or plaque rupture in a single coronary artery. Coronary arteries with smooth contours and without focal diameter reduction, or those with atherosclerotic lesions causing less than 50% stenosis, were classified as "normal". Importantly, patients with normal coronaries or non-obstructive disease were excluded from the analysis. Patients with more than one coronary lesion were likely excluded from the study, based on the standard definition of multi-vessel disease, which is defined as stenosis of ≥50% in more than one major coronary artery on coronary angiography. The rationale behind this exclusion was to focus the analysis on single-vessel disease to maintain homogeneity and to reduce confounding variables related to multi-vessel involvement. Also, by excluding patients with multiple lesions, the study aimed to reduce variability in clinical presentation and treatment responses, thus allowing for clearer analysis and comparison between patients with and without new-onset left bundle branch block. These patients were then treated according to established protocols, which involved the placement of second-generation drug-eluting stents. The PCI was customized to suit the coronary anatomy and clinical condition of each individual patient. Following the PCI, all patients received standard treatment regimens that adhered to established guidelines. This included contemporary antiplatelet therapy and standard-dose statin therapy. After discharge, patients were routinely monitored and followed up at the clinic. This comprehensive approach aimed to provide optimal care and management for patients with STEMI.

2.3. Follow-Up and Outcomes

During the study, all participants were prospectively evaluated over a median follow-up period lasting 9.4 years. Follow-up assessments were conducted through in-person visits to the clinic. All patients were followed until the study's completion. The primary endpoint of the study was the incidence of major adverse cardiac and cerebrovascular events (MACEs), defined as a composite of the following outcomes: cardiac mortality (death attributed to cardiac causes), recurrent myocardial infarction (new infarction occurring in the previously treated target vessel), stroke (including both fatal and non-fatal ischemic strokes), and target vessel revascularization (any repeat percutaneous or surgical intervention on the previously treated vessel) [1–3,9]. The secondary endpoint of the study aimed to assess the predictive significance of the newly acquired LBBB in terms of both mortality and the development of heart failure.

The study adhered to the principles of the Declaration of Helsinki and its subsequent revisions, as approved by the hospital's Ethics Committee. Patient data were anonymized, and informed consent for the use of personal information was obtained at the time of hospital admission, ensuring compliance with ethical standards and safeguarding patient confidentiality throughout the research.

2.4. Statistical Analysis

First, the normality of the distribution of numerical variables was assessed using the Kolmogorov–Smirnov test. Parametric variables were analyzed with an independent sample t-test, while non-parametric variables were evaluated using the Mann–Whitney U test. Categorical data were compared using the chi-square or Fisher's exact test as appropriate. A multivariate Cox proportional hazards regression analysis was conducted to identify independent predictors of MACEs. The analysis incorporated key variables, including the presence of LBBB, left ventricular ejection fraction, pain-to-admission time, age, and relevant comorbidities such as diabetes, hypertension, and chronic kidney disease. Initially, each variable was independently analyzed to determine its association with MACE. Variables with a p-value of less than 0.05 in the univariate analysis were included in the multivariate Cox regression model. The final Cox regression model was employed to identify independent predictors while accounting for potential confounding factors. The results are presented as hazard ratios (HRs) with 95% confidence intervals (CIs). All statistical analyses were performed using the IBM SPSS statistics version 26.

3. Results

Among the 3526 patients admitted with acute myocardial infarction between 1 January 2011 and 31 December 2013, 42 had STEMI with a single coronary lesion and newly diagnosed LBBB. To ensure comparability, a control group of 42 patients with STEMI but without LBBB was randomly selected.

All participants underwent prospective evaluation over a median follow-up period of 9.4 years. During this follow-up, different biological parameters were assessed to investigate the impact of an acute coronary event on lifestyle modifications. Additionally, the study aimed to determine the prognostic significance of newly acquired LBBB in terms of mortality and the development of heart failure.

3.1. Patient Characteristics at Baseline

The demographic characteristics, medical history, and admission hemodynamics of the patients were analyzed to determine if there were any significant differences between the groups. The median age of patients with STEMI and new LBBB was 67 years (range 52–83), while for those without LBBB, it was 66 years (range 40–81) with a p-value of 0.864, indicating no significant difference. The percentage of female patients was 38.9% in the LBBB group and 33.3% in the control group ($p = 0.760$). This balance in gender distribution helps in isolating the effect of LBBB on outcomes, as gender differences in myocardial infarction can influence prognosis.

Regarding the medical history and admission hemodynamics, there were no significant differences, indicating that the groups were comparable at baseline. The median pain-to-admission time for patients was 9 h (interquartile range [IQR]: 3–13 h) in STEMI with new LBBB and 10 h (IQR: 2–15 h) in patients with STEMI without LBBB. This similarity suggests that both patient groups experienced similar delays from the onset of symptoms to hospital admission. Also, there was a consistency in the location of myocardial infarction between the groups, and more than half of the patients had anterior myocardial infarction. In our study, all procedures were performed via the femoral approach. The interventions were carried out by a team of highly trained and experienced interventional cardiologists, ensuring standardized and expert care throughout the study. All patients underwent successful PCI, with drug-eluting stents, and with a procedural success rate of 100%. Only one patient with new LBBB presented a local hematoma as a post-procedural complication, without significant hemoglobin loss. By ensuring that the two patient cohorts are well-matched at baseline, the study provides a robust platform for investigating the specific effects of newly acquired LBBB on the long-term outcomes of STEMI patients.

Table 1 presents the baseline characteristics of the two groups.

Table 1. Patient characteristics at baseline.

Variable	STEMI with New LBBB (n = 42 Patients)	STEMI without LBBB (n = 42 Patients)	p-Value
Demographic characteristics			
Age, median (IQR), years	67 (52–83)	66 (40–81)	0.864
Female	38.09%	33.33%	0.760
Rural area	40.47%	35.71%	0.630
Medical history			
Hypertension	69.04%	66.66%	0.822
Diabetes	28.57%	23.80%	0.869
Dyslipidemia	71.42%	66.66%	0.814
Heart failure	23.80%	16.66%	0.685
Atrial fibrillation	2.38%	4.76%	0.820
Chronic kidney disease	7.14%	9.52%	0.856
Pain-to-admission time (hours)			
<6 h	16.66%	14.28%	0.565
6–12 h	71.42%	76.19%	0.905
>12 h	11.90%	9.52%	0.824
Admission hemodynamics			
Killip > I	23.80%	19.04%	0.855
Anterior location	54.76%	57.14%	0.780
LVEF (%)	43%	45%	0.856
Ventricular arrhythmias	2.38%	4.76%	0.895
In-hospital outcomes			
Median hospital stay (days)	9 (6–11)	6 (5–9)	**0.048**
Atrial fibrillation	7.14%	4.76%	0.780
Third-degree atrioventricular block	2.38%	0%	0.855

LBBB, left bundle branch block; LVEF, left ventricular ejection fraction; STEMI, acute myocardial infarction with ST-segment elevation.

3.2. Laboratory Characteristics

The results reveal notable differences and trends that provide insights into the long-term outcomes and management of these patient groups (Table 2).

The hemoglobin and hematocrit levels showed a general trend of slight decline in both patient groups over time. These trends could suggest a mild, chronic anemia or hemodilution developing over time, potentially due to long-term medication use or underlying chronic conditions. A significant reduction in white blood cell counts was observed in both groups, reflecting a possible reduction in systemic inflammation over time. Platelet counts also declined, which might reflect effects of antiplatelet therapies commonly prescribed to these patients.

Table 2. Laboratory characteristics.

Variable	STEMI with New LBBB (n = 42 Patients) Mean ± S.D.		p-Value	STEMI without LBBB (n = 42 Patients) Mean ± S.D.		p-Value
	Baseline	Follow-Up (Median 9.6 Years)		Baseline	Follow-Up (Median 9.2 Years)	
Hemoglobin (g/dL)	13.80 ± 1.37	13.44 ± 1.44	0.247	14.58 ± 1.28	14.20 ± 1.40	0.201
Hematocrit (%)	43.65 ± 5.6	42.55 ± 6.7	0.419	46.55 ± 4.8	44.50 ± 6.6	0.111
Platelets (mm^3)	285.200 ± 11,500	275,000 ± 10,340	<0.001	245,000 ± 10,680	234,050 ± 10,450	<0.001
White blood cells (mm^3)	14,500 ± 1065	10.230 ± 1050	<0.001	12,350 ± 1055	10,050 ± 1060	<0.001
LDL cholesterol (mg/dL)	116.9 ± 49.5	87.79 ± 31.1	0.002	123.4 ± 49.16	104.19 ± 26.3	0.031
Creatinine (mg/dL)	1.1 ± 0.4	0.9 ± 0.6	0.080	1.2 ± 0.8	1.0 ± 0.5	0.177
Uric acid (mg/dL)	6.9 ± 0.9	6.2 ± 0.8	0.001	7.1 ± 0.8	6.7 ± 0.8	0.027
Glycemia (mg/dL)	123 ± 43	106 ± 23	0.029	107 ± 11	102 ± 31	0.330

LDL, low-density lipoprotein; LBBB, left bundle branch block; STEMI, acute myocardial infarction with ST-segment elevation.

LDL cholesterol levels showed a substantial decrease in both groups, from 116.9 ± 49.5 to 87.79 ± 31.1 mg/dL, $p = 0.002$ in the LBBB group, and from 123.4 ± 49.16 to 104.19 ± 26.3 mg/dL, $p = 0.031$ in the non-LBBB group. This significant reduction highlights the effectiveness of lipid-lowering therapies and dietary modifications in managing cardiovascular risk factors over the long term, with a better control in patients with LBBB.

Both creatinine and uric acid levels decreased over the follow-up period, suggesting improved renal function or better control of metabolic factors through medication and lifestyle changes. This also might reflect better management of conditions like hypertension and gout, often associated with elevated uric acid.

Glycemic control also showed improvement in both groups, which also indicates successful long-term management of blood glucose levels, possibly through medication, diet, and lifestyle interventions.

3.3. Long-Term Outcomes

The presence of new LBBB in STEMI patients significantly influences both therapeutic strategies and prognostic outcomes (Table 3).

3.3.1. Treatment for Heart Failure

Patients with STEMI and new LBBB experienced significant improvements in heart failure management, particularly with the increased use of angiotensin receptor-neprilysin inhibitor/angiotensin-converting enzyme inhibitors/angiotensin II receptor blockers (ARNI/ACEi/ARB) and mineralocorticoid receptor antagonist (MRAs), reflecting a proactive approach in addressing the more severe cardiac dysfunction typically associated with LBBB. The substantial rise in the use of sodium-glucose cotransporter 2 (SGLT2) inhibitors (with 61.90% use for STEMI with new LBBB, $p < 0.001$, and 38.09% use for STEMI without LBBB, $p = 0.028$) in both groups indicates their growing importance in heart failure therapy, underscoring their benefits in reducing hospitalization rates and improving cardiovascular health.

Table 3. Long-term treatment and functional outcomes in patients with STEMI, with and without LBBB.

Variable	STEMI with New LBBB (n = 42 Patients)		p-Value	STEMI without LBBB (n = 42 Patients)		p-Value
	Baseline	Follow-Up (Median 9.6 Years)		Baseline	Follow-Up (Median 9.2 Years)	
Treatment for heart failure						
Beta-blockers	92.85%	85.71%	0.467	78.57%	85.71%	0.238
ARNI/ACEi/ARB	0/33.3/28.57%	42.85/7.14/4.76%	0.040	0/57.14/21.42%	38.09/4.76/19.04%	0.560
MRA	14.28%	21.42%	0.031	11.90%	14.28%	0.670
SGLT2i	0%	61.90%	<0.001	0%	38.09%	0.028
Diuretics	59.52%	40.47%	0.208	14.28%	11.90%	0.450
Left ventricular ejection fraction (%)						
<40%	30.95%	21.42%	<0.001	14.28%	7.14%	<0.001
40–50%	42.85%	52.38%	0.004	64.28%	54.76%	0.003
>50%	28.57%	26.19%	0.456	21.42%	38.09%	0.026
Heart failure						
NYHA I	2.38%	4.76%	0.445	4.76%	7.14%	0.767
NYHA II	30.95%	42.85%	0.003	23.80%	28.57%	0.522
NYHA III	7.14%	4.76%	0.767	4.76%	2.38%	0.445
NYHA IV	2.38%	0%	0.497	2.38%	0%	0.497

ARNI/ACEi/ARBs, angiotensin receptor-neprilysin inhibitor/angiotensin-converting enzyme inhibitors/angiotensin II receptor blockers; LBBB, left bundle branch block; MRA, mineralocorticoid receptor antagonist; NYHA, New York Heart Association; SGLT2i, sodium-glucose cotransporter 2 inhibitors; STEMI, acute myocardial infarction with ST-segment elevation.

The use of beta-blockers remained high in both groups but did not change significantly over time. This indicates that beta-blockers are a consistently integral part of heart failure management in STEMI patients regardless of the presence of LBBB.

3.3.2. Left Ventricular Ejection Fraction

The analysis of LVEF categories reveals significant shifts over the follow-up period, highlighting improvements in cardiac function. There was a significant decrease in the proportion of patients with severely reduced LVEF (<40%) in both groups. This improvement is indicative of successful heart failure management and potentially better myocardial recovery or remodeling. A significant increase in the proportion of patients with moderately reduced LVEF was observed in patients with STEMI and new LBBB (42.85% vs. 52.38%, $p = 0.004$). In the STEMI without LBBB group, the proportion of patients with preserved LVEF significantly increased (21.42% vs. 38.09%, $p = 0.026$). In contrast, no significant change was observed in the STEMI with new LBBB group (28.57% vs. 26.19%, $p = 0.456$). This shift suggests a transition of patients from severely to moderately impaired cardiac function, reflecting therapeutic efficacy and a better overall recovery in ventricular function among patients without LBBB.

Changes in New York Heart Association (NYHA) functional classification revealed an increase in moderate symptoms in STEMI with new LBBB (NYHA II, 30.95% vs. 42.85%, $p = 0.003$) and consistently low severe symptoms (NYHA IV) in both groups over time.

3.3.3. Outcomes

Long-term outcomes highlight significant differences between the two patient groups, reflecting varying degrees of clinical risk and prognosis (Table 4).

Table 4. Comparison of long-term outcomes in patients with STEMI with and without LBBB, at baseline and follow-up.

Variable	STEMI with New LBBB (n = 42 Patients)		p-Value	STEMI without LBBB (n = 42 Patients)		p-Value
	Baseline	Follow-Up (Median 9.6 Years)		Baseline	Follow-Up (Median 9.2 Years)	
			Outcomes			
Myocardial infarction	0	9.52%	<0.001	0	4.76%	0.059
Revascularization	0	9.52%	<0.001	0	4.76%	0.059
Stroke	0	4.76%	0.059	0	2.38%	0.497
Death	0	9.52%	<0.001	0	4.76%	0.059

LBBB, left bundle branch block; STEMI, acute myocardial infarction with ST-segment elevation.

The STEMI with new LBBB group experienced a significant increase in myocardial infarction ($p < 0.001$) and revascularization ($p < 0.001$), compared to the STEMI without LBBB group, indicating a higher risk for recurrent ischemic events and a greater need for interventional strategies. Additionally, there was a trend towards increased stroke incidence ($p = 0.059$) and significantly higher mortality ($p < 0.001$) in the STEMI with new LBBB group, underscoring the severe prognostic implications of new LBBB. In contrast, the STEMI without LBBB group showed no significant changes in these outcomes, suggesting a comparatively lower risk profile.

3.4. Predictors of Major Cardiovascular Event in Patients with STEMI and New LBBB

In patients with STEMI, it is very important to identify factors that may influence long-term outcomes.

A multivariate Cox regression analysis was performed to identify independent predictors of major cardiovascular events among STEMI patients with and without LBBB. Variables included in the model were LBBB presence, LVEF, pain-to-admission time, age, and key comorbidities such as diabetes, hypertension, and chronic kidney disease. Each variable was first evaluated independently to assess its association with major adverse cardiovascular events. Significant predictors ($p < 0.05$) were then included in the multivariate analysis. A Cox regression model was applied to identify independent predictors while adjusting for potential confounders. The analysis demonstrated that LBBB (HR: 2.15, 95% CI: 1.28–3.62, $p = 0.003$), lower LVEF (HR: 1.45, 95% CI: 1.22–1.72, $p < 0.001$), and longer pain-to-admission time (HR: 1.32, 95% CI: 1.09–1.61, $p = 0.008$) were significant independent predictors of adverse outcomes (Table 5).

Table 5. Univariate and multivariate Cox regression analysis to estimate predictors of MACE in STEMI patients with and without LBBB.

Variable	Univariate			Multivariate		
	HR	95% CI	p	HR	95% CI	p
LBBB presence	2.6	1.45–4.68	0.002	2.15	1.28–3.62	**0.003**
LVEF (%)	1.7	1.30–2.21	<0.001	1.45	1.22–1.72	**<0.001**
Pain-to-admission time (hours)	1.4	1.15–1.71	0.004	1.32	1.09–1.61	**0.008**
Age (years)	1.1	0.98–1.25	0.076	1.05	0.94–1.18	0.342
Diabetes	1.6	1.05–2.45	0.031	1.35	0.90–2.02	0.120
Hypertension	1.2	0.78–1.85	0.384	-	-	-
Chronic kidney disease	1.85	1.11–3.08	0.018	1.48	0.90–2.45	0.125

CI, confidence interval; HR, hazard ratio; LBBB, left bundle branch block; LVEF, left ventricular ejection fraction.

4. Discussion

The findings from this study underscore the critical differences in long-term management and outcomes between STEMI patients with new LBBB and those without LBBB. Patients with new LBBB demonstrated significant improvements in heart failure management, particularly with increased use of ARNI/ACEi/ARB and MRAs. However, they also faced higher risks of adverse outcomes, including myocardial infarction, revascularization, and mortality. These results suggest that while therapeutic advancements have improved heart failure management in these patients, the presence of new LBBB remains a marker of poor prognosis, necessitating vigilant monitoring and possibly more aggressive treatment strategies. Conversely, STEMI patients without LBBB showed better overall recovery in ventricular function and lower incidences of adverse outcomes, highlighting a comparatively more favorable long-term prognosis. In the multivariate analysis, the presence of LBBB was independently associated with a higher risk of major adverse cardiovascular events. Moreover, reduced left ventricular ejection fraction and longer pain-to-admission time were also identified as significant independent predictors of poor outcomes.

The baseline characteristics of the two groups were well-balanced, ensuring the reliability of our comparative analyses. There were no significant differences in age, gender distribution, medical history, or admission hemodynamics ($p > 0.05$ for all), which strengthens the reliability of our findings. The balanced distribution of demographic characteristics, comorbid conditions, and initial clinical presentation factors between the groups enhances the reliability of the study's findings regarding the prognostic impact of LBBB in STEMI patients. This thorough baseline matching allows for a clearer interpretation of the impact of LBBB on long-term outcomes, without being confounded by pre-existing differences between the groups. This careful methodological approach strengthens the validity of the study's conclusions and supports the clinical relevance of its findings. A relatively small number of patients present with newly developed LBBB in the context of an acute myocardial infarction. For example, in our study, only 1.2% of patients admitted with acute myocardial infarction had STEMI with a single coronary lesion and newly diagnosed LBBB. In a recent study conducted by the Minneapolis Heart Institute STEMI protocol, 3.3% of the patients had either new or apparently new LBBB. Patients with new LBBB were typically older, predominantly female, had lower ejection fractions, and experienced higher rates of cardiac arrest or heart failure compared to those without newly developed LBBB. Additionally, those with new LBBB had a lower incidence of identifiable culprit arteries (54.2% vs. 86.4%, $p < 0.001$). However, they showed a higher rate of all-cause mortality during the one-year follow-up [12]. We acknowledge that our findings offer valuable insights into the specific subgroup of STEMI patients with newly developed LBBB; however, further validation in larger, multicenter studies is required to confirm the broader applicability of these conclusions to the general STEMI population. Despite the limitation of a smaller sample size, our careful selection process and the well-balanced baseline characteristics between the groups help mitigate some concerns related to sample size, thereby enhancing the internal validity of our results.

Our longitudinal follow-up revealed important trends in laboratory parameters. Both groups exhibited a general decline in white blood cell counts, hemoglobin, hematocrit, and platelet counts, suggesting the potential development of mild chronic anemia, reduction in systemic inflammation, and the effects of long-term antiplatelet therapy. Significant reductions in LDL cholesterol levels ($p = 0.002$ for LBBB group, $p = 0.031$ for non-LBBB group) indicate the effectiveness of lipid-lowering therapies in managing cardiovascular risk over time. Effective lipid management is essential for slowing the progression of coronary artery disease and potentially reducing the need for additional reperfusion procedures, thus maintaining vascular health after STEMI [13–15]. A recent retrospective study evaluated lipid management in post-MI patients based on the 2019 European Society of Cardiology Guidelines for dyslipidemia. The study found that only 14.7% of patients reached the guideline-recommended LDL-C target of <1.4 mmol/L and achieved a $\geq 50\%$ reduction from baseline LDL-C at follow-up. This finding underscores the critical need for improved secondary prevention strategies that align with current guidelines [16]. Additionally, improvements in creatinine and uric acid levels point to enhanced renal function and metabolic control, likely due to optimized management of associated conditions. The significant improvements in lipid profiles, glycemic control, and reductions in inflammatory markers underscore the effectiveness of contemporary treatment strategies, including pharmacotherapy and lifestyle modifications.

Significant improvements were observed in heart failure management among patients with STEMI and new LBBB. The increased use of angiotensin receptor-neprilysin inhibitors, ARBs, ACE inhibitors, MRAs, and SGLT2 inhibitors in this group reflects an advanced therapeutic approach aimed at mitigating the more severe cardiac dysfunction associated with LBBB. The substantial rise in the use of SGLT2 inhibitors, in particular, underscores their growing importance in reducing hospitalization rates and enhancing cardiovascular health. LVEF analysis revealed significant improvements in cardiac function over the follow-up period. There was a significant decrease in the number of patients with severely reduced LVEF, with many improving to moderately impaired or preserved LVEF, especially in those without LBBB. This indicates successful heart failure management and better myocardial recovery in these patients. However, patients with newly diagnosed LBBB demonstrated less improvement in left ventricular ejection fraction, underscoring the importance of strict adherence to treatment protocols and regular follow-up to maintain and enhance the health benefits in STEMI patients [17]. Regarding the role of SGLT2 inhibitors in acute coronary syndrome, recent findings provide mixed insights. While preclinical studies suggest these inhibitors may reduce myocardial infarct size and improve cardiac function, clinical data have yet to establish a clear benefit in the ACS setting. Although some benefits, such as reduced contrast-induced acute kidney injury, have been observed, current evidence does not fully support the use of SGLT2 inhibitors in ACS management, regardless of diabetes status [18]. Larger, well-designed RCTs are necessary to clarify their role in this context and potentially expand the therapeutic indications of these drugs. Furthermore, updated clinical guidelines and new evidence have shaped practice patterns, advocating for more personalized treatment strategies and the incorporation of alternative therapies [1,17,18]. For instance, angiotensin receptor-neprilysin inhibitors have demonstrated significant benefits in patients with heart failure, prompting their increased use in contemporary treatment protocols [19,20].

In our study, all procedures were performed via the femoral approach by a highly experienced interventional cardiology team, resulting in a 100% procedural success rate using drug-eluting stents, with only one minor complication (local hematoma) in a patient with new LBBB. A study by Dudek et al. provides valuable insights into the clinical outcomes, over a 12-month follow-up period, following bioresorbable vascular scaffold

(BVS) implantation in complex coronary lesions, particularly in the context of acute coronary syndrome. The study showed no significant differences in major adverse cardiovascular events between patients with different levels of vessel tortuosity or calcification. However, patients with ACS, particularly those with unstable angina, experienced a higher rate of target lesion revascularization and device-oriented composite endpoints, suggesting that while BVS can be used effectively in ACS cases, careful patient selection and follow-up are crucial [21].

Our multivariate analysis highlights that the presence of LBBB in STEMI patients contributes to worse long-term outcomes, likely due to the resulting electrical and mechanical dyssynchrony that leads to adverse cardiac remodeling. Reduced left ventricular ejection fraction and delayed pain-to-admission time were also identified as significant independent predictors of poor outcomes. Interestingly, comorbidities such as diabetes, hypertension, and chronic kidney disease were not significant predictors in the multivariate analysis after adjusting for other factors, suggesting that the presence of LBBB, LVEF, and admission delay may have a stronger influence on long-term prognosis in this patient cohort. These results highlight the need for vigilant monitoring and aggressive management strategies in STEMI patients with new LBBB to improve long-term outcomes. Further research could help clarify these relationships and potentially guide more effective treatment strategies. In a large retrospective study of 1875 patients undergoing primary PCI, those with LBBB (n = 155, 8.3%) were significantly older, more often female, and had higher rates of prior MI and CABG compared to patients with STEMI. The LBBB group showed significantly lower rates of acute occlusion (12.2% vs. 63%; $p < 0.0001$) and PCI (26% vs. 83%; $p < 0.0001$). Although 30-day mortality was similar between the groups, overall mortality was significantly higher in the LBBB group during the 2-year follow-up (27.8% vs. 13.9%; $p = 0.023$). These findings highlight the need for improved risk stratification and management strategies for LBBB patients referred for primary PCI [22]. Lahti et al. performed research which found that LBBB was linked to higher cardiac mortality even after accounting for clinical risk variables. However, unlike individuals with non-ischemic ventricular conduction delay (NIVCD), this connection disappeared when LVEF was included in the analysis. These findings provide support for the idea that lower left ventricular ejection fraction (LVEF) caused by mechanical dyssynchrony is a significant unfavorable prognostic factor in LBBB [23].

Nevertheless, a worse prognosis after an acute coronary syndrome (ACS) episode may not only be attributed to the mechanical pumping ability of the heart. NIVCD continued to be a significant predictor of cardiac death even after accounting for in-hospital LVEF. Previously, NIVCD has been linked to a high occurrence of cardiac arrests in STEMI patients undergoing treatment [23,24]. Lee et al. found that people with LBBB and non-ischemic cardiomyopathy (NICD) were more likely to end up in the hospital because of HF, cardiovascular mortality, or death from any cause. Among these patients, those with LBBB had the greatest risk of major adverse cardiovascular events [25]. Nevertheless, the frequency of coronary angioplasty was notably lower in patients with BBB compared to those with normal QRS, which is a key contributing factor to the worse outcomes seen in these groups, especially in patients with LBBB [26]. During a 10-year follow-up of patients with ACS, the presence of LBBB, electrocardiographic left ventricular hypertrophy, and Q waves was shown to be linked with a poorer outcome compared to a normal electrocardiogram, RBBB, ST-segment elevation, or ST-segment depression/T-wave inversion. LBBB was correlated with the most elevated death rates [27]. Patients diagnosed with BBB had more unfavorable baseline features, particularly those with LBBB. During the long time of observation, they also had a more unfavorable result, characterized by an elevated rate of death from all causes [24,25,28].

While our study did not directly utilize cardiac MRI due to the lack of availability in our clinic, we recognize the potential of advanced imaging techniques, such as cardiac MRI, in enhancing risk stratification, particularly for high-risk patients like those with new LBBB. MRI parameters like LVEF and late gadolinium enhancement could complement our identified prognostic factors, providing a more comprehensive evaluation of patient prognosis. This highlights the need for future studies to integrate clinical and imaging data and emphasizes the importance of expanding access to advanced imaging in clinical practice. The findings from our study align with and further emphasize the importance of thorough risk stratification in this patient population. In the DERIVATE-ICM registry, a large multicenter study involving 861 patients with ischemic cardiomyopathy and chronic heart failure, the additional use of cardiac magnetic resonance (CMR) was shown to significantly improve risk stratification for major adverse arrhythmic cardiac events compared to standard transthoracic echocardiography (TTE). The study revealed that key CMR parameters, such as left ventricular end-diastolic volume index, CMR-derived LVEF, and late gadolinium enhancement (LGE) mass, were independent predictors of MAACE. Notably, a multiparametric CMR score provided superior predictive accuracy over the conventional TTE-LVEF cutoff of 35%, resulting in a net reclassification improvement (NRI) of 31.7% ($p = 0.007$). These findings underscore the potential role of advanced imaging techniques, such as CMR, in enhancing the precision of risk assessment and guiding appropriate therapeutic strategies, especially in high-risk patients like those with LBBB who are predisposed to adverse cardiovascular events [29].

The results of another recent study indicate that elevated T2 values in the noninfarcted myocardium (NIM) following STEMI are significantly associated with adverse outcomes. Specifically, patients with higher NIM T2 values (>45 ms) exhibited larger infarct sizes, more microvascular obstruction, and greater left ventricular dysfunction compared to those with lower T2 values. During a median follow-up of 17 months, patients with higher NIM T2 values had a markedly increased risk of MACE, predominantly driven by a significantly higher incidence of myocardial reinfarction (26.3% vs. 1.4%, $p < 0.001$). Multivariable analysis confirmed that elevated NIM T2 values independently predicted MACE (HR: 2.824 [95% CI: 1.254–6.361]; $p = 0.012$), highlighting the prognostic value of this imaging marker. These findings suggest that tissue-level inflammation and edema, as captured by higher NIM T2 values, play a critical role in the post-STEMI pathophysiology and could serve as an important risk stratification tool in this patient population [30].

These studies underscore the critical role of advanced imaging techniques, such as cardiac magnetic resonance, in improving risk stratification for cardiovascular events in high-risk populations. These findings highlight the prognostic value of tissue-level assessments in guiding personalized therapeutic strategies and improving long-term outcomes.

This study has some limitations. The results are based on a relatively small sample size from a single tertiary academic hospital in Romania, which may limit the generalizability of the findings to other populations or healthcare settings. Thus, considering the limited number of patients involved, as a result of the very careful selection process to ensure comparability of results, further validation, including an increase in the number of participants, is necessary to strengthen the findings. The reliance on historical patient records from 2011 to 2013, although the study evaluated the patients for a median follow-up period of almost 10 years, may not fully capture recent therapeutic advances or current management practices. Due to limitations in sample size and the complexity of the dataset, advanced multivariate analyses such as Kaplan–Meier curve generation were not performed. This limitation may impact the generalizability of the findings, and future studies with larger cohorts should consider these analyses to further refine the prognostic significance of LBBB in STEMI patients.

Despite its limitations, this study has several strengths that enhance its credibility and contribute meaningfully to the field of cardiovascular disease management, particularly for patients with complex conditions such as STEMI and newly diagnosed LBBB. The prospective data collection likely improves the accuracy and reliability of the findings compared to retrospective studies. The nearly 10-year follow-up offers valuable long-term insights into the management and outcomes of STEMI patients, both with and without LBBB, which is essential for understanding the chronic nature of coronary artery disease. By focusing on patients with newly developed LBBB, the study addresses a subgroup that is often underrepresented in cardiovascular research but may have poor long-term outcomes, providing specific insights that could shape future guidelines and therapeutic strategies.

5. Conclusions

The study highlights the critical prognostic significance of newly acquired LBBB in patients with STEMI. Thus, new-onset LBBB, reduced LVEF, and delayed pain-to-admission time are significant independent predictors of worse long-term outcomes in STEMI patients, highlighting the need for early detection and aggressive management of these factors. Future research should focus on refining therapeutic strategies to improve the prognosis of STEMI patients with LBBB, potentially incorporating advanced heart failure treatments and timely revascularization to mitigate the higher risks observed in this group.

Author Contributions: Conceptualization, L.A.; methodology, L.A.; software, A.T. and B.-S.T.; validation, L.A., R.A.S. and C.S.; formal analysis, L.A., L.-C.B., C.P. and R.R.; investigation, L.A.; data curation, L.A., A.T. and B.-S.T.; writing—original draft preparation, L.A., A.T. and B.-S.T.; writing—review and editing, L.A., L.-C.B., C.P. and R.R.; supervision, R.A.S. and C.S. All authors have read and agreed to the published version of the manuscript.

Funding: This research received no external funding.

Institutional Review Board Statement: The study was conducted in accordance with the Declaration of Helsinki, and approved by the Research Ethics Commission of "Grigore T. Popa" University of Medicine and Pharmacy, Iași, Romania, 206 from 7 June 2016.

Informed Consent Statement: Informed consent was obtained from all subjects involved in the study.

Data Availability Statement: All data generated or analyzed during this study are included in this article.

Conflicts of Interest: The authors declare no conflicts of interest.

References

1. Byrne, R.A.; Rossello, X.; Coughlan, J.J.; Barbato, E.; Berry, C.; Chieffo, A.; Claeys, M.J.; Dan, G.A.; Dweck, M.R.; Galbraith, M.; et al. 2023 ESC Guidelines for the management of acute coronary syndromes. *Eur. Heart J.* **2023**, *44*, 3720–3826. [CrossRef] [PubMed]
2. Vernon, S.T.; Coffey, S.; D'Souza, M.; Chow, C.K.; Kilian, J.; Hyun, K.; Shaw, J.A.; Adams, M.; Roberts-Thomson, P.; Brieger, D.; et al. ST-Segment-Elevation Myocardial Infarction (STEMI) Patients Without Standard Modifiable Cardiovascular Risk Factors-How Common Are They, and What Are Their Outcomes? *J. Am. Heart Assoc.* **2019**, *8*, e013296. [CrossRef] [PubMed]
3. Smith, S.W.; Dodd, K.W.; Henry, T.D.; Dvorak, D.M.; Pearce, L.A. Diagnosis of ST-elevation myocardial infarction in the presence of left bundle branch block with the ST-elevation to S-wave ratio in a modified Sgarbossa rule. *Ann. Emerg. Med.* **2012**, *60*, 766–776. [CrossRef] [PubMed]
4. Meyers, H.P.; Limkakeng, A.T., Jr.; Jaffa, E.J.; Patel, A.; Theiling, B.J.; Rezaie, S.R.; Stewart, T.; Zhuang, C.; Pera, V.K.; Smith, S.W. Validation of the modified Sgarbossa criteria for acute coronary occlusion in the setting of left bundle branch block: A retrospective case-control study. *Am. Heart J.* **2015**, *170*, 1255–1264. [CrossRef] [PubMed]
5. Gulati, M.; Levy, P.D.; Mukherjee, D.; Amsterdam, E.; Bhatt, D.L.; Birtcher, K.K.; Blankstein, R.; Boyd, J.; Bullock-Palmer, R.P.; Conejo, T.; et al. 2021 AHA/ACC/ASE/CHEST/SAEM/SCCT/SCMR Guideline for the Evaluation and Diagnosis of Chest Pain: A Report of the American College of Cardiology/American Heart Association Joint Committee on Clinical Practice Guidelines. *Circulation* **2021**, *144*, e368–e454. [CrossRef] [PubMed]
6. Niknam, R.; Mohammadi, M. Frequency of Left Bundle Branch Block in Patients with Acute Myocardial Infarction; A Cross-Sectional Study. *Galen. Med. J.* **2019**, *8*, e1576. [CrossRef]
7. Wu, A.H.; Parsons, L.; Every, N.R.; Bates, E.R.; Second National Registry of Myocardial, I. Hospital outcomes in patients presenting with congestive heart failure complicating acute myocardial infarction: A report from the Second National Registry of Myocardial Infarction (NRMI-2). *J. Am. Coll. Cardiol.* **2002**, *40*, 1389–1394. [CrossRef]
8. Vernon, S.T.; Coffey, S.; Bhindi, R.; Soo Hoo, S.Y.; Nelson, G.I.; Ward, M.R.; Hansen, P.S.; Asrress, K.N.; Chow, C.K.; Celermajer, D.S.; et al. Increasing proportion of ST elevation myocardial infarction patients with coronary atherosclerosis poorly explained by standard modifiable risk factors. *Eur. J. Prev. Cardiol.* **2017**, *24*, 1824–1830. [CrossRef]
9. Marx, N.; Federici, M.; Schutt, K.; Muller-Wieland, D.; Ajjan, R.A.; Antunes, M.J.; Christodorescu, R.M.; Crawford, C.; Di Angelantonio, E.; Eliasson, B.; et al. 2023 ESC Guidelines for the management of cardiovascular disease in patients with diabetes. *Eur. Heart J.* **2023**, *44*, 4043–4140. [CrossRef]

10. Williams, B.; Mancia, G.; Spiering, W.; Agabiti Rosei, E.; Azizi, M.; Burnier, M.; Clement, D.L.; Coca, A.; de Simone, G.; Dominiczak, A.; et al. 2018 ESC/ESH Guidelines for the management of arterial hypertension. *Eur. Heart J.* **2018**, *39*, 3021–3104. [CrossRef]
11. McDonagh, T.A.; Metra, M.; Adamo, M.; Gardner, R.S.; Baumbach, A.; Bohm, M.; Burri, H.; Butler, J.; Celutkiene, J.; Chioncel, O.; et al. 2021 ESC Guidelines for the diagnosis and treatment of acute and chronic heart failure. *Eur. Heart J.* **2021**, *42*, 3599–3726. [CrossRef] [PubMed]
12. Pera, V.K.; Larson, D.M.; Sharkey, S.W.; Garberich, R.F.; Solie, C.J.; Wang, Y.L.; Traverse, J.H.; Poulose, A.K.; Henry, T.D. New or presumed new left bundle branch block in patients with suspected ST-elevation myocardial infarction. *Eur. Heart J. Acute Cardiovasc. Care* **2018**, *7*, 208–217. [CrossRef] [PubMed]
13. Mach, F.; Baigent, C.; Catapano, A.L.; Koskinas, K.C.; Casula, M.; Badimon, L.; Chapman, M.J.; De Backer, G.G.; Delgado, V.; Ference, B.A.; et al. 2019 ESC/EAS Guidelines for the management of dyslipidaemias: Lipid modification to reduce cardiovascular risk. *Eur. Heart J.* **2020**, *41*, 111–188. [CrossRef] [PubMed]
14. Cannon, C.P.; Blazing, M.A.; Giugliano, R.P.; McCagg, A.; White, J.A.; Theroux, P.; Darius, H.; Lewis, B.S.; Ophuis, T.O.; Jukema, J.W.; et al. Ezetimibe Added to Statin Therapy after Acute Coronary Syndromes. *N. Engl. J. Med.* **2015**, *372*, 2387–2397. [CrossRef] [PubMed]
15. Michaeli, D.T.; Michaeli, J.C.; Albers, S.; Boch, T.; Michaeli, T. Established and Emerging Lipid-Lowering Drugs for Primary and Secondary Cardiovascular Prevention. *Am. J. Cardiovasc. Drugs* **2023**, *23*, 477–495. [CrossRef]
16. Wambua, P.M.; Khan, Z.; Kariuki, C.M.; Ogola, E.N. A Retrospective Study on the Adoption of Lipid Management Guidelines in Post-Myocardial Infarction Patients in a Tertiary Care Centre. *Cureus* **2023**, *15*, e41402. [CrossRef]
17. Escobar, J.; Rawat, A.; Maradiaga, F.; Isaak, A.K.; Zainab, S.; Arusi Dari, M.; Mekonen Gdey, M.; Khan, A. Comparison of Outcomes Between Angiotensin-Converting Enzyme Inhibitors and Angiotensin II Receptor Blockers in Patients With Myocardial Infarction: A Meta-Analysis. *Cureus* **2023**, *15*, e47954. [CrossRef]
18. Karakasis, P.; Fragakis, N.; Kouskouras, K.; Karamitsos, T.; Patoulias, D.; Rizzo, M. Sodium-Glucose Cotransporter-2 Inhibitors in Patients With Acute Coronary Syndrome: A Modern Cinderella? *Clin. Ther.* **2024**, S0149-2918(24)00149-8. [CrossRef]
19. Lee, K.; Han, S.; Lee, M.; Kim, D.W.; Kwon, J.; Park, G.M.; Park, M.W. Evidence-Based Optimal Medical Therapy and Mortality in Patients With Acute Myocardial Infarction After Percutaneous Coronary Intervention. *J. Am. Heart Assoc.* **2023**, *12*, e024370. [CrossRef]
20. Riccardi, M.; Sammartino, A.M.; Piepoli, M.; Adamo, M.; Pagnesi, M.; Rosano, G.; Metra, M.; von Haehling, S.; Tomasoni, D. Heart failure: An update from the last years and a look at the near future. *ESC Heart Fail.* **2022**, *9*, 3667–3693. [CrossRef]
21. Rzeszutko, Ł.; Siudak, Z.; Tokarek, T.; Plens, K.; Włodarczak, A.; Lekston, A.; Ochała, A.; Gil, R.J.; Balak, W.; Dudek, D. Twelve months clinical outcome after bioresorbable vascular scaffold implantation in patients with stable angina and acute coronary syndrome. Data from the Polish National Registry. *Postepy Kardiol. Interwencyjnej* **2016**, *12*, 108–115. [CrossRef] [PubMed]
22. Mannakkara, N.N.; Mozid, A.M.; Showkathali, R.; Sheikh, A.S.; Tang, K.H.; Robinson, N.M.; Kabir, A.M.; Jagathesan, R.O.; Sayer, J.W.; Kelly, P.A.; et al. Comparison of clinical characteristics and outcomes in patients with left bundle branch block versus ST elevation myocardial infarction referred for primary PCI. *Heart* **2013**, *99*, A26–A27. [CrossRef]
23. Lahti, R.; Rankinen, J.; Eskola, M.; Nikus, K.; Hernesniemi, J. Intraventricular conduction delays as a predictor of mortality in acute coronary syndromes. *Eur. Heart J. Acute Cardiovasc. Care* **2023**, *12*, 430–436. [CrossRef] [PubMed]
24. Timoteo, A.T.; Mendonca, T.; Aguiar Rosa, S.; Goncalves, A.; Carvalho, R.; Ferreira, M.L.; Ferreira, R.C. Prognostic impact of bundle branch block after acute coronary syndrome. Does it matter if it is left of right? *Int. J. Cardiol. Heart Vasc.* **2019**, *22*, 31–34. [CrossRef]
25. Lee, W.C.; Fang, Y.N.; Chen, T.Y.; Hsieh, Y.Y.; Tsai, Y.H.; Fang, H.Y.; Wu, P.J.; Chen, H.C.; Liu, P.Y. The Relationship of Conduction Disorder and Prognosis in Patients with Acute Coronary Syndrome. *Int. J. Clin. Pract.* **2022**, *2022*, 9676434. [CrossRef]
26. Wegmann, C.; Pfister, R.; Scholz, S.; Markhof, A.; Wanke, S.; Kuhr, K.; Rudolph, T.; Baldus, S.; Reuter, H. Diagnostic value of left bundle branch block in patients with acute myocardial infarction. A prospective analysis. *Herz* **2015**, *40*, 1107–1114. [CrossRef]
27. Nestelberger, T.; Cullen, L.; Lindahl, B.; Reichlin, T.; Greenslade, J.H.; Giannitsis, E.; Christ, M.; Morawiec, B.; Miro, O.; Martín-Sánchez, F.J.; et al. Diagnosis of acute myocardial infarction in the presence of left bundle branch block. *Heart* **2019**, *105*, 1559–1567. [CrossRef]
28. Avdikos, G.; Michas, G.; Smith, S.W. From Q/Non-Q Myocardial Infarction to STEMI/NSTEMI: Why It's Time to Consider Another Simplified Dichotomy; a Narrative Literature Review. *Arch. Acad. Emerg. Med.* **2022**, *10*, e78. [CrossRef]
29. Pontone, G.; Guaricci, A.I.; Fusini, L.; Baggiano, A.; Guglielmo, M.; Muscogiuri, G.; Volpe, A.; Abete, R.; Aquaro, G.; Barison, A.; et al. Cardiac Magnetic Resonance for Prophylactic Implantable-Cardioverter Defibrillator Therapy in Ischemic Cardiomyopathy: The DERIVATE-ICM International Registry. *JACC Cardiovasc. Imaging* **2023**, *16*, 1387–1400. [CrossRef]
30. Bergamaschi, L.; Landi, A.; Maurizi, N.; Pizzi, C.; Leo, L.A.; Arangalage, D.; Iglesias, J.F.; Eeckhout, E.; Eeckhout, E.; Eeckhout, E.; et al. Acute Response of the Noninfarcted Myocardium and Surrounding Tissue Assessed by T2 Mapping After STEMI. *JACC Cardiovasc. Imaging* **2024**, *17*, 610–621. [CrossRef]

Disclaimer/Publisher's Note: The statements, opinions and data contained in all publications are solely those of the individual author(s) and contributor(s) and not of MDPI and/or the editor(s). MDPI and/or the editor(s) disclaim responsibility for any injury to people or property resulting from any ideas, methods, instructions or products referred to in the content.

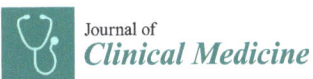

Review

A Dual Challenge: *Coxiella burnetii* Endocarditis in a Patient with Familial Thoracic Aortic Aneurysm—Case Report and Literature Review

Alina-Ramona Cozlac [1,2,3], Caius Glad Streian [1,2,3,*], Marciana Ionela Boca [2], Simina Crisan [1,2,3], Mihai-Andrei Lazar [1,2,3], Mirela-Daniela Virtosu [2,4,5], Adina Ionac [1,2,3], Raluca Elisabeta Staicu [2,5], Daniela-Carmen Dugaci [2], Adela Emandi-Chirita [6], Ana Lascu [2,7,8], Dan Gaita [1,2,3] and Constantin-Tudor Luca [1,2,3]

1. Department VI Cardiology-Cardiovascular Surgery, "Victor Babes" University of Medicine and Pharmacy of Timișoara, Eftimie Murgu Square No. 2, 300041 Timisoara, Romania; alina-ramona.cozlac@umft.ro (A.-R.C.); simina.crisan@umft.ro (S.C.); lazar.mihai@umft.ro (M.-A.L.); adina.ionac@umft.ro (A.I.); dan.gaita@umft.ro (D.G.); constantin.luca@umft.ro (C.-T.L.)
2. Institute for Cardiovascular Diseases of Timisoara, "Victor Babes" University of Medicine and Pharmacy of Timișoara, G. Adam Str. No. 13A, 300310 Timisoara, Romania; boca.marciana@cardiologie.ro (M.I.B.); daniela.cozma@umft.ro (M.-D.V.); raluca.staicu@umft.ro (R.E.S.); dugaci.daniela@cardiologie.ro (D.-C.D.); lascu.ana@umft.ro (A.L.)
3. Advanced Research Center of the Institute for Cardiovascular Diseases, "Victor Babes" University of Medicine and Pharmacy of Timișoara, Eftimie Murgu Square No. 2, 300041 Timisoara, Romania
4. Department VI Cardiology Internal Medicine and Ambulatory Care, Prevention and Cardiovascular Recovery, "Victor Babeș" University of Medicine and Pharmacy of Timișoara, Eftimie Murgu Square No. 2, 300041 Timisoara, Romania
5. Doctoral School Medicine-Pharmacy, "Victor Babes" University of Medicine and Pharmacy of Timișoara, Eftimie Murgu Square No. 2, 300041 Timisoara, Romania
6. Centre of Genomic Medicine, Genetics Discipline, "Victor Babeș" University of Medicine and Pharmacy of Timișoara, 300041 Timisoara, Romania; adela.chirita@umft.ro
7. Department III Functional Sciences—Pathophysiology, "Victor Babes" University of Medicine and Pharmacy of Timișoara, Eftimie Murgu Square No. 2, 300041 Timisoara, Romania
8. Centre for Translational Research and Systems Medicine, "Victor Babes" University of Medicine and Pharmacy of Timișoara, Eftimie Murgu Square No. 2, 300041 Timisoara, Romania
* Correspondence: streian.caius@umft.ro

Abstract: Background/Objectives: Thoracic aortic aneurysms (TAAs) are potentially life-threatening medical conditions, and their etiology involves both genetic and multiple risk factors. *Coxiella burnetii* endocarditis is one of the most frequent causes of blood culture-negative infective endocarditis (BCNIE) in patients with previous cardiac surgery. Our review aims to emphasize the importance of genetic testing in patients with thoracic aortic aneurysms but also the importance of additional testing in patients with suspected endocarditis whose blood cultures remain negative. The reported case has a history of acute DeBakey type I aortic dissection that developed during her second pregnancy, for which the Bentall procedure was performed at that time. Ten years after the surgery, the patient started developing prolonged febrile syndrome with repeatedly negative blood cultures, the serological tests revealing the presence of an infection with *Coxiella burnetii*. Considering her family history and the onset of her aortic pathology at a young age, genetic tests were performed, disclosing a missense variant in the actin alpha-2 (*ACTA2*) gene in heterozygous status. **Methods**: For a better understanding of both conditions, our research was conducted in two directions: one reviewing the literature on patients with *Coxiella burnetii* BCNIE and the other focusing on patients who had a familial thoracic aortic aneurysm (FTAA) due to the *ACTA2* variant. This review incorporates studies found on PubMed and ResearchGate up to August 2024. **Conclusions**: BCNIE represents a condition with several diagnostic challenges and may lead to severe complications if timely treatment is not initiated. Also, diagnosing an FTAA requires genetic testing, enabling better follow-up and management.

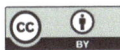

Keywords: thoracic aortic aneurysms; *ACTA2* gene variant; *Coxiella burnetii*; infective endocarditis; chronic Q fever

1. Introduction

Thoracic aortic aneurysms (TAAs) involve the dilation of the vessel caliber, with the aortic diameter thresholds adapting to physical measurements, such as height and weight [1,2]. In addition to the etiology involving inflammatory and infectious diseases or risk factors, such as hypertension and hypercholesterolemia, genetic factors implicated in the physiopathology of vascular wall syndromes have gained significant importance in recent years, leading to improved classification and management of aortic aneurysms [3,4]. The latest AHA Guidelines for the Diagnosis and Management of Aortic Disease recommend routine genetic testing of patients diagnosed with thoracic aortic aneurysm at a young age or having features associated with specific syndromes; additionally, DNA sequencing should be performed on known at-risk relatives of individuals with positive results [2]. FTAAs are caused by their association with variants of either extracellular matrix protein function or vascular smooth muscle proteins [1]. TAAs can be divided into two main subtypes depending on multiorgan damage, the branches being referred to as syndromic or non-syndromic. The syndromic ones include diseases affecting both the vascular system and other connective tissue abnormalities, the most notable examples of this group being Loeys-Dietz syndrome, Marfan syndrome, or vascular Ehlers-Danlos syndrome. Conversely, non-syndromic TAAs are defined by their impact solely on the cardiovascular system [5].

The pathogenic genes involved in the pathway of FTAAs affect proteins that ensure the integrity of the vascular wall, particularly vascular smooth muscle cells. Multiple genes can determine a familial pattern of thoracic aortic aneurysms, most of them having autosomal dominant inheritance, with the highest studied and prominently featured in the academic field being *ACTA2, MYH11, MYLK, PRKG1*, and those involved in the TGF-β pathway [6,7]. Pathogenic variants of the *ACTA2* gene, which encodes α-actin, are some of the most frequent etiologies of FTAAs. Alpha-actin expresses almost half of the total proteins in smooth muscle cells (up to 40%), thus making it the most representative protein at this level [6]. In addition to cardiovascular disorders, pathogenic variants of the *ACTA-2* gene predispose patients to other forms of vascular pathologies, including Moyamoya-like occlusions that can lead to early onset of cerebrovascular events or occlusions of internal carotid arteries or intracranial aneurysms [8–10].

On the other hand, the reported case is one with complex particularities, with several medical specialties being involved and both the patient's genetic and infectious pathology leading to consequences in the cardiovascular system. The infectious disease that the patient contracted during the last few years was an infection with *Coxiella burnetii*. This microorganism is the causative agent of Q fever, being intracellular gram-negative bacteria, and is usually transmitted directly from animals, like goats or sheep, or indirectly by ticks [11,12]. It has been repeatedly indicated as a potential biological threat because it can be transmitted through inhalation, it has a low infective dose, and it has environmental stability [13,14]. The acute onset of the disease manifests as a high fever and flu-like symptoms, for example, a nonproductive cough, but because of the non-specific symptoms, the treatment is not always administered on time, allowing the Q fever to turn into a chronic disease [15,16]. The only method of preventing the disease is through immunization achieved by the Q-vax vaccine, but it is currently only administered in Australia [17].

The most common manifestation of chronic Q fever is blood culture-negative infective endocarditis, but in some cases, the onset form may be represented by hepatitis, osteomyelitis, febrile illness lasting up to fifty days, and even neurological pathology, characterized by encephalitis, meningitis, or peripheral neuropathy [18,19].

The specific treatment of *Coxiella burnetii* infection is the administration of Doxycycline for 14 days for the acute infection, but in the case of chronic Q fever, a combination of Doxycycline and Hydroxychloroquine should be administered for up to 18 months [20,21]. According to the 2023 ESC Guidelines for the management of endocarditis, blood culture-negative infective endocarditis caused by *Coxiella burnetii* should be treated with Doxycycline 200 mg/24 h and Hydroxychloroquine 200–600 mg/24 h for a minimum of 18 months [22].

2. Materials and Methods

The main information sources of the studies examined in this review are PubMed and ResearchGate. The studies were selected based on the inclusion criteria described above, with the selected articles that resemble the reported case including only those published since January 2000. Firstly, the studies selected for the first part of the review, namely patients presenting with BCNIE, had to meet the following criteria: case reports published between January 2000 and August 2024 that include patients currently being diagnosed positive for *Coxiella burnetii* endocarditis but having an aortic valve replacement in their medical history. Article types other than case reports published before 2000 and studies involving non-human participants were excluded. For the second part of the review, the studies included case reports published between January 2000 and August 2024 that describe patients with the *ACTA2* gene causing a familial thoracic aortic aneurysm; the exclusion criteria remained the same as those applied in the first section of the review.

The following keywords were used to maximize search accuracy: "*Coxiella burnetii* infection", "Q fever", "mechanical aortic valve", and "blood culture-negative infective endocarditis" for the first part of the review, and "familial thoracic aortic aneurysm", "*ACTA2* variant/mutation", "aortic dissection", and "*ACTA2* gene", for the second part. The keywords were selected to improve research accuracy and capture the intricate pathologies described in our case report. The MeSH function on PubMed was used to increase the specificity of the research by using combinations of the keywords. The discovered articles were added to the Zotero application, with the ones identified as duplicates being removed. We used Microsoft 365 (Office) software, Microsoft Corporation, Redmond, WA, USA.

Next-generation sequencing (NGS) was performed in the Center for Genomic Medicine, Timișoara, for the patient and one daughter in a panel of 174 genes, using the Illumina TruSight Cardio Sequencing Panel kit and a MiSeq Illumina sequencing platform (Illumina, San Diego, CA, USA). End-to-end bioinformatics algorithms were implemented, using Burrows-Wheeler Aligner (BWAAligner), SAMtools, Genome Analysis Toolkit (GATK-Variant Caller-Broad Institute of MIT and Harvard, Cambridge, MA, USA) and Annovar (as described elsewhere) [23]. Alignment of the sequenced fragments was performed on the human reference genome GRCh37. A tertiary data analysis was performed at the level of current knowledge using online databases and aggregators, including Varsome, ClinVar, gnomAD, DECIPHER, UCSC Genome Browser, OMIM, DGV, and Ensembl. Variants were classified according to the 2015 ACMG guideline [24].

3. Results

The reported case describes a 45-year-old woman known to have multiple cardiovascular conditions and a positive family history, namely her mother died at 36 years old of unknown causes (a possible spontaneous carotid artery dissection). The patient developed acute aortic dissection DeBakey type I during her second pregnancy, which was treated surgically with a Bentall procedure in 2006 by replacing the aortic valve and the ascending aorta with a valved composite graft with re-implantation of the coronary arteries into the graft.

The clinical evolution of the patient was favorable for the first 15 years, followed only by chronic anticoagulant treatment of Acenocumarol 4 mg, adjusted according to the INR test. In December 2021, she started developing prolonged febrile syndrome, which was extensively investigated and treated with antibiotics several times. For two years, the patient was hospitalized in various clinics, and sets of blood cultures were performed repeatedly, all with negative results. After all the investigations were carried out, the established diagnoses were blood culture-negative infective endocarditis on the mechanical aortic valve, anti-neutrophil cytoplasmic antibody (ANCA)-associated systemic vasculitis, chronic glomerulonephritis (nephritic syndrome form) with splenic infarction, and diet-controlled type 2 diabetes.

In June 2024, the patient was admitted to our clinic for suspected intermittent febrile syndrome with subfebrile onset for about 3 months, accompanied by vertigo. The medical examination revealed normal vital signs and pale skin, and the cardiac examination highlighted a systolic murmur, heard loudest in the aortic area with a closing click. The ECG was normal. The pathological blood samples collected at admission revealed an inflammatory syndrome, i.e., highly elevated ESR and C-reactive protein, with positive procalcitonin. The transthoracic echocardiography showed an apparently normal mechanical prosthesis in the aortic position, mild intraprosthetic aortic regurgitation, mild mitral regurgitation, mild functional tricuspid regurgitation, mild secondary pulmonary hypertension, and a roughly 12 mm echo-dense mass surrounding the ascending aorta, also visible on the transesophageal echocardiography, as seen in Figure 1. Transesophageal echocardiography provides additional information on heart morphology, usually being used for a better view of the left atrium and the left atrial appendage in order to detect thrombi, but in our case, it was used for a better view of the aortic valve [25,26].

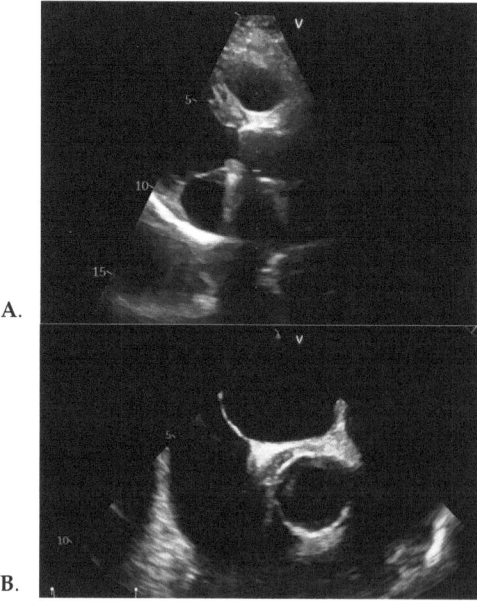

Figure 1. (**A**) Transthoracic and (**B**) transesophageal echocardiographies showing an echo-dense mass surrounding the ascending aorta.

On the second day after admission, the patient experienced a subfebrile episode, which prompted the collection of blood cultures, but the results were negative. Consequently, more specific investigations were performed, and serological tests for infective endocarditis of diverse etiology were acquired, including IgG and IgM antibodies for *Mycoplasma pneumoniae*, *Bartonella henselae*, *Chlamydophila pneumoniae*, *Brucella* spp., *Legionella pneumophila*, and *Coxiella burnetii*. All results were negative, except for *Coxiella burnetii* IgG and IgM phase I and phase II antibodies, and the results of both the phase I and phase II immunofluorescent assay (IFA) highlighted increased antibody titers, as seen in Table 1. Likewise, the PCR for *Coxiella burnetii* in the blood by molecular hybridization with an amplification test also revealed a positive result. Therefore, the diagnosis of acute onset of chronic Q fever as a disease was confirmed, the targeted therapy with Hydroxychloroquine 200 mg tid and Doxycycline 100 mg bid was initiated, and treatment will continue to be administered for 18 months. A relevant reference is the patient's travel history; starting from 2021, the patient had not traveled abroad, and no direct link could be made to a potential source of infection, such as domestic animals. However, from 2006 to 2011, the patient traveled to several African countries for about 3 months/year, and starting in 2012, she traveled several times to Switzerland and Germany.

Table 1. Serology of *Coxiella burnetii* antibodies.

Serology	Value
IgG phase I antibodies	>1:4096
IgM phase I antibodies	1:2024
IgG phase II antibodies	>1:4096
IgM phase II antibodies	1:1024

Consequently, with the echocardiographic images revealing a significant peri-aortic mass, it was decided to perform further investigations. The thorax CT scan detected a multiloculated right semi-circumferential fluid accumulation with iodophilic walls that extends from the level of the aortic valve along the aortic prosthesis to the anterior mediastinum, suggesting a peri-aortic abscess, as seen in Figure 2. Pericardial and pleural fluid collection and mediastinal adenopathies were also found.

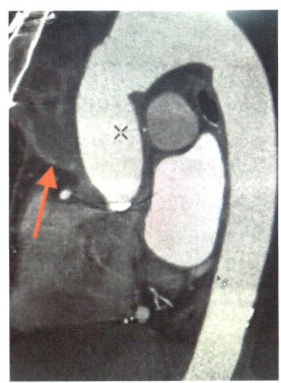 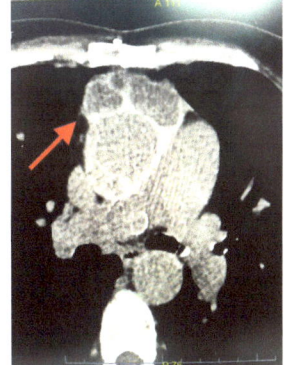

A.   B.

Figure 2. Thorax CT scan images showing the periaortic fluid accumulation (red arrow): (**A**) sagittal and (**B**) axial sections.

The preliminary diagnosis was *Coxiella burnetii* infective endocarditis complicated with mediastinal abscess; thus, a multidisciplinary team, consisting of a cardiologist, cardiovascular surgeon, infectionist, and intensive care physician, decided that the optimal management in this case would be a surgical redo operation with antibiotic protection. The surgery involved the removal of the periaortic fluid mass, with the macroscopic examination suggesting a liquefied chronic hematoma that can be seen in Figure 3. The bacteriological examination of the collected biological products, pericardial fragment, periprosthetic and subprosthetic tissue, and clot fragment revealed no bacterial or fungal growth on the inoculated culture media.

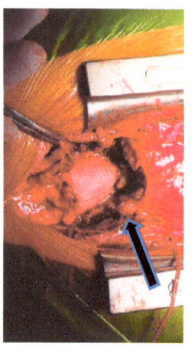 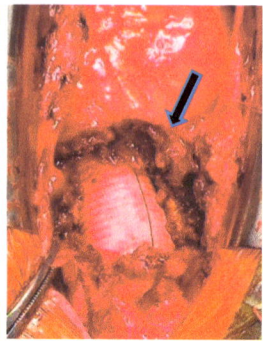

Figure 3. Intraoperative images showing the periaortic fluid accumulation (black arrow).

The post-operative evolution was favorable, and the investigations continued with genetic tests. Genetic testing for a familial aortopathy was proposed considering the positive family history of early cardiovascular-related death, the patient's mother having passed away at the age of 36, possibly due to a spontaneous carotid artery dissection. The patient's onset of the aortic pathology manifested as thoracic aortic dissection at the age of 27, which also constituted one of the factors that prompted the suspicion of a hereditary condition, thereby leading to genetic testing. A missense variant (variant NM_001613.4:c.773G>A, NP_001604.1:p.(Arg258His)) was detected in heterozygous status in the *ACTA2* gene located on chromosome 10q23.31. This variant was identified in several individuals with FTAAs, segregated by phenotype. The variant was classified with pathogenic significance according to the American College of Medical Genetics and Genomics (ACMG) guideline [24]. As a result, the suspicion of a genetic disease was confirmed, establishing the diagnosis of familial thoracic aortic aneurysm 6, part of a non-syndromic FTAA cluster. In some cases, the pathogenic variant of *ACTA2* is associated with intracranial aneurysms and Moyamoya-like cerebrovascular disease, so the patient will be undergoing a cranial CT scan [27]. Subsequently, her two daughters are proposed to be genetically tested and will have follow-up echocardiographic examinations.

To provide a better perspective on the patient's clinical status, paraclinical data, personal and family medical histories, and the treatment have been summarized in Table 2.

Table 2. Significant characteristics of the patient.

Clinical Manifestation	Family History of Aortic Disease	History of Cardiovascular Surgery	Blood Samples	Echocardiography Findings	Fever History	Treatment
-prolonged febrile syndrome -vertigo -pale skin -closing click in the aortic area	Mother died at 36 y (spontaneous carotid artery dissection)	Bentall procedure (for acute DeBakey type I aortic dissection)	-elevated ESR -elevated C-reactive protein -positive procalcitonin -negative blood cultures -elevated phase I and phase II IgG and IgM	-mechanical prosthesis in aortic position -12 mm echo-dense mass surrounding the ascending aorta	2 years	Medical: -antibiotics: Doxycycline (100 mg/bid) and Hydroxychloroquine (200 mg/tid) -Acenocumeral 4 mg -Furosemide/ Spironolactone 20/50 mg/day Surgical: removal of the periaortic hematoma

The patient was discharged with a good general condition and the following diagnosis: blood culture-negative infective endocarditis with *Coxiella burnetii*, liquefied chronic periprosthetic hematoma (surgically treated), status post-Bentall operation, normofunctional double disc mechanical prosthesis in the aortic position, mild mitral regurgitation, mild functional tricuspid regurgitation, mild secondary pulmonary hypertension, NYHA I chronic heart failure with preserved ejection fraction, diet-controlled type 2 diabetes, ANCA-associated systemic vasculitis, chronic glomerulonephritis (nephritic syndrome form), enlarged spleen with subcapsular infarction, and mild normochromic normocytic anemia, and the following treatment being recommended at home: Hydroxychloroquine 200 mg/tid, Doxycycline 100 mg bid, Acenocoumarol 4 mg (dose controlled by INR test in order to maintain a value between 2.5–3.5), diuretics (association between Furosemide/Spironolactone 20/50 mg/day), and a probiotic. The specific antibiotic treatment for *Coxiella burnetii* BCNIE with Hydroxychloroquine and Doxycycline will be administered for 18 months, according to the 2023 ESC Guidelines for the management of endocarditis. This approach is tailored to the patient's clinical course, the prolonged progression of febrile syndrome with multiple recurrences, and the potential complications that could be associated with mediastinal spread of the infection [22]. The only side effects reported by the patient regarding the specific medication for *Coxiella burnetii* were insomnia and tinnitus.

4. Discussion

In order to perform an accurate review starting with the reported case, which included two major significant pathologies, both a genetically inherited disease, the *ACTA2* variant gene leading to a familial thoracic aortic aneurysm and dissection, as well as a rare infectious disease, namely blood culture-negative infective endocarditis on a mechanical aortic valve, the research on the medical literature started by looking for the coexistence of both pathologies, but it failed to identify any patient similar to the case presented above.

Therefore, our research was oriented toward searching separately for the two intricate pathologies, the review encompassing medical articles describing, on one hand, blood culture-negative infective endocarditis with *Coxiella burnetii* on a mechanical aortic valve and, on the other hand, studies presenting patients having familial thoracic aortic aneurysm and/or dissection due to the *ACTA2* disease-causing variant.

Firstly, in the interest of achieving similarities between the described patient's infectious disease with cardiovascular implications and the patients included in the chosen studies, we identified articles published in the medical literature between 2000 and August 2024 available on PubMed and ResearchGate. The inclusion criteria that the selected articles had to meet were patients with a medical history including a surgery replacing the native aortic valve with a prosthetic one; patients diagnosed with *Coxiella burnetii* blood culture-negative infective endocarditis; studies including clear diagnosis and management parameters and having an explicit outcome for the patients; articles published in the target period of time; and studies defined as case reports. The exclusion criteria were studies published before 2000; studies having qualities other than case reports; articles that did not include accurate patient management details; and studies including non-human participants. The research strategy was designed using keywords and phrases closely relevant to the reported case; thus, the keywords included "*Coxiella burnetii* infection", "Q fever", "mechanical aortic valve", and "blood culture-negative infective endocarditis".

There were four identified case reports describing *Coxiella burnetii*-associated blood culture-negative infective endocarditis on a prosthetic aortic valve, as seen in Table 3.

The most frequently described symptom in these patients was fever, and, in most of the cases, febrile symptomatology started about a month before the presentation. In our patient, fever was present for about two and a half years, with periods of remission, subfebrility, or aggravation episodes.

Table 3. Patients presenting *Coxiella burnetii* blood culture-negative endocarditis and their characteristics.

No	First Author/ Year/Reference	No. of Patients/ Gender/Age	History of Cardiovascular Surgery	Fever History	Surgical or Medical Treatment
1	Bozza et al., 2023 [28]	1/M/55	Aortic valve replacement (aortic regurgitation and aneurysm)	1 month	Medical: Doxycycline (100 mg/bid) and Hydroxychloroquine (200 mg/tid)
2	Deyell et al., 2006 [29]	1/M/31	Open valvulotomy for congenital aortic stenosis + mechanical aortic replacement for severe aortic regurgitation	Not described	Surgical: Aortic root replacement of the ascending aorta and aortic valve replacement
3	Afrasiabian et al., 2024 [30]	1/F/67	Aortic valve replacement	1 month	Medical: Levofloxacin-intolerance of Doxycycline
4	Krol et al., 2008 [31]	1/F/43	Aortic valve replacement (bicuspid aortic valve)	Fever history, but no time described	Both; medical: Doxycycline monotherapy

The treatment in two of the cases was exclusively medical, one patient benefited from surgical intervention, and one case was managed through both medical and surgical therapy. One case was treated with a special antibiotic, as Afrasiabian et al. [30] described intolerance to Doxycycline, and thus the antibiotic treatment chosen instead was levofloxacin. Krol et al. [31] also preferred the administration of monotherapy with Doxycycline for 5 months, leading to a favorable result and an improved patient outcome. The treatment preferred by Bozza et al. [28] was the administration of Doxycycline 100 mg/bid in association with Hydroxychloroquine 200 mg/tid for 24 months, with a long-term follow-up of the patient, which proved the efficacy of the chosen antibiotics through a decreasing trend in the serological tests. This combination of antibiotics was also chosen for the patient treated in our clinic, being well tolerated by the patient, without fever remissions.

The characteristics of the *Coxiella burnetii* infection selected to compare with the patient's evolution described in our case report with the literature data represent only a subset of the features associated with this complex disease. *Coxiella burnetii* is defined as an intracellular bacterium causing a zoonotic disease transmitted from animals like sheep, cattle, or goats to humans, with ticks being the main reservoir in nature. The transmission is usually performed through aerosols, but vertical, transplacental, or even nosocomial infection is also possible. In humans, the infection may present many forms, including an asymptomatic course or progression through two distinct phases, acute and chronic disease. Acute infection can manifest as febrile symptomatology or flu-like onset, but it may also appear as hepatitis, pneumonia, or other manifestations. The presence and duration of fever were included in the comparative characteristics evaluated in the patients analyzed in this review. The most common manifestation of chronic Q fever is endocarditis; however, hepatitis, ophthalmological or neurological disorders, and infections of vascular grafts may also be present as forms of the disease.

In addition, a second part of the research was the comparison of the patient's evolution regarding the aortic disease caused by the *ACTA2* variant with the patients described in the chosen articles. The research among the medical literature provided five case reports published between 2000 and August 2024 that describe patients having a thoracic aortic aneurysm with a positive family history and the *ACTA2* variant, as seen in Table 4. The inclusion criteria were patients presenting any type of variant of the *ACTA2* gene expressing vascular smooth muscle cells; studies having the quality of case reports; and studies providing clear evidence of patient management. On the other hand, the exclusion criteria were studies involving non-human participants; studies published before the year 2000;

and studies with characteristics other than case reports. The examination was conducted among the studies found on PubMed and ResearchGate.

The prevalence of the targeted aortic pathology was found to be higher among men, with 57.1% of the patients described in the selected studies being males. Similarly, the ACTA2 disease-causing variant genes were discovered to be more frequent among males with aortic disease. Concerning the average age of patients with familial thoracic aortic aneurysm, the oldest patient experiencing acute onset of the condition was 41 years old, as described by Hoffjan et al. [32], while the youngest was just 15 years old, namely the study published by Ware et al. [33] presenting the twins who developed acute aortic dissection at the same time. In the patients' family history, cases carrying the mutant gene were identified after genetic counseling and testing because they did not experience any clinical manifestation of the disease. Similar to the reported data in the literature, our patient's clinical onset was very early; the acute aortic dissection occurred at the age of 27.

Among the included patients, only two of them presented a notable phenotypic manifestation, namely congenital mydriasis in the twins described by Ware et al. [33]. This clinical expression was also described in the specialized literature as being strongly associated with a particular missense variant in arginine 179 in the ACTA2 gene [5].

The complexity of the reported case arises from the early onset of the aortic disease, the patient being 7 months pregnant when she presented at the hospital for acute aortic dissection. This circumstance is consistent with the documented data regarding the evolution of pregnancies in females with the ACTA2 variant [34]. Thus, Hoffjan et al. [32] described two patients with a history of physiological pregnancy before being diagnosed with mild aortic dilation and acute aortic dissection. The academic literature describes a powerful connection between an underlying aortic disease and an aortic dissection associated with pregnancy. Fluctuations in pregnancy hormone levels, along with the hemodynamic stress experienced by pregnant women, can exacerbate a subjacent aortic condition, particularly during the third trimester [35].

Furthermore, genetic counseling should be the standard practice in all the cases outlined above. This management step is crucial for families where one member has already been identified for the ACTA2 disease-causing variant, as this gene is associated with an increased risk of vascular diseases, as seen in every presented study. Considering the autosomal dominant transmission of the ACTA2 gene, each child of an affected parent has a 50% chance of inheriting the variant; thus, the two daughters of the patient presented in our case report will undergo genetic counseling to facilitate future cardiovascular follow-up and ensure that any potential complication can be managed in time. If a child is found to be a hereditary carrier, management strategies should focus on regular cardiovascular monitoring through echocardiograms or CT scans and implementing lifestyle changes that minimize stress on the cardiovascular system. This might include controlling blood pressure and avoiding heavy lifting or other risk factors, such as smoking. Pregnancy will be monitored closely as it adds additional stress to the aorta. In some cases, preventive surgical options might be discussed if imaging indicates a high risk of vascular events. In addition to medical information, genetic counseling addresses the emotional impact of a genetic diagnosis, providing resources and support for the psychological aspects of living with an inherited condition. Discussing the options for preimplantation genetic or prenatal testing of the ACTA2 variant is included in the genetic counseling.

Table 4. Patients presenting the *ACTA2* gene and their characteristics.

No.	First Author/ Year/Reference	No. of Patients/ Gender/Age	Medical History of Aortic Disease	Family History of Aortic Disease	Clinical Features	Healthy Pregnancy
1.	Hoffjan et al., 2011 [32]	3 patients a. F, 38 b. F, 37 c. M, 41	a. Mild aortic dilation b. Acute aortic dissection c. Thoracic aortic aneurysm	a. 1 brother had ascending aorta aneurysm and died at 46 years old; 1 brother and the father had thoracic aortic aneurysm b. 1 brother died at 29 years old from acute aortic dissection c. no data available	Not described	a. 2 healthy pregnancies b. 2 healthy pregnancies c. -
2.	Keravnou et al., 2018 [36]	1/M/30	Type A aortic dissection	Father had aortic root and ascending aorta aneurysm (Bentall procedure performed) Mother had ascending aortic dilation	Not described	-
3.	Marutani et al., 2023 [37]	1/M/15	Extensive dissection from the ascending aorta to the common iliac artery	Genetic tests not performed	Not described	-
4.	Ware et al., 2014 [33]	1/M/17	Recurrent aortic dissection, severe aortic regurgitation	Twin brother had aortic dissection	Congenital mydriasis (both twins)	-
5.	Delsart et al., 2021 [38]	1/F/29	DeBakey type I aortic dissection	2 siblings had acute aortic dissection Mother died at 49 years old from type B aortic dissection	Not described	No pregnancies

5. Conclusions

To summarize, a familial thoracic aortic aneurysm is a condition with a high mortality rate if it is not properly diagnosed and monitored over time. These findings should encourage more frequent genetic testing in patients with aortic aneurysms, especially those with significant familial medical history or an early onset of the aortic disease. Additionally, a condition of particular importance but meaningful diagnostic and therapeutical challenges is blood culture-negative infective endocarditis. Rare causes should be investigated, and serological testing for infectious agents such as *Coxiella burnetii* ought to be considered. The management of a patient with both a genetic variant already manifested through a cardiovascular complication and a concurrent infectious disease is very particular due to the complexity of the case and requires a comprehensive, multidisciplinary approach focused on surveillance and proactive care. Therefore, regular cardiovascular imaging, blood pressure monitoring, and infection status assessment are essential to detect early signs of complications. Genetic counseling and family screening may also be beneficial for identifying at-risk relatives, enabling timely follow-up.

Author Contributions: Conceptualization, A.-R.C., C.G.S., M.I.B., S.C., M.-A.L., M.-D.V., A.I., R.E.S., D.-C.D., A.E.-C., A.L., D.G. and C.-T.L.; methodology, A.-R.C., C.G.S. and C.-T.L.; software, A.-R.C., C.G.S., M.I.B. and C.-T.L.; validation, A.-R.C., C.G.S., M.I.B., S.C., M.-A.L., M.-D.V., A.I., R.E.S., D.-C.D., A.E.-C., A.L. and C.-T.L.; formal analysis, A.-R.C., C.G.S. and C.-T.L.; investigation, A.-R.C., C.G.S., M.I.B. and C.-T.L.; resources, A.-R.C., C.G.S., M.I.B. and C.-T.L.; data curation, A.-R.C., C.G.S. and C.-T.L.; writing—original draft preparation, A.-R.C., C.G.S., M.I.B., S.C., M.-A.L., M.-D.V., A.I., R.E.S., D.-C.D., A.E.-C., A.L., D.G. and C.-T.L.; writing—review and editing, A.-R.C., C.G.S., M.I.B., A.L. and C.-T.L.; visualization, A.-R.C., C.G.S. and C.-T.L.; supervision, A.-R.C., C.G.S. and C.-T.L.; project administration, A.-R.C., C.G.S. and C.-T.L.; funding acquisition, A.-R.C., C.G.S. and C.-T.L. All authors have read and agreed to the published version of the manuscript.

Funding: This research received no external funding. Internal funding: we would like to acknowledge the "Victor Babes" University of Medicine and Pharmacy, Timisoara, for their support in covering the costs of publication for this research paper.

Institutional Review Board Statement: This study was conducted in accordance with the Declaration of Helsinki and approved by the Ethics Committee of the Institute for Cardiovascular Diseases of Timisoara (Nr. 5300/9 July 2024).

Informed Consent Statement: Written informed consent was obtained from the patient to publish this paper.

Data Availability Statement: All data are mentioned in the manuscript.

Conflicts of Interest: The authors declare no conflicts of interest.

References

1. Goyal, A.; Keramati, A.R.; Czarny, M.J.; Resar, J.R.; Mani, A. The Genetics of Aortopathies in Clinical Cardiology. *Clin. Med. Insights Cardiol.* **2017**, *11*, 1179546817709787. [CrossRef] [PubMed]
2. Isselbacher, E.M.; Preventza, O.; Black, J.H.; Augoustides, J.G.; Beck, A.W.; Bolen, M.A.; Braverman, A.C.; Bray, B.E.; Brown-Zimmerman, M.M.; Chen, E.P.; et al. 2022 ACC/AHA Guideline for the Diagnosis and Management of Aortic Disease: A Report of the American Heart Association/American College of Cardiology Joint Committee on Clinical Practice Guidelines. *Circulation* **2022**, *146*, E334–E482. [CrossRef] [PubMed]
3. Zhou, Z.; Cecchi, A.C.; Prakash, S.K.; Milewicz, D.M. Risk Factors for Thoracic Aortic Dissection. *Genes* **2022**, *13*, 1814. [CrossRef] [PubMed]
4. Ince, H.; Nienaber, C.A. Etiology, pathogenesis and management of thoracic aortic aneurysm. *Nat. Clin. Pr. Cardiovasc. Med.* **2007**, *4*, 418–427. [CrossRef] [PubMed]
5. Isselbacher, E.M.; Cardenas, C.L.L.; Lindsay, M.E. Hereditary Influence in Thoracic Aortic Aneurysm and Dissection. *Circulation* **2016**, *133*, 2516–2528. [CrossRef]
6. Pinard, A.; Jones, G.T.; Milewicz, D.M. Genetics of Thoracic and Abdominal Aortic Diseases: Aneurysms, Dissections, and Ruptures. *Circ. Res.* **2019**, *124*, 588–606. [CrossRef]
7. Renard, M.; Francis, C.; Ghosh, R.; Scott, A.F.; Witmer, P.D.; Adès, L.C.; Andelfinger, G.U.; Arnaud, P.; Boileau, C.; Callewaert, B.L.; et al. Clinical Validity of Genes for Heritable Thoracic Aortic Aneurysm and Dissection. *J. Am. Coll. Cardiol.* **2018**, *72*, 605–615. [CrossRef]
8. Guo, D.-C.; Pannu, H.; Tran-Fadulu, V.; Papke, C.L.; Yu, R.K.; Avidan, N.; Bourgeois, S.; Estrera, A.L.; Safi, H.J.; Sparks, E.; et al. Mutations in smooth muscle α-actin (ACTA2) lead to thoracic aortic aneurysms and dissections. *Nat. Genet.* **2007**, *39*, 1488–1493. [CrossRef]
9. Guo, D.-C.; Papke, C.L.; Tran-Fadulu, V.; Regalado, E.S.; Avidan, N.; Johnson, R.J.; Kim, D.H.; Pannu, H.; Willing, M.C.; Sparks, E.; et al. Mutations in Smooth Muscle Alpha-Actin (ACTA2) Cause Coronary Artery Disease, Stroke, and Moyamoya Disease, Along with Thoracic Aortic Disease. *Am. J. Hum. Genet.* **2009**, *84*, 617–627. [CrossRef]
10. Roder, C.; Peters, V.; Kasuya, H.; Nishizawa, T.; Wakita, S.; Berg, D.; Schulte, C.; Khan, N.; Tatagiba, M.; Krischek, B. Analysis of ACTA2 in European Moyamoya disease patients. *Eur. J. Paediatr. Neurol.* **2011**, *15*, 117–122. [CrossRef]
11. Dragan, A.L.; Voth, D.E. Coxiella burnetii: International pathogen of mystery. *Microbes Infect.* **2019**, *22*, 100–110. [CrossRef] [PubMed]
12. Neupane, K.; Kaswan, D. Coxiella burnetii Infection. In *StatPearls [Internet]*; StatPearls Publishing: Treasure Island, FL, USA, 2024. Available online: http://www.ncbi.nlm.nih.gov/books/NBK557893/ (accessed on 22 October 2024).
13. Madariaga, M.G.; Rezai, K.; Trenholme, G.M.; Weinstein, R.A. Q fever: A biological weapon in your backyard. *Lancet Infect. Dis.* **2003**, *3*, 709–721. [CrossRef] [PubMed]
14. Oyston, P.C.F.; Davies, C. Q fever: The neglected biothreat agent. *J. Med. Microbiol.* **2011**, *60*, 9–21. [CrossRef] [PubMed]
15. Cherry, C.C.; Nichols Heitman, K.; Bestul, N.C.; Kersh, G.J. Acute and chronic Q fever national surveillance—United States, 2008–2017. *Zoonoses Public Health* **2022**, *69*, 73–82. [CrossRef] [PubMed]

16. España, P.P.; Uranga, A.; Cillóniz, C.; Torres, A. Q Fever (*Coxiella burnetii*). *Semin. Respir. Crit. Care Med.* **2020**, *41*, 509–521. [CrossRef]
17. Chiu, C.K.; Durrheim, D.N. A review of the efficacy of human Q fever vaccine registered in Australia. *New South Wales Public Health Bull.* **2007**, *18*, 133–136. [CrossRef]
18. Raoult, D.; Tissot-Dupont, H.; Foucault, C.; Gouvernet, J.; Fournier, P.E.; Bernit, E.; Stein, A.; Nesri, M.; Harle, J.R.; Weiller, P.J. Q Fever 1985-1998: Clinical and Epidemiologic Features of 1383 Infections. *Medicine* **2000**, *79*, 109–123. [CrossRef]
19. Kofteridis, D.P.; Mazokopakis, E.E.; Tselentis, Y.; Gikas, A. Neurological complications of acute Q fever infection. *Eur. J. Epidemiol.* **2004**, *19*, 1051–1054. [CrossRef]
20. Million, M.; Lepidi, H.; Raoult, D.; Fièvre, Q. Actualités diagnostiques et thérapeutiques. *Méd. Mal. Infect.* **2009**, *39*, 82–94. [CrossRef]
21. Raoult, D.; Houpikian, P.; Dupont, H.T.; Riss, J.M.; Arditi-Djiane, J.; Brouqui, P. Treatment of Q Fever Endocarditis: Comparison of 2 Regimens Containing Doxycycline and Ofloxacin or Hydroxychloroquine. *Arch. Intern. Med.* **1999**, *159*, 167. [CrossRef]
22. Delgado, V.; Marsan, N.A.; de Waha, S.; Bonaros, N.; Brida, M.; Burri, H.; Caselli, S.; Doenst, T.; Ederhy, S.; Erba, P.A.; et al. Correction to: 2023 ESC Guidelines for the management of endocarditis: Developed by the task force on the management of endocarditis of the European Society of Cardiology (ESC) Endorsed by the European Association for Cardio-Thoracic Surgery (EACTS) and the European Association of Nuclear Medicine (EANM). *Eur. Heart J.* **2023**, *44*, 3948–4042. [CrossRef] [PubMed]
23. Chirita-Emandi, A.; Andreescu, N.; Zimbru, C.G.; Tutac, P.; Arghirescu, S.; Serban, M.; Puiu, M. Challenges in reporting pathogenic/potentially pathogenic variants in 94 cancer predisposing genes—In pediatric patients screened with NGS panels. *Sci. Rep.* **2020**, *10*, 223. [CrossRef] [PubMed]
24. Richards, S.; Aziz, N.; Bale, S.; Bick, D.; Das, S.; Gastier-Foster, J.; Grody, W.W.; Hegde, M.; Lyon, E.; Spector, E.; et al. Standards and guidelines for the interpretation of sequence variants: A joint consensus recommendation of the American College of Medical Genetics and Genomics and the Association for Molecular Pathology. *Genet. Med.* **2015**, *17*, 405–424. [CrossRef] [PubMed]
25. Cozma, D.; Streian, C.G.; Vacarescu, C.; Mornos, C. Back to sinus rhythm from atrial flutter or fibrillation: Dabigatran is safe without transoesophageal control. *Kardiologia Polska* **2016**, *74*, 425–430. [CrossRef]
26. Arnautu, S.F.; Arnautu, D.A.; Lascu, A.; Hajevschi, A.A.; Rosca, C.I.I.; Sharma, A.; Jianu, D.C. A Review of the Role of Transthoracic and Transesophageal Echocardiography, Computed Tomography, and Magnetic Resonance Imaging in Cardioembolic Stroke. *Med. Sci. Monit.* **2022**, *28*, e936365-1. [CrossRef]
27. Roder, C.; Nayak, N.R.; Khan, N.; Tatagiba, M.; Inoue, I.; Krischek, B. Genetics of Moyamoya disease. *J. Hum. Genet.* **2010**, *55*, 711–716. [CrossRef]
28. Bozza, S.; Graziani, A.; Borghi, M.; Marini, D.; Duranti, M.; Camilloni, B. Case report: Coxiella burnetii endocarditis in the absence of evident exposure. *Front. Med.* **2023**, *10*, 1220205. [CrossRef]
29. Deyell, M.W.; Chiu, B.; Ross, D.B.; Alvarez, N. Q fever endocarditis: A case report and review of the literature. *Can. J. Cardiol.* **2006**, *22*, 781–785. [CrossRef]
30. Afrasiabian, S.; Esmaeili, S.; Hajibagheri, K.; Hadizadeh, N.; Lotfi, G.; Veysi, A. Endocarditis Caused by *Coxiella burnetii*: A Case Report in Western Iran. *J. Arthropod-Borne Dis.* **2024**, *18*, 78–83. [CrossRef]
31. Krol, V.; Kogan, V.; Cunha, B.A. Q fever bioprosthetic aortic valve endocarditis (PVE) successfully treated with doxycycline monotherapy. *Heart Lung* **2008**, *37*, 157–160. [CrossRef]
32. Hoffjan, S.; Waldmüller, S.; Blankenfeldt, W.; Kötting, J.; Gehle, P.; Binner, P.; Epplen, J.T.; Scheffold, T. Three novel mutations in the ACTA2 gene in German patients with thoracic aortic aneurysms and dissections. *Eur. J. Hum. Genet.* **2011**, *19*, 520–524. [CrossRef] [PubMed]
33. Ware, S.M.; Shikany, A.; Landis, B.J.; James, J.F.; Hinton, R.B. Twins With Progressive Thoracic Aortic Aneurysm, Recurrent Dissection and *ACTA2* Mutation. *Pediatrics* **2014**, *134*, e1218–e1223. [CrossRef] [PubMed]
34. Coulon, C. Thoracic aortic aneurysms and pregnancy. *Presse Médicale* **2015**, *44*, 1126–1135. [CrossRef] [PubMed]
35. Braverman, A.C.; Mittauer, E.; Harris, K.M.; Evangelista, A.; Pyeritz, R.E.; Brinster, D.; Conklin, L.; Suzuki, T.; Fanola, C.; Ouzounian, M.; et al. Clinical Features and Outcomes of Pregnancy-Related Acute Aortic Dissection. *JAMA Cardiol.* **2021**, *6*, 58–66. [CrossRef]
36. Keravnou, A.; Bashiardes, E.; Michailidou, K.; Soteriou, M.; Moushi, A.; Cariolou, M. Novel variants in the ACTA2 and MYH11 genes in a Cypriot family with thoracic aortic aneurysms: A case report. *BMC Med. Genet.* **2018**, *19*, 208. [CrossRef]
37. Marutani, S.; Nishino, T.; Shimokawa, O.; Pooh, R.K.; Morisaki, H.; Inamura, N. Aortic Dissection and a Previously Unreported *ACTA2* Missense Variant Mutation in a Young Patient: A Case Report. *Pediatr. Dev. Pathol.* **2023**, *26*, 494–498. [CrossRef]
38. Delsart, P.; Vanlerberghe, C.; Juthier, F.; Sobocinski, J.; Domanski, O.; Longere, B.; Hanna, N.; Arnaud, P.; Marsili, L. The natural history of a family with aortic dissection associated with a novel ACTA2 variant. *Ann. Vasc. Surg.* **2021**, *77*, 348.e7–348.e11. [CrossRef]

Disclaimer/Publisher's Note: The statements, opinions and data contained in all publications are solely those of the individual author(s) and contributor(s) and not of MDPI and/or the editor(s). MDPI and/or the editor(s) disclaim responsibility for any injury to people or property resulting from any ideas, methods, instructions or products referred to in the content.

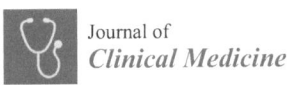

Article

The Interplay between Severe Cirrhosis and Heart: A Focus on Diastolic Dysfunction

Dragoș Lupu [1,2], Laurențiu Nedelcu [1,*] and Diana Țînț [2,3]

1 Department of Fundamental, Prophylactic, and Clinical Disciplines, Transilvania University of Brasov, 500036 Brașov, Romania; dragos182@yahoo.com
2 ICCO Clinics Brasov, Transilvania University of Brasov, 500059 Brașov, Romania; dianatint@gmail.com
3 Department of Medical and Surgical Specialties, Transilvania University of Brasov, 500036 Brașov, Romania
* Correspondence: laurnedelcu@yahoo.com; Tel.: +40-7-2273-0846

Abstract: Background/Objectives: Cardiovascular involvement in severe cirrhosis presents diagnostic challenges and carries significant prognostic implications. This study aims to evaluate the relationship between liver disease severity and portal hypertension with the burden of diastolic dysfunction. **Methods**: We prospectively enrolled patients with hepatic cirrhosis, classified according to the Child–Pugh criteria. Of the 102 patients included, 65 were classified as Group A (non-severe cirrhosis: Child–Pugh Classes A and B) and 37 as Group B (severe cirrhosis: Child–Pugh Class C). Portal vein and spleen diameters were assessed using abdominal ultrasound. All patients underwent echocardiographic evaluation. LV systolic function was assessed by measuring ejection fraction, while diastolic function was evaluated using three parameters: E/Em ratio, E/Vp ratio, and indexed left atrial volume. **Results**: We observed a significantly greater burden of diastolic dysfunction in Group B compared to Group A. Specifically, the E/Vp ratio was 2.2 ± 0.4 in Group B versus 1.9 ± 0.3 in Group A ($p < 0.001$); the indexed LA volume was 34.5 ± 3.2 mL/m^2 in Group B versus 30.1 ± 2.9 mL/m^2 in Group A ($p < 0.001$); and the E/Em ratio was 17.0 ± 3.0 in Group B versus 11.5 ± 2.8 in Group A ($p < 0.001$). Additionally, the mean diameters of the portal vein and spleen were larger in Group B, with measurements of 14.3 ± 2.1 mm versus 11.5 ± 1.6 mm for the portal vein and 15.0 ± 1.2 mm versus 11.7 ± 1.5 mm for the spleen ($p < 0.001$), which correlated with the extent of diastolic dysfunction. **Conclusions**: Diastolic dysfunction was prevalent in 55% of patients with liver cirrhosis. The burden of diastolic dysfunction was higher in patients with severe hepatic cirrhosis compared to those with milder forms, and it correlated with the severity of portal hypertension, as assessed by measuring portal vein diameter and spleen diameter.

Keywords: diastolic dysfunction; cirrhotic cardiomyopathy; echocardiography; hepatic cirrhosis

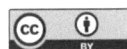

1. Introduction

Liver cirrhosis is a severe condition characterized by the progressive scarring of liver tissue. It can arise from various causes, including viral infections (such as hepatitis B and C), chronic alcohol consumption, obesity, and metabolic diseases. As the global prevalence of cirrhosis increases, it poses significant challenges not only to individual health, but also to healthcare systems, increasing the demand for treatments, hospitalizations, and other medical resources. Complications of cirrhosis include liver failure, gastrointestinal hemorrhages, heightened risk of liver cancer, and heart failure. Patients with liver cirrhosis exhibit well-documented hemodynamic alterations, including elevated cardiac output and reduced systemic vascular resistance [1,2]. The vasodilation that occurs in patients with cirrhosis can mask early systolic cardiac dysfunction and the initial decrease in contractility by reducing afterload and increasing preload, which in turn increases cardiac output. Resting diastolic evaluation may be inadequate for patients whose symptoms are limited to exertional dyspnea, as the increase in left ventricular filling pressures and pulmonary congestion in these individuals may only manifest during exercise [3]. Over the past three decades, research has highlighted a phenomenon known as "cirrhotic cardiomyopathy", which includes impaired myocardial contractility, altered diastolic relaxation, and electrophysiological abnormalities in the absence of overt heart disease [4–7].

While the exact prevalence of cirrhotic cardiomyopathy remains unclear, estimates suggest that around 50% of cirrhotic patients may develop this type of cardiomyopathy at some stage in their illness [8]. Cirrhotic cardiomyopathy is often under-recognized in clinical practice, as it may only become apparent under stress, making diagnosis challenging.

The presence of cirrhotic cardiomyopathy, marked by left ventricular diastolic dysfunction, is associated with accelerated disease progression and a poorer prognosis. Increased stiffness of the cirrhotic heart can lead to reduced compliance, resulting in diastolic dysfunction. This condition can be assessed using transmitral Doppler echocardiography, tissue Doppler echocardiography, and cardiac magnetic resonance imaging. Additionally, there seems to be a correlation between diastolic dysfunction and the severity of liver dysfunction, as well as the presence of ascites [9].

In 2019, the Cirrhotic Cardiomyopathy Consortium redefined the diagnostic criteria for cirrhotic cardiomyopathy, incorporating the latest recommendations from the American Society of Echocardiography (ASE) and the European Association of Cardiovascular Imaging (EACVI) for assessing systolic and diastolic function. This update superseded the diagnostic recommendations from the 2005 World Congress of Gastroenterology [10]. Diastolic dysfunction is frequently observed in cirrhotic patients, with prevalence rates ranging from 43% to 70%, even when left ventricular ejection fraction (LVEF) remains normal [11].

The Consortium recommends using parameters such as the septal velocity of the Em wave, the E/Em ratio, indexed left atrial (LA) volume, and tricuspid regurgitation velocity for evaluating diastolic function.

While specific guidelines on whether the diastolic function should be assessed at rest or during exercise are lacking, it is crucial to recognize that diastolic abnormalities may not manifest at rest. Diastolic dysfunction symptoms often appear only during exercise, as left ventricular filling pressure may be normal at rest, but increases with physical activity due to the heart's inability to increase cardiac output without increasing filling pressure [12].

Diastolic dysfunction has proven to be the most sensitive indicator for diagnosing cirrhotic cardiomyopathy, as it is the earliest parameter to be affected. Atroush and colleagues utilized tissue Doppler imaging and speckle tracking to evaluate diastolic function in patients with end-stage liver disease, investigating the correlation between cardiac dysfunction and the Child–Pugh classification of liver cell failure. The study identified a high prevalence of diastolic dysfunction (87.5%) among patients with end-stage liver disease by measuring the E/É ratio using tissue Doppler imaging (TDI), which was found to be more accurate than the E/A ratio. Although the study did not find a correlation between cardiac dysfunction and the severity of liver disease, it is important to note that it had a small sample size, consisting of only 40 patients who were followed for three months [13].

A meta-analysis by Stundiene et al., encompassing 16 studies, found that approximately 51% of cirrhotic patients have diastolic dysfunction [14]. However, these findings are limited by the use of less specific parameters, such as the E/A ratio and the inclusion of patients with potential ventricular relaxation impairment from other causes. As noted by Prekumar et al. and Ruíz-del-Árbol et al., inadequate detection of diastolic dysfunction may lead to adverse clinical outcomes. Therefore, early and accurate identification of this condition is crucial for improving patient prognosis [15,16].

The presence of cirrhotic cardiomyopathy and impaired diastolic function represent critical factors, especially for patients following liver transplantation. Ershoff et al. conducted a retrospective cohort study involving 254 liver transplant recipients to evaluate the impact of diastolic dysfunction on mortality. The LA volume index was used as a key parameter for assessment. The study concluded that this condition is associated with increased mortality in post-liver transplant patients, particularly those with a high Model for End-Stage Liver Disease (MELD) score [17]. Similarly, a 2022 study by Vetrugno et al., which included 83 orthotopic liver transplant recipients, explored the relationship between preoperative diastolic dysfunction and the risk of early allograft dysfunction. The study found that patients with impaired diastolic function were more likely to develop early allograft dysfunction after orthotopic liver transplantation [18].

This study aimed to analyze the correlation between the severity of liver disease (severe Child–Pugh C vs. non-severe Child–Pugh A and B) and the burden of diastolic dysfunction measured after exercise using a combination of parameters. Additionally, it sought to evaluate the potential correlation between diastolic dysfunction and the severity of portal hypertension, as assessed by abdominal ultrasonography parameters, specifically portal vein and spleen diameters.

2. Materials and Methods

We conducted an observational, prospective study involving 102 patients with hepatic cirrhosis, classified according to Child–Pugh criteria. Patient recruitment and subsequent clinical, laboratory, and abdominal ultrasound evaluations were conducted at the internal medicine clinic from November 2021 to March 2024. Within the first 15 days after inclusion, participants underwent cardiac ultrasound evaluations at a cardiology outpatient clinic. The inclusion and exclusion criteria are detailed in Table 1.

Table 1. Inclusion and exclusion criteria.

Inclusion Criteria	Exclusion Criteria
Age over 18 years	Age under 18 years
Diagnosis of hepatic cirrhosis	Heart failure from any cause other than CCM
Written informed consent	Persistent or permanent atrial fibrillation
	Significant ventricular arrhythmia
	Uncontrolled hypertension
	Acute coronary syndrome
	Ch Chronic kidney disease in hemodialysis stage
	Sequelae of ischemic or hemorrhagic stroke
	Inability to perform physical exertion

CCM = cirrhotic cardiomyopathy.

This study was approved by the Ethics Committee of Transilvania University of Brașov (approval number no.5, approval date: 26 February 2020), and all participants provided informed consent prior to enrollment.

Laboratory tests were performed to assess blood cell count, liver function (bilirubin, AST, ALT, GGT, LDH), renal function (creatinine, urea), coagulation status (INR), plasma albumin, and glucose levels. Additionally, the glomerular filtration rate (GFR) was calculated for all patients. Abdominal ultrasound evaluations focused on the dimensions of the liver, spleen, portal vein, and splenic vein, as well as the presence or absence of ascitic fluid.

The Child–Pugh score was assessed for each patient, following the classification system described in the MSD Manual (https://www.msdmanuals.com/professional/multimedia/clinical-calculator/child-pugh-classification-for-severity-of-liver-disease, accessed on: 30 July 2024). This score typically categorizes patients into three groups based on liver function severity: Class A (score of 5–6), Class B (score of 7–9), and Class C (score of 10–15). For our study, patients were divided into two groups: Group A (non-severe cirrhosis, encompassing Child–Pugh Classes A and B) and Group B (severe cirrhosis, Child–Pugh Class C).

Regarding cirrhosis etiology, the majority of patients had alcoholic cirrhosis (77 patients, representing 75% of the total). Eighteen patients had viral etiology (17%), while seven patients were classified under other etiologies (6%).

To assess systolic and diastolic function, all participants performed five squats and were subsequently evaluated via echocardiography.

Modern echocardiographic techniques are used to evaluate systolic and diastolic function for diagnosing cirrhotic cardiomyopathy. Left ventricular (LV) systolic function is commonly assessed by measuring the LV ejection fraction (LVEF), with values below 50% considered abnormal. For the assessment of diastolic function, four echocardiographic parameters may be used: septal and lateral mitral annular peak early diastolic velocity (e'), the ratio of the peak velocity of mitral inflow during early diastole (E) to the average of septal and lateral e' (E/e'), LA volume indexed to body surface area, and tricuspid regurgitation velocity [3].

In our study, cardiac ultrasound was performed using a General Electric Vivid E9 machine with a 4.2 MHz cardiac transducer. A thorough examination was carried out, which included measurements of the dimensions of the aorta, left atrium, left ventricle, right atrium, right ventricle, interventricular septum, and posterior wall. The assessment also encompassed valve functionality, systolic pulmonary artery pressures, and evaluation of the pericardium. Systolic function was measured by calculating the LVEF using the Simpson method. Diastolic function was assessed using the following parameters:

E/Em Ratio: The ratio of E, the velocity of early mitral inflow measured by pulsed Doppler, to Em, the early diastolic mitral annular tissue velocity. Normal values are <15.

E/Vp Ratio: The ratio of E to Vp, where Vp represents the propagation of early diastolic trans-mitral velocity assessed by M-mode echocardiography. Normal values are <2, with values >2.5 linked to pulmonary capillary wedge pressures above 15 mmHg [19].

Indexed Left Atrial (LA) Volume: Normal values are <34 mL/m^2.

Peak E wave velocity was evaluated in the apical four-chamber view using color flow imaging to achieve optimal alignment of PW Doppler with the mitral flow. We analyzed the peak modal velocity during late diastole (following the P wave on the ECG) at the leading edge of the spectral waveform.

Pulsed-wave tissue Doppler imaging (TDI) e' velocity (cm/s) was measured in the four-chamber view using a pulsed-wave sample volume positioned at the lateral and septal basal regions, facilitating the calculation of the average e' velocity. We assessed the peak modal velocity during early diastole at the leading edge of the spectral waveform.

For E/Vp acquisition, we used color M-mode in the apical four-chamber view, utilizing color flow imaging to guide M-mode cursor positioning. The color baseline was adjusted toward the mitral valve inflow to lower the velocity scale, enhancing the red/yellow inflow velocity profile. We then analyzed the slope of the inflow from the mitral valve plane into the left ventricular chamber during early diastole at a 4 cm distance.

To obtain the indexed LA volume, we used the apical four- and two-chamber views, capturing freeze frames before the mitral valve (MV) opening. The area–length method was utilized, with the left atrial appendage and pulmonary veins excluded from the tracings. The values were adjusted for body surface area.

An example of echocardiographic parameters used for evaluating diastolic function is displayed in Figure 1.

The physical exertion was supervised by medical staff, and echocardiography was performed immediately afterward. Following the evaluation, diastolic function parameters obtained from all three measurements were compared between the two study groups. Additionally, correlations were analyzed between diastolic function parameters and the diameters of the portal vein and spleen as measured with abdominal ultrasound.

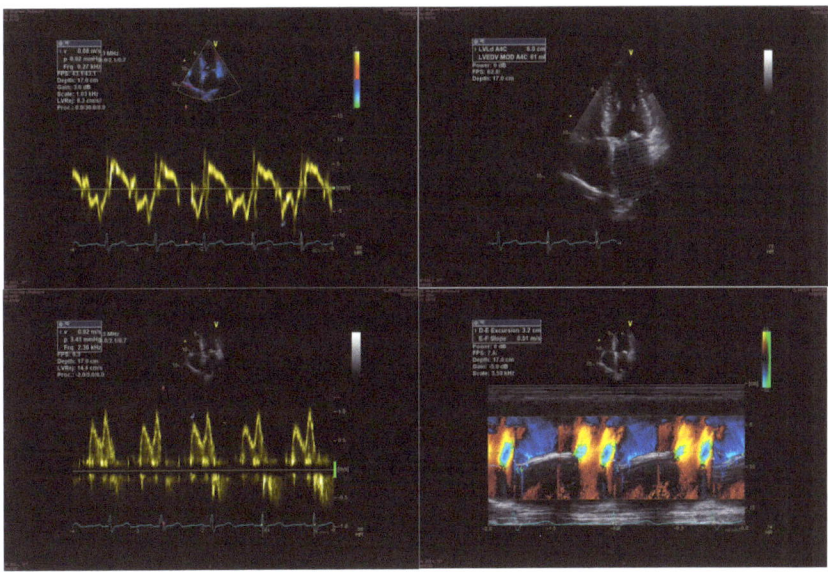

Figure 1. Diastolic function parameters measured by echocardiography: the upper left image shows the Em wave, the upper right image shows the LA volume, the bottom left image shows the E wave, and the bottom right image shows the Vp measurement.

Statistical Analysis

Statistical analyses were conducted using Python 3.4 (PSF, Wilmington, DE, USA). Variables were reported as mean ± SD. Gender, smoking status, hypertension, dyslipidemia, and diabetes mellitus were recorded as dichotomous variables. The Chi-squared test was employed to compare the frequency of nominal variables. For continuous variables, the Independent-Samples *t*-test was used to compare means, while the Mann–Whitney U-test analyzed mean rank differences for ordinal variables. A two-sided *p*-value of <0.05 was considered statistically significant.

3. Results

Out of the 102 study participants, sixty-five patients had non-severe cirrhosis (Child–Pugh Classes A and B), while thirty-seven patients had severe cirrhosis (Child–Pugh Class C). Factors influencing diastolic function were similarly prevalent in both groups, regardless of the severity of hepatic disease (Table 2). Baseline characteristics were comparable between the two groups, with no significant differences in age, hypertension, dyslipidemia, coronary artery disease, or obesity. However, the prevalence of diabetes was notably higher in the severe cirrhosis group.

All patients were prescribed cardiovascular medication as shown in Table 3.

Significant differences were observed in medication prescriptions between patients with varying levels of hepatic function impairment. Beta-blockers were prescribed to all patients in the severe cirrhosis group, compared to only 46.2% in the non-severe group. Additionally, spironolactone and furosemide were more frequently administered in the severe group (91.9% vs. 3.1%, $p < 0.001$, and 86.5% vs. 3.1%, $p < 0.001$, respectively). In contrast, angiotensin-converting enzyme inhibitors were exclusively used in the non-severe group (24.6%). The dosage of furosemide ranged from 20 to 40 mg, while spironolactone was administered at doses between 25 and 50 mg. A total of ten patients were treated with SGLT2 inhibitors (dapagliflozin or empagliflozin), including four with non-severe cirrhosis and six with severe cirrhosis, all of whom had diabetes mellitus.

Table 2. Characteristics and comorbidities of the groups with non-severe cirrhosis compared to the severe cirrhosis group.

Characteristic	Non-Severe Cirrhosis n = 65	Severe Cirrhosis n = 37	p
Age, mean ± SD [years]	65.5 ± 10.9	64.5 ± 11.6	0.69
Male, n (%)	44 (67.7)	22 (59.5)	0.68
Hypertension	32 (49)	17 (45)	0.74
Diabetes mellitus	8 (12)	11 (29)	**0.03**
Chronic coronary syndrome	5 (7)	4 (10)	0.45
Dyslipidemia, n (%)	12 (18)	9 (23)	0.34
Smoking, n (%)	23 (34.3)	15 (40.5)	0.61
BMI, mean ± SD [kg/m^2]	24.2 ± 3.9	23.8 ± 4.5	0.84

BMI = Body mass index; GFR = estimated Glomerular Filtration Ratio; SD = standard deviation. Bold: statistical significance.

Table 3. Cardiovascular medication.

Medication	Non-Severe Cirrhosis n = 65	Severe Cirrhosis n = 37	p
Beta-blockers, n (%)	30 (46.2)	37 (100)	**<0.001**
Spironolactone, n (%)	2 (3.1)	34 (91.9)	**<0.001**
Furosemide, n (%)	22 (3.1)	32 (86.5)	**<0.001**
SGLT2 inhibitors, n (%)	4 (6)	6 (16)	0.1003
Angiotensin-converting enzyme inhibitors, n (%)	16 (24.6)	0 (0)	

SGLT2 = sodium-glucose transport protein 2. Bold: statistical significance.

While LVEF was comparable between the two groups, significant differences were noted in diastolic function measurements between patients with non-severe and severe cirrhosis. Specifically, the E/Vp ratio was 1.9 ± 0.3 in the non-severe cirrhosis group versus 2.2 ± 0.4 in the severe cirrhosis group ($p < 0.001$); the indexed LA volume was 30.1 ± 2.9 mL/m^2 compared to 34.5 ± 3.2 mL/m^2 ($p < 0.001$); and the E/Em ratio was 11.5 ± 2.8 versus 17.0 ± 3.0 ($p < 0.001$).

Diastolic dysfunction was present in the majority of patients with severe cirrhosis, affecting 26 individuals (70%). Conversely, 34 patients in the non-severe group did not have this condition, leading to a lower prevalence in that group (47%). Overall, the prevalence of diastolic dysfunction across the entire study population was 55%.

Abdominal ultrasound parameters indicative of portal hypertension severity were markedly altered in patients with severe cirrhosis. The mean portal vein diameter was 14.3 ± 2.1 mm in the severe cirrhosis compared to 11.5 ± 1.6 mm in the non-severe cirrhosis group, group ($p < 0.001$). Additionally, the mean spleen diameter was significantly greater in the severe cirrhosis group (15.0 ± 1.2 mm vs. 11.7 ± 1.5 mm; $p < 0.001$), as shown in Table 4.

We also examined the relationship between the severity of portal hypertension and LV diastolic function. Moderate and statistically significant correlations were found between the portal vein diameter and two diastolic function parameters (Figure 2a,b), as well as between the spleen diameter and all three diastolic function parameters (Figure 3a–c).

Table 4. Comparison of cardiac and abdominal parameters assessed with ultrasound between the two patient groups.

Parameter	Non-Severe Cirrhosis n = 65	Severe Cirrhosis n = 37	p
LV Ejection fraction, mean ± SD [%]	56.9 ± 6.2	58.9 ± 3.9	0.06
E/VP, mean ± SD	1.9 ± 0.3	2.2 ± 0.4	**<0.001**
Indexed LA volume, mean ± SD [mL/m^2]	30.1 ± 2.9	34.5 ± 3.2	**<0.001**
E/Em, mean ± SD	11.5 ± 2.8	17.0 ± 3.0	**<0.001**
PV, mean ± SD [mm]	11.5 ± 1.6	14.3 ± 2.1	**<0.001**
Spleen diameter, mean ± SD [mm]	11.7 ± 1.5	15.0 ± 1.2	**<0.001**

E = velocity of the early phase of mitral inflow; Em = early diastolic mitral annular tissue velocity LA = left atrium; LV = Left ventricle; PV = portal vein; VP = propagation of early diastolic trans-mitral velocity; SD = standard deviation. Bold: statistical significance.

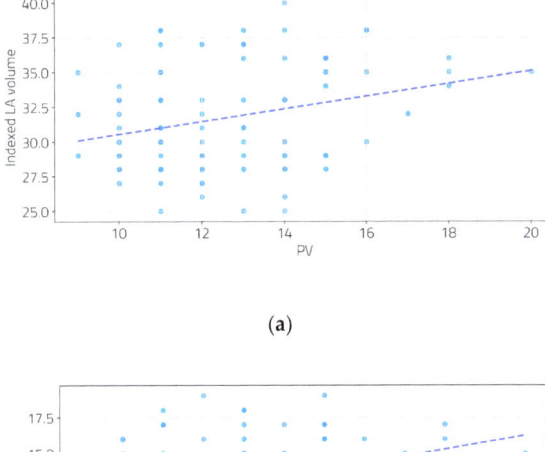

(a)

(b)

Figure 2. Correlation between PV and indexed LA volume (**a**) and E/EM (**b**). [(**a**) r = 0.28, p = 0.004; (**b**) r = 0.34, p < 0.001].

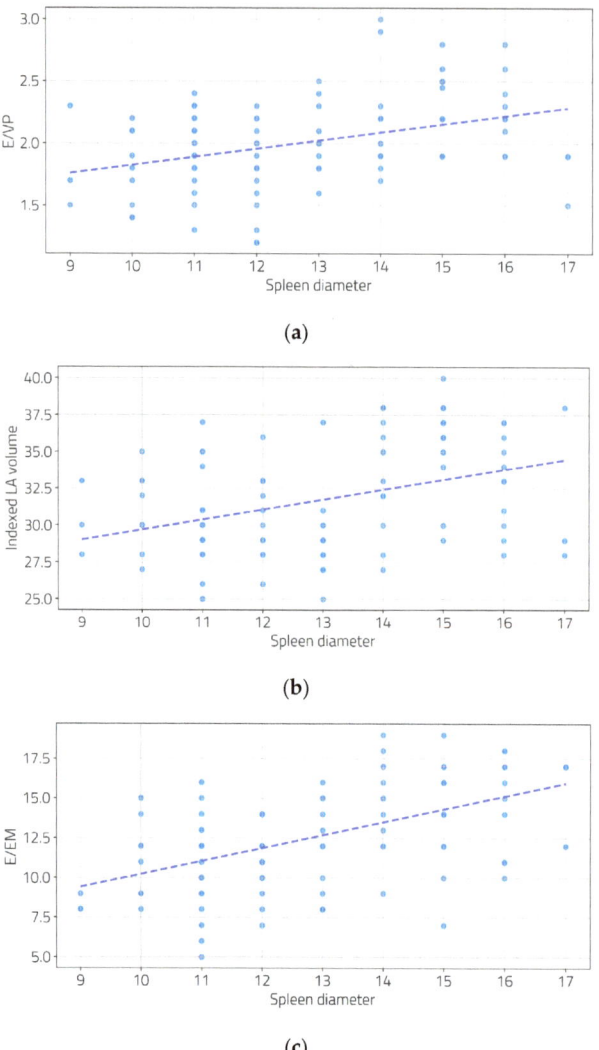

Figure 3. Correlations between spleen diameters and E/Vp (**a**), indexed LA volume (**b**), and E/Em (**c**). ((**a**) r = 0.39, $p < 0.001$; (**b**) r = 0.39, $p < 0.001$, and (**c**) r = 0.53, $p < 0.001$).

4. Discussion

The clinical significance of diastolic dysfunction has gained considerable attention in recent years, with substantial evidence demonstrating its profound impact on both the quality of life and the prognosis of affected patients [20–22]. A meta-analysis by Ladeiras-Lopes et al. revealed that impaired diastolic function is associated with a 3.53-fold increased risk of cardiovascular events or death [23]. Similarly, research by Kosmala et al. indicated that asymptomatic LV diastolic dysfunction in patients with preserved systolic function is linked to the development of heart failure and decreased survival [24].

These findings underscore the importance of early detection and accurate assessment of diastolic dysfunction, particularly in patients with hepatic cirrhosis. Proper evaluation is crucial as it can significantly influence the prognosis of patients with impaired diastolic function, even when systolic function appears normal.

However, the presence and implications of diastolic dysfunction in patients with normal systolic function within the context of hepatic cirrhosis are less well-explored. Current studies are often limited by small sample sizes and inconsistent results, highlighting the need for further research in this area. Table 5 below summarizes the key studies on diastolic dysfunction in cirrhotic patients.

Table 5. Main studies on diastolic dysfunction in cirrhotic patients.

Clinical Study	Number of Patients Enrolled	Aim	Results
A case-cohort study of left ventricular diastolic dysfunction in patients with cirrhosis: the liver–heart axis [25]	203	Assessment of the association of diastolic dysfunction with the factors affecting cirrhosis patients' severity, complications, and survival	Higher Child–Pugh class, prolonged QTc, higher ascitic fluid protein levels, and poor survival are significantly associated with diastolic dysfunction
Cardiac dysfunction in cirrhotic portal hypertension with or without ascites [26]	60	To evaluate cardiac systolic and diastolic functions in liver cirrhosis patients with or without ascites	Diastolic dysfunction is commonly associated with advancement of hepatic dysfunction
Ultrasonographic Prevalence and Factors Predicting Left Ventricular Diastolic Dysfunction in Patients with Liver Cirrhosis: Is There a Correlation between the Grade of Diastolic Dysfunction and the Grade of Liver Disease? [27]	92	To assess the echocardiographic prevalence of diastolic dysfunction among a population of cirrhotic patients and to investigate whether a correlation between stage of cardiac dysfunction and stage of liver disease could be established	Diastolic dysfunction stage 1 is fairly prevalent among all CTP classes, whereas diastolic dysfunction stage 2 seems to be characteristic of the advanced liver disease (CTP-class C)
Diastolic myocardial dysfunction does not affect survival in patients with cirrhosis [28]	76	To investigate if diastolic dysfunction is associated with severity and etiology of cirrhosis and mortality	Diastolic dysfunction is more frequent in patients with ascites and does not link to mortality
Cardiac dysfunction in cirrhosis is not associated with the severity of liver disease [29]	74	To investigate factors associated with cardiac dysfunction in cirrhotic patients	No association between severity of liver disease and cardiac dysfunction
Systolic and diastolic impairment in cirrhotic cardiomyopathy: insights from a cross-sectional study [30]	68	To investigate the prevalence of systolic and diastolic function in patients with cirrhotic cardiomyopathy	Remarkable prevalence of cirrhotic cardiomyopathy Lack of correlation with the severity of liver cirrhosis

CTP = Child–Turcotte–Pugh, QTc—corrected QT interval.

Our study conducted a comprehensive evaluation of diastolic function by incorporating three advanced parameters, including two (E/Em and indexed LA volume) recommended by the Cirrhotic Cardiomyopathy Consortium. Previous research has identified E/Em as a highly specific marker for elevated left ventricular filling pressure, while indexed LA volume serves as an indicator of chronically increased end-diastolic LV pressure, though it does not strongly correlate with LA pressure [31]. The third parameter, E/Vp, also proved to be valuable in assessing diastolic function [32]. Garcia et al. demonstrated that E/Vp is less dependent on left ventricular filling conditions; by combining Vp (an index of ventricular relaxation) with the E wave velocity (reflecting left atrial pressure), E/Vp is particularly useful for estimating left ventricular filling pressures [33]. To the best of our knowledge, our research is the first to utilize these three parameters to define diastolic dysfunction in cirrhotic patients.

Our findings revealed no significant differences in LV systolic function between the two groups, which aligns with the existing literature [34,35]. However, all three parameters used to define diastolic function were significantly more altered in patients with advanced hepatic disease, partially in line with findings from other studies [25–28]. While some previous studies have shown a link between diastolic dysfunction and the severity of cirrhotic disease, others, such as the research by Merli et al., found no such association [29,30].

By combining these three parameters, we were able to highlight the pressure changes in all three components: left ventricle, left atrium, and pulmonary capillary, reflecting the progression of these cardiac changes in parallel with the worsening of liver disease. Moreover, to support this hypothesis, we were able to show the correlation between the severity of portal hypertension and diastolic dysfunction. In our research, the degree of diastolic dysfunction correlates with both the portal vein diameter and spleen diameter.

Similar results were published in the literature. Thus, in a recent study, Behera et al. found that Child C patients with portal hypertension had a higher prevalence of cirrhotic cardiomyopathy and diastolic dysfunction [36]. Also, Marconi et al. concluded in their 2017 study that diastolic dysfunction, measured by Em and LA volume, worsens as portal pressures increase [37].

Since the focus of this research was on diastolic dysfunction, systolic function was assessed solely through the LVEF determined by the Simpson method, which revealed no statistically significant differences between the two groups. It is important to note that previous studies have demonstrated that global longitudinal strain (GLS) [38] and S wave velocity measured with tissue Doppler [39] are more effective methods for evaluating systolic function compared to ejection fraction.

Our study uniquely utilizes three distinct high-fidelity parameters: E/Vp, E/Em, and indexed LA volume to estimate diastolic function, correlating these measures with the severity of liver disease and assessing diastolic dysfunction after brief exercise. This approach allows us to uncover diastolic abnormalities that may not be evident under resting conditions. Furthermore, E/Vp has not been previously utilized as a marker for diastolic dysfunction in the context of hepatic cirrhosis.

Given that liver cirrhosis is associated with comorbidities such as malnutrition, muscle mass loss, reduced exercise capacity, and decreased muscle strength, we opted to use a non-standardized exercise test. This involved performing five squats, immediately followed by an assessment of diastolic function parameters.

To the best of our knowledge, this is the first study to utilize these three parameters to define diastolic dysfunction and to analyze them after exercise in patients with cirrhosis.

This study involved interdisciplinary collaboration, with patient enrollment conducted at an internal medicine clinic after a thorough evaluation and diagnosis. Cardiac assessments were performed separately in an outpatient cardiology clinic. Additionally, we implemented a novel approach by categorizing patients according to the severity of their cirrhosis—severe versus non-severe.

Our findings indicate that diastolic dysfunction, as a marker of heart failure, warrants consideration of specific interventions, particularly for patients with severe cirrhosis who have limited treatment options [40]. Thus, early recognition of diastolic dysfunction as a sign of heart failure (in conjunction with natriuretic peptides) could expand the therapeutic options by incorporating SGLT2 inhibitors into the treatment regimen. These drugs are now included in the guidelines with a Class I recommendation for the entire spectrum of heart failure, including heart failure with preserved LVEF [41]. Furthermore, earlier integration into a palliative care program should be considered, as it offers significant benefits for these patients [42].

The diagnosis of diastolic dysfunction is also critically important in post-liver transplant patients, as numerous studies have demonstrated an association with increased morbidity and mortality [43,44].

5. Conclusions

In our study, diastolic dysfunction was less prevalent in patients with non-severe cirrhosis, while the majority of patients with severe cirrhosis exhibited this condition.

The overall prevalence of diastolic dysfunction among patients with liver cirrhosis was found to be 55%. Severe hepatic cirrhosis (Child–Pugh Class C) was also associated with a more pronounced degree of diastolic dysfunction compared to milder forms of the disease. This dysfunction was significantly correlated with the severity of portal hypertension, as reflected by surrogate parameters such as portal vein and spleen diameters. Spleen diameter was the sole factor that demonstrated a significant correlation with all three evaluated parameters of diastolic function. These findings underscore the importance of monitoring diastolic function in cirrhotic patients, particularly those with advanced disease, as early identification and management of diastolic dysfunction could potentially improve clinical outcomes.

5.1. Study Limitations

Our study has several limitations. The relatively small sample size may have impacted the thoroughness and significance of the results. Additionally, follow-up visits could have offered better insights into symptom progression and the development of diastolic dysfunction. Furthermore, measuring natriuretic peptides and examining their correlation with diastolic function and the severity of cirrhosis, along with the use of tissue Doppler ultrasound for GLS or S wave analysis, could significantly improve our understanding of these conditions.

5.2. Future Directions

Recognizing the importance of the early detection of diastolic dysfunction in reducing cardiovascular events after liver transplantation, a paradigm shift is essential. This shift involves incorporating diastolic function evaluated through modern diagnostic parameters into pre-liver transplant risk stratification, which has traditionally focused on ejection fraction and right-sided cardiac pressures.

Author Contributions: Conceptualization, D.Ț. and D.L.; Methodology, D.L.; Formal Analysis, L.N.; Investigation, D.L.; Resources, D.L.; Data Curation, D.L.; Writing—Original Draft Preparation, D.L.; Writing—Review and Editing, D.Ț.; Visualization, L.N.; Supervision, D.Ț.; Project Administration, D.L. and D.Ț. All authors have read and agreed to the published version of the manuscript.

Funding: This research received no external funding.

Institutional Review Board Statement: This study was conducted in accordance with the Declaration of Helsinki and approved by the Ethics Committee of the Transilvania University of Brasov, no.5, approval date: 26 February 2020.

Informed Consent Statement: Informed consent was obtained from all subjects involved in this study.

Data Availability Statement: Dataset available on request from the authors.

Acknowledgments: We would like to thank Andreea Popescu for her valuable support with the statistical analysis.

Conflicts of Interest: The authors declare no conflicts of interest.

References

1. Kowalski, H.; Abelmann, W. The cardiac output at rest in Laennec's cirrhosis. *J. Clin. Investig.* **1953**, *32*, 1025–1033. [CrossRef] [PubMed] [PubMed Central]
2. Schrier, R.W.; Arroyo, V.; Bernardi, M.; Epstein, M.; Henriksen, J.H.; Rodés, J. Peripheral arterial vasodilation hypothesis: A proposal for the initiation of renal sodium and water retention in cirrhosis. *Hepatology* **1988**, *8*, 1151–1157. [CrossRef] [PubMed]
3. Liu, H.; Naser, J.A.; Lin, G.; Lee, S.S. Cardiomyopathy in cirrhosis: From pathophysiology to clinical care. *JHEP Rep.* **2023**, *6*, 100911. [CrossRef] [PubMed] [PubMed Central]
4. Kalluru, R.; Gadde, S.; Chikatimalla, R.; Dasaradhan, T.; Koneti, J.; priya Cherukuri, S. Cirrhotic Cardiomyopathy: The Interplay Between Liver and Heart. *Cureus* **2022**, *14*, e27969. [CrossRef] [PubMed] [PubMed Central]
5. Lee, S.S. Cardiac abnormalities in liver cirrhosis. *West. J. Med.* **1989**, *151*, 530–535. [PubMed] [PubMed Central]
6. Liu, H.; Song, D.; Lee, S.S. Cirrhotic cardiomyopathy. *Gastroenterol. Clin. Biol.* **2002**, *26*, 842–847. [PubMed]
7. Alqahtani, S.A.; Fouad, T.R.; Lee, S.S. Cirrhotic cardiomyopathy. *Semin. Liver Dis.* **2008**, *28*, 59–69. [CrossRef] [PubMed]

8. Razpotnik, M.; Bota, S.; Wimmer, P.; Hackl, M.; Lesnik, G.; Alber, H.; Peck-Radosavljevic, M. The prevalence of cirrhotic cardiomyopathy according to different diagnostic criteria. *Liver Int.* **2021**, *41*, 1058–1069. [CrossRef]
9. Møller, S.; Wiese, S.; Halgreen, H.; Hove, J.D. Diastolic dysfunction in cirrhosis. *Heart Fail. Rev.* **2016**, *21*, 599–610. [CrossRef] [PubMed]
10. Izzy, M.; VanWagner, L.B.; Lin, G.; Altieri, M.; Findlay, J.Y.; Oh, J.K.; Watt, K.D.; Lee, S.S.; Cirrhotic Cardiomyopathy Consortium. Redefining Cirrhotic Cardiomyopathy for the Modern Era. *Hepatology* **2020**, *71*, 334–345, Erratum in *Hepatology* **2020**, *72*, 1161. [CrossRef] [PubMed] [PubMed Central]
11. Kaur, H.; Premkumar, M. Diagnosis and Management of Cirrhotic Cardiomyopathy. *J. Clin. Exp. Hepatol.* **2022**, *12*, 186–199. [CrossRef] [PubMed] [PubMed Central]
12. Ha, J.W.; Andersen, O.S.; Smiseth, O.A. Diastolic Stress Test: Invasive and Noninvasive Testing. *JACC Cardiovasc. Imaging* **2020**, *13 Pt 2*, 272–282. [CrossRef] [PubMed]
13. Al Atroush, H.H.; Mohammed, K.H.; Nasr, F.M.; Al Desouky, M.I.; Rabie, M.A. Cardiac dysfunction in patients with end-stage liver disease, prevalence, and impact on outcome: A comparative prospective cohort study. *Egypt. Liver J.* **2022**, *12*, 37. [CrossRef]
14. Stundiene, I.; Sarnelyte, J.; Norkute, A.; Aidietiene, S.; Liakina, V.; Masalaite, L.; Valantinas, J. Liver cirrhosis and left ventricle diastolic dysfunction: Systematic review. *World J. Gastroenterol.* **2019**, *25*, 4779–4795. [CrossRef] [PubMed] [PubMed Central]
15. Premkumar, M.; Devurgowda, D.; Vyas, T.; Shasthry, S.M.; Khumuckham, J.S.; Goyal, R.; Thomas, S.S.; Kumar, G. Left Ventricular Diastolic Dysfunction is Associated with Renal Dysfunction, Poor Survival and Low Health Related Quality of Life in Cirrhosis. *J. Clin. Exp. Hepatol.* **2019**, *9*, 324–333. [CrossRef] [PubMed] [PubMed Central]
16. Ruíz-del-Árbol, L.; Achécar, L.; Serradilla, R.; Rodríguez-Gandía, M.Á.; Rivero, M.; Garrido, E.; Natcher, J.J. Diastolic dysfunction is a predictor of poor outcomes in patients with cirrhosis, portal hypertension, and a normal creatinine. *Hepatology* **2013**, *58*, 1732–1741. [CrossRef] [PubMed]
17. Ershoff, B.D.; Gordin, J.S.; Vorobiof, G.; Elashoff, D.; Steadman, R.H.; Scovotti, J.C.; Wray, C.L. Improving the Prediction of Mortality in the High Model for End-Stage Liver Disease Score Liver Transplant Recipient: A Role for the Left Atrial Volume Index. *Transpl. Transplant. Proc.* **2018**, *50*, 1407–1412. [CrossRef] [PubMed]
18. Vetrugno, L.; Cherchi, V.; Zanini, V.; Cotrozzi, S.; Ventin, M.; Terrosu, G.; Baccarani, U.; Bove, T. Association between preoperative diastolic dysfunction and early allograft dysfunction after orthotopic liver transplantation. An observational study. *Echocardiography* **2022**, *39*, 561–567. [CrossRef]
19. Dokainish, H. Left ventricular diastolic function and dysfunction: Central role of echocardiography. *Glob. Cardiol. Sci. Pract.* **2015**, *2015*, 3. [CrossRef] [PubMed] [PubMed Central]
20. Nagueh, S.F. Classification of left ventricular diastolic dysfunction and heart failure diagnosis and prognosis. *J. Am. Soc. Echocardiogr.* **2018**, *31*, 1209–1211. [CrossRef]
21. Halley, C.M.; Houghtaling, P.L.; Khalil, M.K.; Thomas, J.D.; Jaber, W.A. Mortality rate in patients with diastolic dysfunction and normal systolic function. *Arch. Intern. Med.* **2011**, *171*, 1082–1087. [CrossRef] [PubMed]
22. Nagueh, S.F. Left ventricular diastolic dysfunction: Diagnostic and prognostic perspectives. *J. Am. Soc. Echocardiogr.* **2023**, *36*, 307–309. [CrossRef] [PubMed]
23. Ladeiras-Lopes, R.; Araújo, M.; Sampaio, F.; Leite-Moreira, A.; Fontes-Carvalho, R. The impact of diastolic dysfunction as a predictor of cardiovascular events: A systematic review and meta-analysis. *Rev. Port. Cardiol.* **2019**, *38*, 789–804. [CrossRef] [PubMed]
24. Kosmala, W.; Marwick, T. Asymptomatic Left Ventricular Diastolic Dysfunction: Predicting Progression to Symptomatic Heart Failure. *JACC Cardiovasc. Imaging* **2020**. [CrossRef] [PubMed]
25. Solanki, R.; Sreesh, S.; Attumalil, T.V.; Mohapatra, S.D.; Narayanan, V.; Madhu, D.; Chakravorty, A.; Pal, R.; Nair, A.N.K.K.; Devadas, K. A case-cohort study of left ventricular diastolic dysfunction in patients with cirrhosis: The liver-heart axis. *Ann. Gastroenterol.* **2023**, *36*, 678–685. [CrossRef] [PubMed] [PubMed Central]
26. Dadhich, S.; Goswami, A.; Jain, V.K.; Gahlot, A.; Kulamarva, G.; Bhargava, N. Cardiac dysfunction in cirrhotic portal hypertension with or without ascites. *Ann. Gastroenterol.* **2014**, *27*, 244–249. [PubMed] [PubMed Central]
27. Papastergiou, V.; Skorda, L.; Lisgos, P.; Papakonstantinou, N.; Giakoumakis, T.; Ntousikos, K.; Karatapanis, S. Ultrasonographic prevalence and factors predicting left ventricular diastolic dysfunction in patients with liver cirrhosis: Is there a correlation between the grade of diastolic dysfunction and the grade of liver disease? *Sci. World J.* **2012**, *2012*, 615057. [CrossRef] [PubMed] [PubMed Central]
28. Alexopoulou, A.; Papatheodoridis, G.; Pouriki, S.; Chrysohoou, C.; Raftopoulos, L.; Stefanadis, C.; Pectasides, D. Diastolic myocardial dysfunction does not affect survival in patients with cirrhosis. *Transpl. Transplant. Int.* **2012**, *25*, 1174–1181. [CrossRef] [PubMed]
29. Merli, M.; Calicchia, A.; Ruffa, A.; Pellicori, P.; Riggio, O.; Giusto, M.; Gaudio, C.; Torromeo, C. Cardiac dysfunction in cirrhosis is not associated with the severity of liver disease. *Eur. J. Intern. Med.* **2013**, *24*, 172–176. [CrossRef] [PubMed]
30. Mansoor, H.; Khizer, M.; Afreen, A.; Sadiq, N.M.; Habib, A.; Ali, S.; Raza, A.; Hafeez, T. Systolic and diastolic impairment in cirrhotic cardiomyopathy: Insights from a cross-sectional study. *Egypt. Liver J.* **2024**, *14*, 60. [CrossRef]
31. Andersen, O.S.; Smiseth, O.A.; Dokainish, H.; Abudiab, M.M.; Schutt, R.C.; Kumar, A.; Sato, K.; Harb, S.; Gude, E.; Remme, E.W.; et al. Estimating Left Ventricular Filling Pressure by Echocardiography. *J. Am. Coll. Cardiol.* **2017**, *69*, 1937–1948. [CrossRef] [PubMed]

32. Robinson, S.; Ring, L.; Oxborough, D.; Harkness, A.; Bennett, S.; Rana, B.; Sutaria, N.; Lo Giudice, F.; Shun-Shin, M.; Paton, M.; et al. The assessment of left ventricular diastolic function: Guidance and recommendations from the British Society of Echocardiography. *Echo Res. Pract.* **2024**, *11*, 16. [CrossRef] [PubMed] [PubMed Central]
33. Garcia, M.J.; Ares, M.A.; Asher, C.; Rodriguez, L.; Vandervoort, P.; Thomas, J.D. An index of early left ventricular filling that combined with pulsed Doppler peak E velocity may estimate capillary wedge pressure. *J. Am. Coll. Cardiol.* **1997**, *29*, 448–454. [CrossRef] [PubMed]
34. Yap, E.M.L.; Supe, M.G.S.; Yu, I.I. Cardiac Profile of Filipino Patients with Liver Cirrhosis: A 10-Year Study. *Cardiol. Res.* **2018**, *9*, 358–363. [CrossRef] [PubMed] [PubMed Central]
35. Poojary, M.S.; Samanth, J.; Nayak, K.; Shetty, S.; Nayak, S.K.; Rao, M.S. Evaluation of subclinical left ventricular systolic dysfunction using two-dimensional speckle-tracking echocardiography in patients with Child-Pugh A and B cirrhosis: A case-control study. *Indian. J. Gastroenterol.* **2022**, *41*, 567–575. [CrossRef] [PubMed]
36. Behera, S.K.; Behera, P.; Behera, J.R.; Behera, G. Study of Cardiac Dysfunction in Portal Hypertension: A Single-Center Experience from Eastern India. *Cureus* **2023**, *15*, e51399. [CrossRef] [PubMed] [PubMed Central]
37. Marconi, C.; Bellan, M.; Giarda, P.; Minisini, R.; Favretto, S.; Burlone, M.E.; Franzosi, L.; Pirisi, M. Cardiac dysfunction as an early predictor of portal hypertension in chronic hepatitis C. *Ann. Gastroenterol.* **2017**, *30*, 675–681. [CrossRef] [PubMed] [PubMed Central]
38. Gherbesi, E.; Gianstefani, S.; Angeli, F.; Ryabenko, K.; Bergamaschi, L.; Armillotta, M.; Guerra, E.; Tuttolomondo, D.; Gaibazzi, N.; Squeri, A.; et al. Myocardial strain of the left ventricle by speckle tracking echocardiography: From physics to clinical practice. *Echocardiography* **2024**, *41*, e15753. [CrossRef] [PubMed]
39. Suran, D.; Sinkovic, A.; Naji, F. Tissue Doppler imaging is a sensitive echocardiographic technique to detect subclinical systolic and diastolic dysfunction of both ventricles in type 1 diabetes mellitus. *BMC Cardiovasc. Disord.* **2016**, *16*, 72. [CrossRef] [PubMed] [PubMed Central]
40. Ottosen, C.I.; Nadruz, W.; Inciardi, R.M.; Johansen, N.D.; Fudim, M.; Biering-Sørensen, T. Diastolic Dysfunction in Hypertension: A Comprehensive Review of Pathophysiology, Diagnosis, and Treatment. *Eur. Heart J. Cardiovasc. Imaging* **2024**, *17*, jeae178. [CrossRef] [PubMed]
41. McDonagh, T.A.; Metra, M.; Adamo, M.; Gardner, R.S.; Baumbach, A.; Böhm, M.; Burri, H.; Butler, J.; Čelutkienė, J.; Chioncel, O.; et al. ESC Scientific Document Group. 2023 Focused Update of the 2021 ESC Guidelines for the diagnosis and treatment of acute and chronic heart failure. *Eur. Heart J.* **2023**, *44*, 3627–3639, Erratum in *Eur. Heart J.* **2024**, *45*, 53. [CrossRef] [PubMed]
42. Mosoiu, D.; Rogozea, L.; Landon, A.; Bisoc, A.; Tint, D. Palliative Care in Heart Failure: A Public Health Emergency. *Am. J. Ther.* **2020**, *27*, e204–e223. [CrossRef] [PubMed]
43. Spann, A.; Coe, C.; Ajayi, T.; Montgomery, G.; Shwetar, M.; Oje, A.; Annis, J.; Slaughter, J.C.; Alexopoulos, S.; Brittain, E.; et al. Cirrhotic cardiomyopathy: Appraisal of the original and revised criteria in predicting posttransplant cardiac outcomes. *Liver Transpl.* **2022**, *28*, 1321–1331. [CrossRef] [PubMed] [PubMed Central]
44. Izzy, M.; Soldatova, A.; Sun, X.; Angirekula, M.; Mara, K.; Lin, G.; Watt, K.D. Cirrhotic Cardiomyopathy Predicts Posttransplant Cardiovascular Disease: Revelations of the New Diagnostic Criteria. *Liver Transpl.* **2021**, *27*, 876–886. [CrossRef] [PubMed]

Disclaimer/Publisher's Note: The statements, opinions and data contained in all publications are solely those of the individual author(s) and contributor(s) and not of MDPI and/or the editor(s). MDPI and/or the editor(s) disclaim responsibility for any injury to people or property resulting from any ideas, methods, instructions or products referred to in the content.

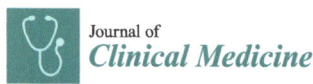

Review

Non-Pharmacological Therapy in Heart Failure and Management of Heart Failure in Special Populations—A Review

Jasmine K. Dugal [1], Arpinder S. Malhi [1], Noyan Ramazani [1], Brianna Yee [1,*], Michael V. DiCaro [1] and KaChon Lei [1,2]

[1] Department of Internal Medicine, University of Nevada Las Vegas, 1701 W. Charleston Blvd., Las Vegas, NV 89102, USA; jasmine.dugal@unlv.edu (J.K.D.); arpinder.malhi@unlv.edu (A.S.M.); noyan.ramazani@unlv.edu (N.R.); michael.dicaro@unlv.edu (M.V.D.); kachon.lei@unlv.edu (K.L.)
[2] Division of Cardiovascular Medicine, University of Nevada Las Vegas, 1701 W. Charleston Blvd., Las Vegas, NV 89102, USA
* Correspondence: brianna.yee@unlv.edu

Abstract: Non-pharmacological therapies play an essential role in the management of heart failure, complementing pharmacological treatments to mitigate disease progression and improve patient outcomes. This review provides an updated perspective on non-pharmacological interventions with a focus on lifestyle modifications, device therapies, and the management of heart failure in special populations, such as the elderly, women, and patients with comorbid conditions like renal dysfunction and diabetes. Key lifestyle interventions, including sodium and fluid restriction, dietary changes, and physical activity, are explored for their impact on symptom reduction, hospital readmissions, and quality of life. Device therapies like cardiac resynchronization therapy (CRT) and implantable cardioverter defibrillators (ICD) are also evaluated for their effectiveness in reducing mortality in patients with advanced HF. Special attention is given to vulnerable populations, emphasizing the need for individualized approaches tailored to specific pathophysiological mechanisms and socioeconomic factors. By integrating these strategies, healthcare providers can optimize care and enhance patient adherence, reducing the overall burden of heart failure.

Keywords: heart failure; lifestyle modification; diet; exercise; diabetes; chronic kidney disease

Citation: Dugal, J.K.; Malhi, A.S.; Ramazani, N.; Yee, B.; DiCaro, M.V.; Lei, K. Non-Pharmacological Therapy in Heart Failure and Management of Heart Failure in Special Populations—A Review. *J. Clin. Med.* **2024**, *13*, 6993. https://doi.org/10.3390/jcm13226993

Academic Editors: Cristina Tudoran and Larisa Anghel

Received: 8 October 2024
Revised: 31 October 2024
Accepted: 5 November 2024
Published: 20 November 2024

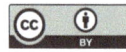

Copyright: © 2024 by the authors. Licensee MDPI, Basel, Switzerland. This article is an open access article distributed under the terms and conditions of the Creative Commons Attribution (CC BY) license (https://creativecommons.org/licenses/by/4.0/).

1. Introduction

Heart failure (HF), a complex clinical syndrome characterized by the inability of the heart to pump blood effectively, remains a significant public health challenge, with increasing prevalence and associated morbidity and mortality. Specifically, HF refers to cardiac dysfunction linked to structural and/or functional incapabilities, either during ventricular filling or ventricular ejection [1]. In industrialized and high-income countries, the prevalence of heart failure (HF) is approximately 1–2% in the adult population, which increases to 10% when sub-stratifying the population of adults over 70 years of age [2]. Based on the guidelines of management of HF, the AHA/ACC/Heart Failure Society of America (HFSA) has classified HF into four main variations: heart failure with preserved ejection fraction (HFpEF), heart failure with reduced ejection fraction (HFrEF), heart failure with mildly reduced ejection fraction (HFmrEF), and heart failure with improved ejection fraction (HFimpEF) [1,2].

A guideline-directed medical therapy (GDMT) has been well studied and established as the mainstay of treatment. Yet, non-pharmacological management of HF is equally as important to mitigate and decrease the complications that arise from HF. However, poor compliance has been reported in the HF population, especially in the elderly, which results in an increased risk for mortality and HF readmissions [3]. The four core tenets of non-pharmacological management of HF include (1) adopting a lifestyle where patients follow a low sodium diet, (2) restricting the amount of fluid consumption, (3) weighing themselves daily, and (4) abiding with the recommendations and guidelines set for them by their physicians regarding exercise therapy and activity training [3]. Patients who were compliant with one modality (i.e., made modifications to diet and exercise) were also more eager and motivated to adopt secondary behavioral changes, such as decreasing consumption of alcohol and cigarette smoke [3]. This intrinsic behavioral modification among this class of patients caused a decrease in hospital readmission rates related to HF complications.

This review aims to provide an in-depth analysis of the current non-pharmacological interventions for HF, focusing on their effectiveness in diverse populations. Special attention will be given to particularly vulnerable groups, such as the elderly, women during pregnancy, and individuals with concomitant renal dysfunction or diabetes. Moreover, this review will explore the impact of HF across different socioeconomic and financial statuses and between various population classes, racial backgrounds, and age groups. This manuscript provides a more comprehensive approach to the non-pharmacological management of HF that encompasses the many facets of preventative measures and treatment regimens and discusses the importance of compliance and adherence to such therapies and interventions.

2. Lifestyle Modifications

Effective lifestyle modifications are an integral component in the management of HF, complementing GDMT by reducing symptom burden and hospitalizations and concomitantly improving quality of life. The interplay between cardiac, renal, and endocrine systems, termed cardio–kidney–metabolic (CKM) syndrome, requires a multifaceted approach to HF treatment. The major tenets of lifestyle modification include sodium restriction, fluid restriction, dietary adjustments, physical activity, and weight management.

2.1. Sodium Restriction

The mechanism of sodium restriction improvement has been a subject of debate, particularly regarding sodium stimulation of the neurohormonal system. Increased salt retention by kidneys leads to worsening edema and congestion and stimulates increased sympathetic activity. This results in peripheral vasoconstriction of the afferent renal artery and decreased blood flow to the juxtaglomerular apparatus in the kidneys, thereby activating the renin–angiotensin–aldosterone system (RAAS). Angiotensin II (ATII) directly causes sodium retention in the proximal tubules, while aldosterone leads to increased sodium resorption in the distal tubule and plays a key role in worsening heart failure [4].

It has also been shown that water retention and volume overload in acute heart failure exacerbation are primarily driven by sodium retention [5]. However, experts have suggested sodium restriction in patients with poor nutritional status may lead to poorer results in heart failure patients due to reduced appetite and food intake, exacerbating malnutrition. In fact, a systematic review and meta-analysis of 10 randomized controlled trials were performed (1011 participants with HF) to evaluate the effects of dietary sodium restriction on quality of life (QoL), and the results showed that sodium restriction did not improve QoL over long term (>30 days) ($p = 0.61$). The pooled results also showed that sodium restriction might increase mortality risk ($p < 0.00001$). Lastly, it also showed that it did not reduce the readmission rate within the short term ($\leq$30 days) ($p = 0.78$) and, on the contrary, increased the readmission rate over the long term ($p = 0.0003$) [6]. Despite its controversy, sodium restriction has been internationally acknowledged as a method of lifestyle modification in HF patients.

Dietary sodium restriction in heart failure patients has been recommended by many different guidelines. The Korean Society of Heart Failure (KSHF), European Society of Cardiology (ESC), and American Heart Association/American College of Cardiology (AHA/ACC) all recommend sodium restriction. However, the consensus among the societies varies. The Korean heart failure guidelines recommend sodium restriction to <2 g per day in moderate to severe heart failure [7], while European guidelines recommend avoiding excessive sodium (>5 g/day) [8]. Per AHA/ACC guidelines, patients should avoid excessive sodium to reduce congestive symptoms [9]. Even though guidelines have recommendations regarding sodium restriction in HF patients, there is a disagreement among experts about sodium restriction, especially in malnourished patients. Because of the variability in recommendations and patient responses, an individualized approach to sodium restriction, particularly in patients with comorbid conditions or malnutrition risk, may be more beneficial than a one-size-fits-all approach.

2.2. Fluid Restriction

The benefit of fluid restriction in HF patients is similarly a subject of debate, with inconsistent evidence supporting its routine use [5]. A small single blind study was carried out by Travers et al. to investigate the clinical impact of fluid restriction in class IV heart failure patients during their hospitalization. The study showed no significant difference in time to clinical stability, discontinuation of IV diuretic therapy, or stabilization of serum urea, serum creatinine, natriuretic peptides, or sodium in fluid-restricted patients ($n = 34$) versus free-fluid patients ($n = 33$) [10]. A key study examining the outcomes with 1 L fluid restriction in patients found that quality of life improved, though it did not find any differences in HF rehospitalization or all-cause mortality [11]. Given the limited data on fluid restriction, new randomized control studies are needed to adequately determine the utility and effectiveness of fluid restriction.

Subsequently, there are no clear recommendations in clinical guidelines for fluid restriction. KSHF guidelines suggest educating patients about fluid restriction at discharge following a hospitalization for heart failure [7]. However, KSHF does not specify an exact amount of fluid restriction in the guidelines. Conversely, ESC guidelines recommend considering a fluid restriction of 1.5 to 2 L in patients with severe heart failure/hyponatremia to relieve symptoms and congestion, taking note to increase fluid intake during periods of high heat/humidity and/or nausea/vomiting [8]. AHA/ACC guidelines make a 2b recommendation regarding fluid restriction in heart failure patients as the benefit of fluid restriction to reduce congestive symptoms is uncertain [9]. Ultimately, fluid restriction should be considered on a case-by-case basis, with careful attention to patient-specific factors such as comorbid conditions and symptomatology.

2.3. Dietary Changes

Dietary interventions are essential in managing heart failure, particularly in patients with comorbid obesity or metabolic syndrome. A healthy diet should be adapted to the specific needs of each patient. Nutrition with restricted caloric intake designed for weight loss is recommended in overweight or obese HF patients. Patients who are overweight or obese have a significantly increased risk of developing HF, suffering from more frequent HF exacerbations, and experiencing progression of HF. Particularly, the increased cardiac work required to maintain cardiac output in such individuals increases ventricular strain, leading to earlier onset and worsening of HF [12]. The newly termed CKM syndrome has emerging evidence on the risk of cardiovascular disease (CVD), including HF [9,13]. Risk calculators such as PREVENT for the staging of CKM may help providers evaluate an individual's risk for the development of CVD and guide management accordingly. This model includes considerations of sex, age, comorbidities such as diabetes and CKD, and lifestyle habits including tobacco use [13].

While neither the KSHF nor the ESC provides specific dietary recommendations, the AHA/ACC guidelines recommend adherence to heart-healthy, evidence-based diets such as the Dietary Approaches to Stop Hypertension (DASH) diet and the Mediterranean diet. The DASH diet focuses on reducing sodium intake and increasing consumption of fruits, vegetables, and low-fat dairy products. The DASH diet, through the original DASH trial, was shown to substantially reduce blood pressure compared with a diet that is low in these foods [14,15]. Furthermore, consistent compliance with diets that are low in sodium and high in fruits, vegetables, low-fat dairy products, antioxidants, and potassium may be linked to decreased heart failure hospitalizations [16]. The Mediterranean diet, a generic term used to describe a dietary pattern consisting of fruits, vegetables, unsalted nuts, whole grains, lean proteins, and extra-virgin olive oil, has been shown through multiple studies to reduce blood pressure and improve overall cardiovascular health [17,18].

Elderly HF patients, particularly those who are frail, often face barriers to maintaining a heart-healthy diet as they are more likely to be dependent on caregivers for meal preparation. A study of 40 patients found that both patients and caregivers consume poor-quality diets, which suggests that even though the Mediterranean diet and DASH diet have beneficial effects, the focus should be placed on household modifications for heart failure patients to have any success [9].

In patients with advanced HF (AHA/ACC stage C and D), unintentional weight loss, sarcopenia, and cardiac cachexia are common, which further complicates the management of nutritional intake. These conditions are associated with lower caloric intake and higher micronutrient deficiencies compared with age- and sex-matched healthy adults [19]. Additional weight loss to address obesity may exacerbate these conditions. Dietary changes need professional guidance and counseling on adapting a diet to reduce weight loss that is driven by malnutrition to avoid sarcopenia and cardiac cachexia. Strategic treatment for sarcopenia includes resistance training exercises to improve overall muscle strength and mass with focused nutritional support in protein intake. Cardiac cachexia is a complex metabolic syndrome that can be addressed through high-calorie, high-protein diets. At times, appetite stimulants may also be required, especially in end-stage heart failure. Both sarcopenia and cardiac cachexia are factors associated with worsened prognosis in heart failure [20].

2.4. Physical Activity

Physical activity has been linked to increased quality of life, exercise capacity, and decreased hospitalizations. Exercise-based cardiac rehabilitation programs have been shown to significantly enhance functional status, as measured by the 6 min walk test and reduce all-cause and HF-related hospitalizations [21]. Such classes have tailored exercises for cardiac patients to improve heart health. Current guidelines strongly recommend cardiac rehabilitation programs (CRP) for all eligible heart failure patients though practical data show low participation rates [21]. A CRP is primarily based on physical exercise; however, a comprehensive CRP also includes educational sessions that focus on risk factors, lifestyle modification, nutritional advice, psychosocial support, smoking cessation, regulation of body weight, and optimization of blood pressure, lipid levels, and glycemic control [22]. General exercise and physical activity are still highly recommended, particularly for patients who do not qualify for CRP or where CRP is not available. Patients who have completed CRP are also recommended to continue physical activity, utilizing learned skills for future habits. Guidelines recommend exercise as a non-pharmacological treatment for heart failure but do not specify intensity or duration. KSHF guidelines recommend promoting exercise-related activities, along with an exercise prescriber, in a multidisciplinary team that handles heart failure patients [7]. ESC recommends exercise for all patients who are capable of doing so [8]. The 2022 AHA/ACC Heart Failure Guidelines also recommend exercise training or regular physical activity to improve functional status, exercise performance, and quality of life in heart failure patients who can participate in the exercise training [9].

2.5. Weight Management

Obesity can lead to heart failure directly (through the effects on the myocardium) and indirectly (through obesity-related comorbidities). Obesity can lead to hemodynamic changes, including increased blood volume and cardiac output through activating RAAS. Apart from hypertension, it can also increase the risk of diabetes and hyperlipidemia, all of which are risk factors for developing heart failure. Obesity can also directly affect the heart through fat accumulation in the myocardium, which can lead to fibrosis and the development of heart failure [23]. In fact, a study performed by Kenchaiah et al.

investigated the relation between body mass index (BMI) and the incidence of heart failure among 5881 participants and found that after adjustment for established risk factors, there was an increase in the risk of heart failure of 5 percent for men and 7 percent for women for each increment of 1 in BMI increase. Compared with participants with normal BMI, obese participants had a doubling of the risk of developing heart failure [24].

Weight loss is recommended to help prevent heart failure; however, in patients with established heart failure, the efficacy of weight loss is less clear [5]. Even though obesity increases the risk of heart failure, it has a protective effect in patients already diagnosed with heart failure as a lower body mass index (BMI) is associated with a higher risk of mortality. This phenomenon has been called the "obesity paradox". The obesity paradox is typically observed in mild obesity and seems to lose any potential survival benefit in severely obese patients [25].

Weight loss has been shown to reduce the incidence of heart failure, but in patients with known heart failure, unintentional weight loss can be detrimental. This even includes patients with mild heart failure as weight loss >5% over one year was a significant predictor of cardiovascular death or hospitalization with heart failure exacerbation [26]. The 2016 ESC guidelines stated that in patients with heart failure and moderate obesity (BMI <35 kg/m^2), weight loss cannot be recommended. Patients with a BMI of 35–45 kg/m^2 may consider weight loss for symptom management and exercise capacity [25]. The ACC/AHA guidelines also have a class 1 recommendation stating that conditions that may lead to or contribute to heart failure, such as obesity, should be controlled [25]. However, due to the paucity of data, firm guidance regarding the management of obesity in heart failure patients is lacking.

2.6. Substance Use Cessation

Substance use, particularly alcohol, tobacco, cannabis, and cocaine, is strongly linked to the onset and progression of HF. Moderate alcohol may reduce the incidence of heart failure, but heavy alcohol usage (>5 drinks per day) is strongly associated with dilated cardiomyopathy [27]. In addition, tobacco usage also increases the risk of heart failure by increasing the risk of coronary artery disease (CAD), along with other comorbidities that contribute to CAD, including hypertension, diabetes mellitus, and hyperlipidemia [5,28]. Smoking has a direct effect on the heart as the chemicals that are inhaled damage the blood vessels and form plaque in the coronary arteries, leading to CAD. Figure 1 below summarizes the effects of smoking and alcohol as well as the benefits of smoking and alcohol cessation.

Patients who engage in heavy drinking or smoking should be strongly advised to stay away from heavy and binge drinking [5]. Specifically, smoking cessation has been shown to lower the incidence of serious adverse events, such as myocardial infarction, heart failure, stroke, and death [27]. Healthcare providers should emphasize the importance of substance use cessation as part of comprehensive lifestyle modification strategies for HF patients.

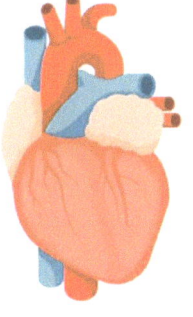
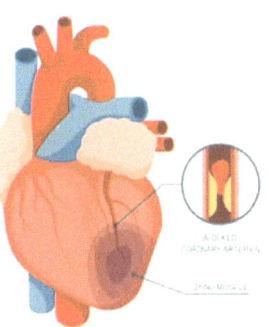

Alcohol Use

Heavy alcohol use (>5 drinks/day) is strongly associated with dilated cardiomyopathy leading to HF.

Patients with continued heavy drinking have worse prognosis and complete cessation or reduction should be recommended.

Tobacco Use

Tobacco increases the risk of heart failure through direct effects on the heart as well as by increasing likelihood of major risk factors associated with HF

Continued smoking worsens outcomes for those with HF.

Smoking cessation decreased the risk of MI, stroke, and death.

Figure 1. The effects of alcohol and tobacco on the heart. Heart failure (HF). Myocardial infarction (MI).

2.7. Weight Monitoring and Education

Regular weight monitoring in patients is critical, particularly in detecting fluid retention, which may indicate worsening heart failure. The WHARF trial, a large randomized controlled study, investigated patients with NYHA class III or IV heart failure and LVEF $\leq$ 35%. It compared heart failure outcomes between those receiving standard care and those receiving standard care alongside access to the AlereNet System, a technology-based monitoring system designed to track daily weight and symptoms in heart failure patients. The results revealed a 56.2% reduction in mortality ($p < 0.003$) for patients in the AlereNet group [29].

A sudden increase in weight often indicates fluid overload, which can occur even in patients compliant with treatment regimens and lifestyle modifications [9]. Accordingly, patients are advised that an increase of two to three pounds per day, or five pounds in one week, will require adjustment to their medication regimen. Recognition of these bodily changes empowers patients to engage in their care, adjust lifestyle factors, and recognize when to seek prompt medical advice to reduce hospital admissions for heart failure exacerbations.

To ensure the accuracy of the daily weight monitoring, providers should educate patients to weigh themselves at the same time every morning, preferably after using the restroom and before eating or drinking [9]. Patients are advised to use the same scale and wear similar clothing daily. These daily weights should be logged, and any concerning trends should be promptly discussed with the healthcare provider. This allows patients to play an active role in managing their heart failure condition, leading to improved outcomes and fewer heart failure exacerbations [9].

3. Advance Interventions: Devices and Surgery

In addition to lifestyle modifications, device therapy, and surgery present another avenue of evidence-based non-pharmacological management of heart failure, especially in severely reduced HF and advanced HF. Cardiac resynchronization therapy (CRT) and implantable cardioverter defibrillators (ICD) are viable options for helping patients with HF reduce overall mortality and prevent sudden cardiac death (SCD).

CRT assists with coordinating cardiac contractions in the lower chambers of the heart and has also been found to decrease the incidence of life-threatening arrhythmias like ventricular tachycardia (V-Tach) and ventricular fibrillation [30]. Relevant indications for

CRT include HFrEF with LVEF ≤ 35%, symptomatic heart failure NYHA class II, II, or ambulatory IV despite optimal medical therapy, and prolonged QRS ≥ 130 milliseconds (Table 1) [31]. CRT is a viable option for treatment in HF patients who have a conduction system abnormality. Even with a substantial non-responder rate of 30%, CRT can lengthen the time to heart transplantation and left ventricular assist device placement in patients with HF [32]. The MIRACLE Trial of 2002 showed the following improvements for patients on CRT versus traditional control groups on standard conventional therapy with heart failure: improved distance walked in six minutes, decreased need for peak oxygen consumption, and improved NYHA class [33].

Table 1. Key aspects of CRT and ICD therapies, including purpose, indications, long-term outcomes, and potential complications. Heart failure with reduced ejection fraction (HfrEF). Left ventricular ejection fraction (LVEF). Heart failure New York Heart Association (HF NYHA). QRS complex (QRS). Ventricular fibrillation (V-fib). Ventricular tachycardia (V-tach). Myocardial infarction (MI).

	Cardiac Resynchronization Therapy (CRT)	Implantable Cardioverter Defibrillator (ICD)
Purpose	• Coordinates cardiac contractions, reduces mortality, prevents arrhythmias and sudden cardiac death (SCD)	• Monitors heart rhythm, delivers shocks to prevent SCD
Indications	• HfrEF with LVEF ≤ 35% • Symptomatic HF NYHA class II, III, or ambulatory IV despite optimal therapy • Prolonged QRS ≥ 130 ms	• LVEF ≤ 35% • Symptomatic HF • History of V-fib or sustained V-tach • Recent MI (within 40 days) with LVEF ≤ 35% and symptomatic HF • Nonischemic cardiomyopathy with LVEF ≤ 35% • Long-standing symptomatic HF despite optimal therapy
Long-term Outcomes	• Lengthens time to heart transplantation and left ventricular assist device placement	• Lower incidence of SCD in the ICD group, more pronounced in patients <70 years
Potential Complications	• Perioperative complications (pneumothorax, bleeding, cardiac perforation)	• Inappropriate shocks • Device-related infection • Fear of appropriate shocks • Impact on quality of life

ICD, which can be an additional feature of CRT, is a device utilized to monitor the heart rhythm and deliver a coordinated shock to prevent SCD caused only by ventricular tachyarrhythmia, severe bradycardia, or complete heart block [34]. HF patients with indication for ICDs include those with LVEF ≤ 35%, symptomatic HF, history of V-fib or sustained V-tach, recent MI within last 40 days with LVEF ≤ 35% and symptomatic HF, nonischemic cardiomyopathy and LVEF ≤ 35%, and long-standing symptomatic HF despite optimal medical therapy (Table 1) [35]. An association was found between reduced all-cause mortality when substratified for age, such that patients who were <70 years of age and had nonischemic systolic heart failure benefited from ICD implantation [27]. In a study on long-term follow-up, patients in the DANISH trial showed that the ICD group had a lower incidence of SCD. This impact was more pronounced in patients ≤70 years of age, but not in the group of patients >70 [36].

Potential complications or risks associated with device usage include perioperative complications such as pneumothorax, bleeding, and cardiac perforation, and late complications associated with ICD treatment such as inappropriate shocks, device-related infection, the fear of appropriate shocks, and quality of life [34]. Key aspects of CRT and ICD therapies are discussed in Table 1 below.

In patients diagnosed with NYHA functional classes II–IV secondary to mitral regurgitation, MitraClip implantation lowered 2-year mortality rates or heart failure-related hospitalizations compared with only providing GDMT. MitraClip valve repair also improved quality of life at two years compared with GDMT alone, independent of baseline functional status [37].

Ischemic cardiomyopathy leading to HfrEF may be reversible and can improve with revascularization. Evidence surrounding PCI versus coronary artery bypass grafting (CABG) has shown that CABG offers substantial survival benefits and significant reduction in myocardial infarction and the need for repeat revascularization in multivessel CAD (MVCAD), particularly in diabetic patients with intermediate and high severity disease [38]. Additionally, patients who underwent coronary artery bypass grafting (CABG) surgery had substantially less risk of mortality from any cardiovascular cause compared with those only receiving traditional medical therapy [39].

4. HF Management in Special Populations

Special populations within HF, such as the elderly, women, and patients with comorbid conditions, face unique challenges that require tailored strategies to optimize outcomes. Understanding the personalized challenges within and between groups allows providers to connect with their patients on an individual level and provide precise, personalized care. This section highlights the fundamental mechanisms, management strategies, and population-specific considerations to aid providers in treating special populations of people with HF. Important takeaways and key considerations for HF management in special populations are summarized in Table 2.

Table 2. HF management in special populations, including general principles and key considerations. Guideline-directed medical therapy (GDMT). Angiotensin-converting enzyme-inhibitor (ACEi). Angiotensin receptor blocker (ARB). Angiotensin receptor-neprilysin inhibitor (ARNI). Mineralocorticoid receptor antagonist (MRA). Heart failure (HF). Cardiac defibrillator therapy (CRT). Implantable cardioverter defibrillator (ICD). Chronic kidney disease (CKD). Sudden cardiac death (SCD). Estimated glomerular filtration rate (eGFR). Sodium-glucose cotransporter-2 inhibitor (SGLTi). Sodium-glucose cotransporter-2 (SGLT2). Glucagon-like peptide-1 (GLP-1). Dipeptidyl peptidase-4 (DPP-4).

Special Population	General Principle	Key Considerations
Elderly patients	Elderly patients with HF have similar GDMT recommendations as the general population but require tailored approaches due to increased sensitivity to medications and changes in intravascular volume.	• Noncompliance: financial issues, social isolation, and cognitive impairments • Medication sensitivity: requires nuanced medication selection 　○ Beta blockers and ACEi/ARBs/ARNIs are the most effective. 　○ MRAs are also beneficial. 　○ Diuretics effectively manage congestive symptoms. • Exercise: improves muscle mass and strength • Patient education and support: improve adherence and monitoring, potentially reducing disparity.
Female patients	Sex-specific research is limited, but certain lifestyle and physiological factors in women affect HF risk and management.	• Diet: 　○ Plant-based diets are associated with a lower HF risk in women. 　○ Southern dietary patterns increase HF risk. • Treat comorbidities: obesity, anemia, depression. • Hormone therapy: estrogen therapy is generally not recommended due to the potential for thrombosis and worsening HF.

Table 2. Cont.

Special Population	General Principle	Key Considerations

Patients with renal dysfunction	Both device-driven and pharmacological therapies are effective in managing HF with renal dysfunction, with specific interventions benefiting across different eGFR levels.	• Device therapy:
		  ○ CRT: reduces mortality, HF hospitalizations, and incidence of VT.
		  ○ ICD: CKD patients have an increased risk of SCD.
		• Pharmacological therapy:
		  ○ Standard GDMT medications: prioritize ACEi/ARB/ARNI and SGLT2i.
		  ○ Nonselective SGLTi: new data support use in CKD.

Patients with diabetes	Exercise and specific antihyperglycemic agents improve HF outcomes in patients with diabetes.	• Exercise:
		  ○ Improves functional capacity and reverses cardiac stiffness.
		• Antihyperglycemic agents
		  ○ SGLT2 inhibitors: improve cardiovascular outcomes (benefits seen even in patients without diabetes).
		  ○ GLP-1 agonists and DPP-4 inhibitors: improve weight loss, glycemic control, and cardiovascular health.

Ethnic and racial minority patients	Socioeconomic factors heavily influence HF outcomes, with financial barriers leading to later-stage HF presentation and reduced adherence.	• Healthcare costs: HF-related hospitalizations are very costly, thus affecting compliance and HF outcomes.
		• Medication accessibility:
		  ○ Cost-effective medication choices: consider ACEi/ARB over ARNI and metoprolol succinate over carvedilol to reduce upfront costs.
		  ○ Medication selection: spironolactone is suggested as an early GDMT medication, with SGLT2 inhibitors used after confirming affordability.

4.1. Heart Failure in Elderly Patients

4.1.1. Mechanism of Heart Failure in Elderly Patients

Aging is a normal process that leads to decreased cardioprotective systems and increased disease processes that may lead to heart failure [40]. Even though aging does not cause heart failure, it lowers the threshold for disease manifestation [40]. The elderly population has an increased prevalence of comorbid conditions that increase cardiovascular risk, such as hypertension, hyperlipidemia, and coronary artery disease, resulting in increased risk for heart failure. Older patients with HF also experience a high burden of polypharmacy, frailty, and cognitive impairment [41]. Changes in arterial vessels and consequences with advanced age involve increased oxidative stress, endothelial dysfunction, inflammation, matrix metalloproteases, and vascular cell proliferation [40]. This leads to changes in arterial walls through decreased elastin content, increased collagen production, cross-linking and glycosylation, decreased collagen degradation, and increased intima medial wall thickness [40]. The hemodynamic consequences of this change result in increased diameter of central arteries, systolic pressure, pulse pressure, LV afterload, and oxygen requirements, as well as a decrease in coronary filling pressures and LV early diastolic filling [40]. Table 3 below provides a summary of age-related changes.

Table 3. The mechanisms, arterial changes, and hemodynamic consequences of aging in the cardiovascular system. Advanced glycation end products (AGEs). Left ventricular (LV). Matrix metalloproteases (MMPs).

Mechanisms	The mechanisms of aging, including increasing oxidative stress, endothelial dysfunction, chronic inflammation, activity of MMPs, and dysregulated vascular cell proliferation, collectively contribute to tissue damage, vascular aging, and the development of age-related diseases.
Changes in Arterial Wall	The changes in the arterial wall with aging include a decrease in elastin content, an increase in collagen production, cross-linking, and glycosylation, a decrease in collagen degradation, an increase in AGEs, and an increase in intima-medial thickness.
Hemodynamic Consequences	The hemodynamic consequences of aging include an increase in the diameter of central arteries, systolic pressure, pulse pressure, LV afterload, contraction, and oxygen requirements, along with a decrease in coronary filling pressure and LV early diastolic filling.

4.1.2. Management Considerations in the Elderly Population

Noncompliance proves to be a large barrier to improvement for HF patients, and the elderly population remains especially vulnerable due to financial difficulties, social isolation, and cognitive impairments that preclude complex medication regimens, among others [40]. Older individuals who are diagnosed with HF have similar recommendations for GDMT to the general population; however, each of these medications has specific, unique mechanistic effects that can be utilized to the advantage of the patients and their comorbidities.

Given that the elderly population is more sensitive to small changes in intravascular volume, diuretics have been proven effective in reducing congestive symptoms [40]. The ultimate effect of beta blockers is to inhibit the sympathetic nervous system, which is often upregulated in heart failure. By reducing heart rate and myocardial oxygen demand, beta-blockers improve left ventricular function and reduce mortality and hospitalization rates [9]. MRAs block the effects of aldosterone, thereby reducing sodium retention, myocardial fibrosis, and ventricular remodeling, leading to improved survival and reduced hospitalizations [42]. ACEis, ARBs, and ARNIs reduce the detrimental effects of RAAS activation, thereby reducing vasoconstriction, sodium retention, and myocardial fibrosis, consequently decreasing afterload and reducing ventricular remodeling [9]. HF in elderly patients is associated with increased activation of the sympathetic system as well as the RAAS; as such, beta-blocker therapy and ACE inhibitor therapy are helpful in the elderly population. Elderly patients tend to exhibit more sensitivity to GDMT, and careful titration of GDMT should be considered to avoid significant hypotension and/or bradycardia.

Exercise training can also be generalized to older patients, as the disease process is associated with decreased muscle mass and strength. Although advances in pharmacological therapies available for heart failure exist, up to 40% of patients with HF will die within one year of their first hospitalization [41]. We emphasize the importance of rigorous patient education, close monitoring, and social support to help reduce the disparity.

4.2. Heart Failure in Females

Heart failure phenotypes can differ based on sex. HfpEF is more prevalent among females, and HfrEF is higher among males [43]. Hypertension (HTN) and diabetes contribute to the risk for HF in females, whereas ischemia is the leading cause of HF in males [44]. Sudden cardiac death, which can be caused by HF, is also more common in males compared with female counterparts, primarily attributed to the fatal arrhythmias associated with HfrEF that may not be seen in HfpEF [45].

4.2.1. Mechanism of Heart Failure in Females

Over the last decade, the hallmark of HfpEF in females has been described by the increased stiffness and smaller size of the left ventricle compared with males. Consequently, females require a greater resting heart rate than males to maintain cardiac output. With HfpEF and aging, an overall increased stiffness of the LV and stroke volume reduction occur, leading to dependence on increased heart rates to compensate for cardiac output.

Although less prevalent, women with HfrEF may present with increased morbidity compared with their male counterparts. One study found that women with severe HfrEF had lower exercise tolerance, worse pulmonary function, and worse kidney function than males of similar age and ejection fraction [44]. The PREVENT model for HF incorporates sex into consideration of the overall risk for HF development.

4.2.2. Females with Comorbid Diabetes

Growing evidence indicates that women with diabetes experience more pronounced endothelial, coronary microvascular, and diastolic abnormalities than men with diabetes. The exact mechanisms behind the heightened risk of heart failure in diabetic women remain unclear. Still, factors such as sex hormones, variations in cardiovascular risk profiles, and potential differences in treatment patterns between men and women might contribute [46].

4.2.3. Pregnancy and Heart Failure

Pregnancy has a known association with peripartum cardiomyopathy (PPCM) and can be a life-threatening syndrome in women. As pregnant patients near the end of pregnancy and in the weeks to months after delivery, left ventricular systolic dysfunction is observed and leads to an increased risk for heart failure. The potential etiology includes inflammation and angiogenic dysregulation, causing vascular damage. Patients usually present with an ejection fraction (EF) of <45% [44].

4.2.4. Management Considerations for Female Patients

There is not much known regarding the sex-specific aspects in the prevention or treatment of HF; however, a prospective study that followed adults with five types of dietary patterns noticed that adherence to a plant-based dietary pattern, more frequently found in women, was inversely associated with incident HF risk. In contrast, the Southern dietary pattern was positively associated with incident HF risk [47]. Obesity, anemia, and depression are more prevalent in females with heart failure, and as such, treating these conditions effectively can help manage heart failure. Current research has not found a benefit to estrogen therapy though targeting hormonal changes during and after menopause may also be considered in the future. Although the loss of estrogen is linked to an increased cardiovascular risk, hormone replacement therapy (HRT) is generally not recommended in women with heart failure due to concerns about clotting and worsening heart failure.

4.2.5. Management Consideration for Pregnant Females

Management of heart failure in pregnancy aims to relieve symptoms, optimize hemodynamic status, improve long-term outcomes with continuation or initiation of therapies for chronic conditions, and treat other precipitating factors such as anemia, thyroid imbalance, infections, and arrhythmias [48]. Chronic heart failure in pregnancy warrants lifestyle modifications, vaccinations, and, possibly, even device therapy such as cardiac resynchronization and/or implantable cardioverter defibrillator therapy [48]. Non-pharmacological management of acute and refractory heart failure in pregnancy includes supplemental oxygen therapy and temporary mechanical circulatory support [46].

4.3. Heart Failure in Renal Dysfunction

4.3.1. Mechanism of Heart Failure in Renal Dysfunction

Heart failure can exacerbate renal dysfunction and vice versa, as third-spacing of fluid in congestive heart failure (CHF) can induce acute kidney injury (AKI), leading to further depletion of intravascular volume. The Acute Decompensated Heart Failure National Registry (ADHERE) calculated that approximately one-third of all patients who have been hospitalized in the past for acute decompensated HF have acute or chronic renal insufficiency [49]. The classic interplay between heart failure and kidney disease, termed cardio-renal syndrome, has three significant comprehensive interactions: (1) hemodynamic mechanisms, (2) neurohormonal mechanisms, and (3) CVD-associated mechanisms [49].

Due to low systemic perfusion rates as a consequence of acute HF exacerbation, the nephron can temporarily avoid damage by activating the RAAS pathway initiated by the glomeruli in this reactive state. This temporary sub-optimal state will eventually lead to exhaustion and depletion of homeostasis and to overt kidney damage, surpassing a simple AKI. HF with 'forward failure,' or a drastic decrease in cardiac output due to HfrEF, can lead to renal tubule hypoxia and acute tubular necrosis [49]. Continuous and recurring insult to the kidneys leads to the development of chronic kidney disease (CKD), severe electrolyte derangements, rise in creatinine and blood urea nitrogen levels (BUN), and elevation of other chemical and enzymatic biomarkers in the blood, causing an overall toxic environment.

4.3.2. Management Strategies for Renal Dysfunction

The specific management strategies of renal dysfunction in the setting of HF encompass both a non-pharmacological device-driven therapeutic approach and a pharmacological approach. The value of cardiac resynchronization therapy (CRT) as an intervention in patients with an eGFR < 60 mL/min has been just as advantageous and efficacious as in patients with an eGFR > 60 mL/min [50]. As such, the usage of CRT, regardless of eGFR in CKD patients, may have equal benefits for reduction in death and HF hospitalizations. Accordingly, CRT-D therapy demonstrated a significantly lower risk of mortality and heart failure hospitalizations compared with ICD [51].

Placement of an ICD as a primary prevention against sudden cardiac death (SCD) may prove to be beneficial for patients with CKD stage 3 and concomitant HfrEF [52]. The risk for SCD in patients with advanced CKD or dialysis is higher than either risk factor alone [53]. However, recommendations remain to implant ICDs in patients with EF < 35% as risk for infection in dialysis patients proves to be a significant consideration.

Pharmacological interventions in patients with HfrEF and CKD are vast and include standard GDMT, with a focus on angiotensin-converting enzyme inhibitors (ACEi), angiotensin receptor blockers (ARBs), hyperpolarization-activated cyclic nucleotide-gated (HCN) channel blockers like Ivabradine, angiotensin receptor/neprilysin inhibitors (ARNI), and sodium-glucose co-transporter-2 (SGLT-2) inhibitors. For African American patients with NYHA class III-IV HfrEF, hydralazine and isosorbide dinitrate reduce morbidity and mortality [54].

Targeting the RAAS pathway with ACEi, ARB, and ARNIs has been most utilized in patients with CKD given its mechanistic effects, as explained previously. GDMT initiation becomes most effective when proactively planning the regimen based on future transitions to other classes. Transitions between two classes of medications, such as ARBs, then transitioning to ARNIs is preferred to transitioning from ACEi to ARNIs due to the presence of a 36 h washout period that is needed for this particular transition. The high prevalence of side effects such as angioedema and cough are common complaints among patients who are on ACEi, which also makes ARBs/ARNIs more optimal. However, landmark trials do not establish a specific order of GDMT administration that is preferred over another.

SGLT2is, initially developed for diabetes, reduces HF hospitalizations and cardiovascular mortality through mechanisms such as natriuresis and reduction in preload and afterload [42]. Newly emerging data from the SCORED trial have linked improvement in mortality and heart failure hospitalizations with sotagliflozin, which is a nonselective SGLT inhibitor [55]. Though not implemented in guidelines yet, we highlight this as a potential consideration for patients with CKD as a possible medication during early GDMT titration.

Ivabradine, another GDMT option, selectively inhibits I_f (funny) channels in a concentration-dependent manner, reducing HR [56]. Ivabradine has a selective advantage in CKD patients as its clearance through the renal tubules only contributes to 20% of the total metabolism of the drug [56]. Careful initiation must be considered for patients with concomitant liver conditions as serum concentration of ivabradine can be increased in chronic liver and cirrhosis patients. Research has shown that patients with a Child–Pugh score ≤ 7 can have increased concentration of ivabradine levels, but generally, there are limited data on studies with patients diagnosed with moderate or severe hepatic impairment [56].

4.4. Heart Failure in Diabetes

4.4.1. Mechanism of Heart Failure in Diabetes

Diabetic patients have over twice the risk of developing HF than patients without diabetes. Diabetes mellitus is associated with increased myocardial fatty acid utilization, decreased glucose utilization (glycolysis and glucose oxidation), increased myocardial oxygen consumption, and decreased cardiac efficiency. In diabetes, fatty acid oxidation occurs at an increased rate, but triglycerides and other lipid metabolites tend to accumulate in the diabetic heart. It is suggested that diabetes increases the risk of heart failure up to twofold in males and fivefold in females. This increased incidence persists despite adjusting for risk factors such as age, HTN, HLD, and CAD [57].

4.4.2. Management Considerations in Diabetes

An important aspect of heart failure management with concurrent diabetes consists of dietary and lifestyle modifications, which are similar to the lifestyle modifications discussed above. In general, patients are recommended to take a multi-lifestyle approach through the "Life's Essential 8" [58]. The ideal Life's Essential eight components include nonsmoking, body mass index <25 kg/m^2, ideal physical activity, ideal diet score, serum cholesterol <200 mg/dL without medication, blood pressure <120/<80 mmHg without medication, sleep health, and fasting glucose <100 mg/dL without medication [58,59].

Nutrition plays a vital role in HF and diabetes; however, dietary plans must be tailored according to personal and cultural food preferences, required caloric intake, comorbidities, current medications, and need for weight loss. Regardless, for those with diabetes and HF, minimizing alcohol intake and avoidance of smoking are always recommended [46].

HF is associated with physical inactivity and low fitness; given the high prevalence of concomitant HF and diabetes, exercise therapy can and should be directed to this population as well. Cardiac stiffness, the mainstay of HfpEF, accelerates in midlife but can be reversed by aerobic exercise [46]. One study consisting of 2331 patients, 32% with diabetes, was randomized to an aerobic exercise training program or standard of care for HF and then followed for 2.5 years. It was noted that although all individuals had a baseline lower functional capacity at the start of the study, those who completed the exercise program had significant improvement in their peak oxygen consumption and distance covered in the six-minute walk test compared with those who received only the standard care without any exercise training. The patients enrolled in this study who also had diabetes accounted for a large portion of the sample and, therefore, support the recommendations for exercise therapy to improve functional capacity in both heart failure and diabetes alike [60].

Several agents that demonstrate cardiovascular safety and improved outcomes also serve as effective antihyperglycemic agents, specifically those studied in heart failure patients. These include dipeptidyl peptidase-4 (DPP-4) inhibitors, glucagon-like peptide-1 (GLP-1) agonists, and sodium-glucose cotransporter-2 (SGLT2) inhibitors [61]. DPP-4 inhibitors increase the concentration of GLP-1. Small human studies with GLP-1 agonists exhibited similar results, with an overall increase in LVEF and functional status noted within the participants [62]. GLP-1 agonists have shown promise in HF treatment not only due to their beneficial effects on cardiovascular outcomes but also by managing other organ systems that relate to HF morbidity, including targeting weight loss and glycemic control, which work through the reduction of metabolic complications associated with obesity and HF, MACE, and HF symptoms [63]. The multisystem approach through GLP-1 agonists has led to a new topic of discussion about its effectiveness in HF, along with other medications for diabetes management. SGLT2 inhibitors have been shown to improve blood pressure control, arterial stiffness, vascular resistance, and microvascular remodeling—all occurring via multiple proposed mechanisms, including the beneficial effects on ion homeostasis, calcium handling, reduction of cardiac oxidative stress, and vascular inflammation. Myocardial metabolism utilizes ketone bodies as an energy-efficient source instead of glucose and lipid oxidation, which leads to improved cardiac contractility and confers cardiovascular protection.

As SGLT2i has been incorporated into GDMT, patients with diabetes are recommended to start empagliflozin or dapagliflozin earlier rather than later for optimal benefits. The DAPA-HF trial found that the risk of worsening heart failure or death from cardiovascular etiologies was lower in patients on dapagliflozin therapy compared with those who received placebo, regardless of the presence or absence of diabetes [64]. Another relevant trial that proved the cardiac benefits of early SGLT2-i is the EMPEROR-preserved trial, which showed that empagliflozin reduced the combined risk of cardiovascular death or hospitalization for patients with HFpEF [65]. Incretin-based therapies such as DPP-4 inhibitors and GLP-1 agonists should also be prioritized in diabetes management in these patients, possibly adjusting patients' diabetes regimen to include either class. Figure 2 below denotes recommendations for stepwise antihyperglycemic therapy based on heart failure stages A through D, indicated at each arrow [61].

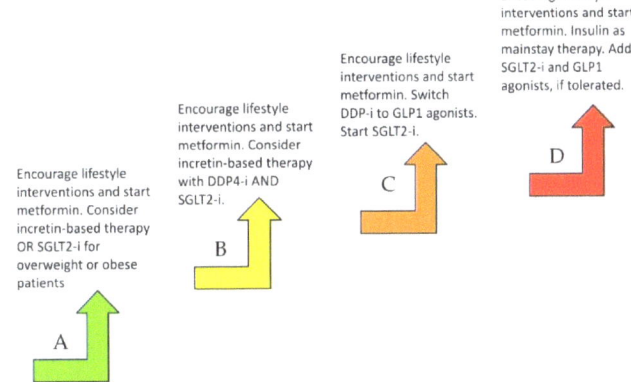

Figure 2. The recommendations for antihyperglycemic therapy based on the heart failure stage. Sodium-glucose cotransporter-2 (SGLT2). Glucagon-like peptide-1 (GLP-1). Dipeptidyl peptidase-4 (DPP-4).

Briefly mentioned above, nonselective SGLT inhibitors may also play a role in diabetes patients with HF. The SOLOIST-WHF trial, which enrolled patients with diabetes and recent worsening heart failure, noted that sotagliflozin (SGLT1 and 2 inhibitors) therapy significantly lowered total number of deaths from cardiovascular causes and decreased the number of hospitalizations and urgent visits for heart failure compared with placebo when the medication was initiated before or shortly after discharge [55].

4.5. Ethnic and Racial Minorities and Heart Failure

Broadly, HF prevalence varies depending on the racial communities; African Americans have a higher hazard ratio of HF, followed by Latin X/Latinos, Caucasians, and Asian communities [66]. HFpEF is more prevalent in non-African American demographics [43]. Comorbidities appear to primarily affect the presence of HF. African Americans exhibit a higher burden of hypertension (HTN), and Hispanics have more complications of diabetes mellitus (DM), both of which are increased risk factors for HF [66]. Thus, the management and prevention of HF are rooted in managing comorbidities, as addressed in previous sections.

4.6. Social Determinants of Health (SDOH), Socioeconomics, and Heart Failure

HF patients experiencing SDOH, particularly those from low-income or underserved populations, face numerous barriers to implementing non-pharmacological therapies for HF management. These barriers are primarily related to a lack of access to care in the form of cost and transportation issues, which increases the likelihood of poor HF outcomes over time due to more frequent symptom exacerbations and recurrent hospital admissions [66]. A significant challenge for this population is the cost associated with managing complex chronic illnesses, including medication and healthcare appointments [67].

Current models that capture the impact of SDOH on HF care include the World Health Organization (WHO) and vulnerable population conceptual frameworks [66]. These models emphasize the interplay between available resources—such as community support, geographic factors, and individual-level healthcare access—and the significance of personal, social, and behavioral factors, including relative risk and the overall health status of HF patients. Based on these frameworks, vulnerable patients facing significant SDOH can benefit from socioeconomic and environmental resources within their communities, which influence health through individual lifestyles, cultural behaviors, and value systems [67]. These resources encompass a range of services, from pharmacies to social and rehabilitation services to telehealth [67].

Patients face real-world challenges when implementing lifestyle changes, particularly those with financial difficulties or limited access to healthcare resources. These challenges can negatively impact survival, quality of life, and readmission rates [67]. Individuals experiencing SDOH benefit from a dedicated team that facilitates their transition to post-acute care facilities, often through a transitional care coordinator. This team also helps improve access to prescribed medication regimens via various patient assistance programs or the Dispensary of Hope, a national charitable medication distributor [67].

However, uninsured patients may struggle to secure an appropriate outpatient follow-up for heart failure management. These individuals require resources to access care at local indigent clinics, federally funded clinics, or county hospitals as viable options for long-term care [67].

The economic burden of HF, like other diseases, is measured on many facets rooted in the financial burdens of direct and indirect costs [2]. Direct costs of HF include hospitalization, outpatient care, medications, rehabilitation, nursing care, and informal care [2]. Indirect costs are those associated with the total societal productivity loss based on standards such as 'presenteeism', or the lack of productivity from employees due to illness or disease even though they are physically present at work, sick leave, early retirement, and premature mortality [2]. In the PURE study, socioeconomic status (SES) and risk of cardiovascular disease in 20 low-income, middle-income, and high-income countries showed that hypertension, diabetes, and secondary prevention and care management were lower in people with the lowest levels of educational attainment among low-income countries [68]. However, less marked differences in cardiovascular health were found in healthcare disparities when comparing educational attainment among middle-income and high-income countries [68]. Possible explanations may include the allocation of budget spending on healthcare each fiscal year in various countries. Thus, low educational attainment in low-income countries equates to poor healthcare outcomes compared with high educational attainment in the same low-income country.

The inpatient cost of hospitalization for HF-related complications is by far the highest expenditure of all. The highest cost of hospitalization in any nation was noted in the US healthcare system, which approximated USD 125,000 per patient per year [69]. In most European countries, those hospitalization costs range from USD 5000 to as close as USD 18,000 per patient per year [69].

Economic disparities and increasing healthcare costs translate to immediate effects on compliance. Lower SES communities tend to present in later-stage HF due to avoidance of healthcare costs [70]. In an effort to address such disparities, risk calculators have begun incorporating factors related to SES, including zip codes within the US. With repeat and large-cost hospitalizations, patients accumulate a debt that results in difficulty optimizing care and future healthcare visits. This healthcare debt spiral leads to worsening HF outcomes [70].

In cases of low SES, lifestyle changes may be of utmost importance. Additional medical therapies that offer high efficacy and low cost should be considered. Initial medication therapy is crucial as patients are less likely to adhere to medication regimens if presented with initial high costs, even if subsequent therapies are more affordable [70]. Thus, we recommend opting for ACEi/ARB over ARNI and choosing metoprolol succinate before carvedilol in these patients. In a head-to-head trial of valsartan (ARB) to captopril (ACEi), ARB was shown to be non-inferior, but not superior, to ACEi [71]. As such, we suggest a selection of ACEi, reserving utilization of ARB if a patient demonstrates side effects of ACEi. Starting spironolactone as an earlier medication in GDMT may also be a consideration, with SGLT2i therapy used after confirming a patient can afford it.

5. Challenges and Considerations

The barriers to implementation and the challenges patients with HF face include both compliance and adherence to both non-pharmacological and pharmacological therapies. Generally speaking, patients who were more compliant with medications in various studies also adhered to effective lifestyle modifications, such as exercise, limited alcohol consumption, and smoking cessation, which all resulted in better outcomes [3].

The explanation of this cohesion among patients with HF and their successful adherence and compliance with non-pharmacological modifications also spills over to pharmacy-driven interventions. In one study, HF patients who were compliant with their non-pharmacological treatment regimen were more likely to also be compliant with medication and pharmacy interventions, which, when combined, led to a better prognosis for patients. Out of the four core non-pharmacological interventions mentioned prior (i.e., daily weighing, diet modification, management of fluid consumption, and exercise programs), compliance with an exercise program recommendation in the HF population was the lowest, nearing 60% [3].

Bridging the gap of noncompliance requires a multifaceted approach, particularly in addressing the underlying cause for the inability to adhere to their regimen [72]. Noncompliance rooted in medical illiteracy can be combated with aggressive education and social support. In contrast, financial noncompliance requires a more tailored approach to management that considers affordability and efficacy in therapies, as noted above.

Educational attainment plays a significant role in how many CRP sessions would be completed by the patient. Patients with at least a 4-year college degree were more likely to complete CR interventions than patients with either a high school or less than a high school/GED diploma with a p value of <0.001 [73].

6. Discussion and Future Directions

The ubiquity of HF affecting multiple organ systems and spanning different populations contributes to the complexity of HF management. Although a well-studied field, growing evidence regarding HF management continues to be a topic of discussion, both in management modalities and nuances in patient-centered care. Particularly, there are varying strengths of data in the management of HF in special populations, with more populations studied compared with others. Clinicians are left to create a personalized approach for each patient using their empiric experiences in combination with existing care algorithms. There appears to be a paucity of evidence-based data on management prioritization in the female population, marking an area of potential growth. Additionally, socioeconomic status proves to be a large consideration in HF management in practice, yet structured approaches to medication titration, compliance, and lifestyle education remain insufficient. Thus, managing such populations continues to be a challenge, warranting further research and guideline-directed approaches.

Broadly speaking, new methods for heart failure management continue to be evaluated, including targeted physical exercise, dietary benefits, and medications. Innovations in the field of HF have led to discoveries of targeted drug therapies intended for other diseases, which can now be generalized to the HF population. In turn, HF management can undergo a paradigm shift, with a transition toward a multisystem and holistic approach as opposed to managing HF as a separate entity. GLP-1 antagonists, in addition to SGLTi, are among some of the examples of emerging drugs as potential HF therapies. Nonselective medications are also a hot topic of research for classes of drugs within GDMT. With further investigation, such therapies may become incorporated into GDMT in the near future.

Interventional management of HF also serves as a new and innovative avenue for heart failure. CardioMems to guide medical therapy has been a relatively new approach. Though beyond the scope of this paper, therapies such as IVC occluders, interatrial septal shunting, renal denervation, and BaroStim are emerging and may grow in popularity for interventional approaches to HF management.

7. Conclusions

Heart failure is a complex syndrome with high morbidity and mortality, and it requires a multidisciplinary approach. Non-pharmacological therapies and heart failure management include patient education, lifestyle modifications, dietary changes, increased physical activity, psychosocial support, and specialized cardiac rehabilitation programs. A continuous educational program is vital for chronic heart failure patients, covering CHF causes, symptoms, diet, salt/fluid restrictions, medication adherence, and lifestyle adjustments. A multidisciplinary team of dietitians, physical therapists, psychologists, nurses, and social workers is recommended to improve patient well-being and reduce healthcare costs. These measures, when used in conjunction with medical therapy, provide a comprehensive approach to managing heart failure, empowering patients to actively participate in their care and achieve better health outcomes.

Funding: This research received no external funding.

Data Availability Statement: No new data were created or analyzed in this study. Data sharing is not applicable to this article.

Conflicts of Interest: The authors declare no conflicts of interest.

References

1. Ranek, M.J.; Berthiaume, J.M.; Kirk, J.A.; Lyon, R.C.; Sheikh, F.; Jensen, B.C.; Hoit, B.D.; Butany, J.; Tolend, M.; Rao, V.; et al. Chapter 5—Pathophysiology of heart failure and an overview of therapies. In *Cardiovascular Pathology*, 5th ed.; Academic Press: Cambridge, MA, USA, 2022; pp. 149–221.
2. Hessel, F.P. Overview of the socio-economic consequences of heart failure. *Cardiovasc. Diagn. Ther.* **2021**, *11*, 254–262. [CrossRef] [PubMed]
3. Van der Wal, M.H.; van Veldhuisen, D.J.; Veeger, N.J.; Rutten, F.H.; Jaarsma, T. Compliance with non-pharmacological recommendations and outcome in heart failure patients. *Eur. Hearth J.* **2010**, *31*, 1486–1493. [CrossRef] [PubMed]
4. Hartupee, J.; Mann, D.L. Neurohormonal activation in heart failure with reduced ejection fraction. *Nat. Rev. Cardiol.* **2017**, *14*, 30–38. [CrossRef] [PubMed] [PubMed Central]
5. Camafort, M.; Park, S.-M.; Kang, S.-M. Lifestyle Modification in Heart Failure Management: Are We Using Evidence-Based Recommendations in Real World Practice? *Int. J. Hearth Fail.* **2023**, *5*, 21–33. [CrossRef]
6. Zhu, C.M.; Cheng, M.M.; Su, Y.M.; Ma, T.M.; Lei, X.M.; Hou, Y. Effect of Dietary Sodium Restriction on the Quality of Life of Patients with Heart Failure: A Systematic Review of Randomized Controlled Trials. *J. Cardiovasc. Nurs.* **2022**, *37*, 570–580. [CrossRef]
7. Kim, M.-S.; Lee, J.-H.; Kim, E.J.; Park, D.-G.; Park, S.-J.; Park, J.J.; Shin, M.-S.; Yoo, B.S.; Youn, J.-C.; Lee, S.E.; et al. Korean guidelines for diagnosis and management of chronic heart failure. *Korean Circ. J.* **2017**, *47*, 555–643. [CrossRef]
8. McDonagh, T.A.; Metra, M.; Adamo, M.; Gardner, R.S.; Baumbach, A.; Böhm, M.; Burri, H.; Butler, J.; Čelutkienė, J.; Chioncel, O.; et al. 2021 ESC Guidelines for the diagnosis and treatment of acute and chronic heart failure: Developed by the Task Force for the diagnosis and treatment of acute and chronic heart failure of the European Society of Cardiology (ESC) With the special contribution of the Heart Failure Association (HFA) of the ESC. *Eur. Heart J.* **2021**, *42*, 3599–3726, Erratum in: *Eur. Heart J.* **2021**, *42*, 4901. https://doi.org/10.1093/eurheartj/ehab670. [CrossRef] [PubMed]

9. Heidenreich, P.A.; Bozkurt, B.; Aguilar, D.; Allen, L.A.; Byun, J.J.; Colvin, M.M.; Deswal, A.L.; Drazner, M.H.; Dunlay, S.M.; Evers, L.R.; et al. 2022 AHA/ACC/HFSA guideline for the management of heart failure: A report of the American College of Cardiology/American Heart Association Joint Committee on Clinical Practice Guidelines. *J. Am. Coll. Cardiol.* **2022**, *79*, e263–e421.
10. Travers, B.; O'Loughlin, C.; Murphy, N.F.; Ryder, M.; Conlon, C.; Ledwidge, M.; McDonald, K. Fluid restriction in the management of decompensated heart failure: No impact on time to clinical stability. *J. Card. Fail.* **2007**, *13*, 128–132. [CrossRef] [PubMed]
11. Albert, N.M.; Nutter, B.; Forney, J.; Slifcak, E.; Tang, W.H.W. A randomized controlled pilot study of outcomes of strict allowance of fluid therapy in hyponatremic heart failure (SALT-HF). *J. Card. Fail.* **2013**, *19*, 1–9. [CrossRef] [PubMed]
12. Ebong, I.A.; Goff, D.C.; Rodriguez, C.J.; Chen, H.; Bertoni, A.G. Mechanisms of heart failure in obesity. *Obes. Res. Clin. Pr.* **2014**, *8*, e540–e548. [CrossRef] [PubMed] [PubMed Central]
13. Khan, S.S.; Coresh, J.; Pencina, M.J.; Ndumele, C.E.; Rangaswami, J.; Chow, S.L.; Palaniappan, L.P.; Sperling, L.S.; Virani, S.S.; Ho, J.E.; et al. Novel Prediction Equations for Absolute Risk Assessment of Total Cardiovascular Disease Incorporating Cardiovascular-Kidney-Metabolic Health: A Scientific Statement from the American Heart Association. *Circulation* **2023**, *148*, 1982–2004. [CrossRef] [PubMed]
14. Appel, L.J.; Moore, T.J.; Obarzanek, E.; Vollmer, W.M.; Svetkey, L.P.; Sacks, F.M.; Bray, G.A.; Vogt, T.M.; Cutler, J.A.; Windhauser, M.M.; et al. A Clinical Trial of the Effects of Dietary Patterns on Blood Pressure. *N. Engl. J. Med.* **1997**, *336*, 1117–1124. [CrossRef] [PubMed]
15. Sacks, F.M.; Svetkey, L.P.; Vollmer, W.M.; Appel, L.J.; Bray, G.A.; Harsha, D.; Obarzanek, E.; Conlin, P.R.; Miller, E.R.; Simons-Morton, D.G.; et al. Effects on Blood Pressure of Reduced Dietary Sodium and the Dietary Approaches to Stop Hypertension (DASH) Diet. *N. Engl. J. Med.* **2001**, *344*, 3–10. [CrossRef]
16. Wickman, B.E.; Enkhmaa, B.; Ridberg, R.; Romero, E.; Cadeiras, M.; Meyers, F.; Steinberg, F. Dietary management of heart failure: Dash diet and precision nutrition perspectives. *Nutrients* **2021**, *13*, 4424. [CrossRef]
17. Ros, E. The PREDIMED study. *Endocrinol. Diabetes Nutr.* **2017**, *64*, 63–66. [CrossRef]
18. Delgado-Lista, J.; Alcala-Diaz, J.F.; Torres-Peña, J.D.; Quintana-Navarro, G.M.; Fuentes, F.; Garcia-Rios, A.; Ortiz-Morales, A.M.; I Gonzalez-Requero, A.; I Perez-Caballero, A.; Yubero-Serrano, E.M.; et al. Long-term secondary prevention of cardiovascular disease with a Mediterranean diet and a low-fat diet (CORDIOPREV): A randomised controlled trial. *Lancet* **2022**, *399*, 1876–1885. [CrossRef]
19. Kang, J.; Moser, D.K.; Biddle, M.J.; Oh, G.; Lennie, T.A. Age- and sex-matched comparison of diet quality in patients with heart failure to similarly aged healthy older adults. *J. Nutr. Sci.* **2021**, *10*, e65. [CrossRef] [PubMed] [PubMed Central]
20. Soto, M.E.; Pérez-Torres, I.; Rubio-Ruiz, M.E.; Manzano-Pech, L.; Guarner-Lans, V. Interconnection between Cardiac Cachexia and Heart Failure-Protective Role of Cardiac Obesity. *Cells* **2022**, *11*, 1039. [CrossRef] [PubMed] [PubMed Central]
21. Taylor, R.S.; Long, L.; Mordi, I.R.; Madsen, M.T.; Davies, E.J.; Dalal, H.; Rees, K.; Singh, S.J. Exercise-based rehabilitation for heart failure: Cochrane systematic review, meta-analysis, and trial sequential analysis. *JACC Heart Fail.* **2019**, *7*, 691–705. [CrossRef]
22. Winnige, P.; Vysoky, R.; Dosbaba, F.; Batalik, L. Cardiac rehabilitation and its essential role in the secondary prevention of cardiovascular diseases. *World J. Clin. Cases* **2021**, *9*, 1761–1784. [CrossRef] [PubMed] [PubMed Central]
23. Powell-Wiley, T.M.; Poirier, P.; Burke, L.E.; Després, J.-P.; Gordon-Larsen, P.; Lavie, C.J.; Lear, S.A.; Ndumele, C.E.; Neeland, I.J.; Sanders, P.; et al. Obesity and Cardiovascular Disease: A Scientific Statement from the American Heart Association. *Circulation* **2021**, *143*, e984–e1010. [CrossRef]
24. Kenchaiah, S.; Evans, J.C.; Levy, D.; Wilson, P.W.; Benjamin, E.J.; Larson, M.G.; Kannel, W.B.; Vasan, R.S. Obesity and the Risk of Heart Failure. *N. Engl. J. Med.* **2002**, *347*, 305–313. [CrossRef]
25. Elagizi, A.; Carbone, S.; Lavie, C.J.; Mehra, M.R.; Ventura, H.O. Implications of obesity across the heart failure continuum. *Prog. Cardiovasc. Dis.* **2020**, *63*, 561–569. [CrossRef] [PubMed] [PubMed Central]
26. Okuhara, Y.; Asakura, M.; Orihara, Y.; Naito, Y.; Tsujino, T.; Ishihara, M.; Masuyama, T. Effects of Weight Loss in Outpatients with Mild Chronic Heart Failure: Findings From the J-MELODIC Study. *J. Card. Fail.* **2019**, *25*, 44–50. [CrossRef]
27. Grubb, A.F.; Greene, S.J.; Fudim, M.; Dewald, T.; Mentz, R.J. Drugs of Abuse and Heart Failure. *J. Card. Fail.* **2021**, *27*, 1260–1275. [CrossRef]
28. Centers for Disease Control and Prevention (US); National Center for Chronic Disease Prevention and Health Promotion (US); Office on Smoking and Health (US). Chapter 6—Cardiovascular Diseases. In *How Tobacco Smoke Causes Disease: The Biology and Behavioral Basis for Smoking-Attributable Disease: A Report of the Surgeon General*; Centers for Disease Control and Prevention: Atlanta, GA, USA, 2010. Available online: https://www.ncbi.nlm.nih.gov/books/NBK53012/ (accessed on 5 October 2024).
29. Goldberg, L.R.; Piette, J.D.; Walsh, M.N.; A Frank, T.; E Jaski, B.; Smith, A.L.; Rodriguez, R.; Mancini, D.M.; A Hopton, L.; Orav, E.; et al. Randomized trial of a daily electronic home monitoring system in patients with advanced heart failure: The Weight Monitoring in Heart Failure (WHARF) trial. *Am. Hearth J.* **2003**, *146*, 705–712. [CrossRef]
30. Sapp, J.L.; Parkash, R.; Wells, G.A.; Yetisir, E.; Gardner, M.J.; Healey, J.S.; Thibault, B.; Sterns, L.D.; Birnie, D.; Nery, P.B.; et al. Cardiac Resynchronization Therapy Reduces Ventricular Arrhythmias in Primary but Not Secondary Prophylactic Implantable Cardioverter Defibrillator Patients: Insight from the Resynchronization in Ambulatory Heart Failure Trial. *Circ. Arrhythmia Electrophysiol.* **2017**, *10*, e004875. [CrossRef]
31. Bristow, M.R.; Saxon, L.A.; Boehmer, J.; Krueger, S.; Kass, D.A.; De Marco, T.; Carson, P.; DiCarlo, L.; DeMets, D.; White, B.G.; et al. Cardiac-Resynchronization Therapy with or without an Implantable Defibrillator in Advanced Chronic Heart Failure. *N. Engl. J. Med.* **2004**, *350*, 2140–2150. [CrossRef]

32. Nakai, T.; Ikeya, Y.; Kogawa, R.; Okumura, Y. Cardiac resynchronization therapy: Current status and near-future prospects. *J. Cardiol.* **2022**, *79*, 352–357. [CrossRef]
33. Abraham, W.T.; Fisher, W.G.; Smith, A.L.; Delurgio, D.B.; Leon, A.R.; Loh, E.; Kocovic, D.Z.; Packer, M.; Clavell, A.L.; Hayes, D.L.; et al. Cardiac resynchronization in chronic heart failure. *N. Engl. J. Med.* **2002**, *346*, 1845–1853. [CrossRef] [PubMed]
34. Elming, M.B.; Nielsen, J.C.; Haarbo, J.; Videbæk, L.; Korup, E.; Signorovitch, J.; Olesen, L.L.; Hildebrandt, P.; Steffensen, F.H.; Bruun, N.E.; et al. Age and outcomes of primary prevention implantable cardioverter-defibrillators in patients with nonischemic systolic heart failure. *Circulation* **2017**, *136*, 1772–1780. [CrossRef] [PubMed]
35. Ghzally, Y.; Mahajan, K. "Implantable Defibrillator". National Library of Medicine. 3 October 2022. Available online: https://www.ncbi.nlm.nih.gov/books/NBK459196/ (accessed on 5 October 2024).
36. Yafasova, A.; Butt, J.H.; Elming, M.B.; Nielsen, J.C.; Haarbo, J.; Videbæk, L.; Olesen, L.L.; Steffensen, F.H.; Bruun, N.E.; Eiskjær, H.; et al. Long-term follow-up of DANISH (the Danish study to assess the efficacy of ICDs in patients with nonischemic systolic heart failure on mortality). *Circulation* **2022**, *145*, 427–436. [CrossRef] [PubMed]
37. Giustino, G.; Lindenfeld, J.; Abraham, W.T.; Kar, S.; Lim, D.S.; Grayburn, P.A.; Kapadia, S.R.; Cohen, D.J.; Kotinkaduwa, L.N.; Weissman, N.J.; et al. NYHA functional classification and outcomes after transcatheter mitral valve repair in heart failure: The COAPT trial. *Cardiovasc. Interv.* **2020**, *13*, 2317–2328. [CrossRef] [PubMed]
38. Taggart, D.P. PCI versus CABG in coronary artery disease. *Vasc. Pharmacol.* **2024**, *155*, 107367. [CrossRef] [PubMed]
39. Velazquez, E.J.; Lee, K.L.; Jones, R.H.; Al-Khalidi, H.R.; Hill, J.A.; Panza, J.A.; Michler, R.E.; Bonow, R.O.; Doenst, T.; Petrie, M.C.; et al. Coronary-artery bypass surgery in patients with ischemic cardiomyopathy. *N. Engl. J. Med.* **2016**, *374*, 1511–1520. [CrossRef]
40. Strait, J.B.; Lakatta, E.G. Aging-associated cardiovascular changes and their relationship to heart failure. *Heart Fail. Clin.* **2012**, *8*, 143–164. [CrossRef] [PubMed] [PubMed Central]
41. Warner, V.; Nguyen, D.; Bayles, T.; Hopper, I. Management of heart failure in older people. *J. Pharm. Pr. Res.* **2022**, *52*, 72–79. [CrossRef]
42. Rahamim, E.; Nachman, D.; Yagel, O.; Yarkoni, M.; Elbaz-Greener, G.; Amir, O.; Asleh, R. Contemporary Pillars of Heart Failure with Reduced Ejection Fraction Medical Therapy. *J. Clin. Med.* **2021**, *10*, 4409. [CrossRef] [PubMed] [PubMed Central]
43. Pandey, A.; Omar, W.; Ayers, C.; LaMonte, M.; Klein, L.; Allen, N.B.; Kuller, L.H.; Greenland, P.; Eaton, C.B.; Gottdiener, J.S.; et al. Sex and Race Differences in Lifetime Risk of Heart Failure with Preserved Ejection Fraction and Heart Failure with Reduced Ejection Fraction. *Circulation* **2018**, *137*, 1814–1823. [CrossRef]
44. Regitz-Zagrosek, V. Sex and Gender Differences in Heart Failure. *Int. J. Hearth Fail.* **2020**, *2*, 157–181. [CrossRef] [PubMed]
45. Miyakoshi, C.; Morimoto, T.; Yaku, H.; Murai, R.; Kaji, S.; Furukawa, Y.; Inuzuka, Y.; Nagao, K.; Tamaki, Y.; Yamamoto, E.; et al. Mode of Death Among Japanese Adults with Heart Failure with Preserved, Midrange, and Reduced Ejection Fraction. *JAMA Netw. Open* **2020**, *3*, e204296. [CrossRef]
46. Pop-Busui, R.; Januzzi, J.L.; Bruemmer, D.; Butalia, S.; Green, J.B.; Horton, W.B.; Knight, C.; Levi, M.; Rasouli, N.; Richardson, C.R. Heart Failure: An Underappreciated Complication of Diabetes. A Consensus Report of the American Diabetes Association. *Diabetes Care* **2022**, *45*, 1670–1690. [CrossRef] [PubMed]
47. Roberts, A. Insights from the REGARDS study. *Nat. Rev. Cardiol.* **2014**, *11*, 3. [CrossRef]
48. DeCara, J.M.; Lang, R.M.; Foley, M. *Management of Heart Failure During Pregnancy*; UpToDate: Waltham, MS, USA, 2023. Available online: www.uptodate.com/contents/management-of-heart-failure-during-pregnancy#H7 (accessed on 5 October 2024).
49. Schefold, J.C.; Filippatos, G.; Hasenfuss, G.; Anker, S.D.; Von Haehling, S. Heart failure and kidney dysfunction: Epidemiology, mechanisms and management. *Nat. Rev. Nephrol.* **2016**, *12*, 610–623. [CrossRef]
50. Tang, A.S.; Wells, G.A.; Talajic, M.; Arnold, M.O.; Sheldon, R.; Connolly, S.; Hohnloser, S.H.; Nichol, G.; Birnie, D.H.; Sapp, J.L.; et al. Cardiac-resynchronization therapy for mild-to-moderate heart failure. *N. Engl. J. Med.* **2010**, *363*, 2385–2395. [CrossRef]
51. Friedman, D.J.; Singh, J.P.; Curtis, J.P.; Tang, W.W.; Bao, H.; Spatz, E.S.; Hernandez, A.F.; Patel, U.D.; Al-Khatib, S.M. Comparative Effectiveness of CRT-D Versus Defibrillator Alone in HF Patients with Moderate-to-Severe Chronic Kidney Disease. *J. Am. Coll. Cardiol.* **2015**, *66*, 2618–2629. [CrossRef] [PubMed]
52. Bardy, G.H.; Lee, K.L.; Mark, D.B.; Poole, J.E.; Packer, D.L.; Boineau, R.; Domanski, M.; Troutman, C.; Anderson, J.; Johnson, G.; et al. Amiodarone or an implantable cardioverter-defibrillator for congestive heart failure. *N. Engl. J. Med.* **2005**, *352*, 225–237. [CrossRef]
53. Turakhia, M.P.; Blankestijn, P.J.; Carrero, J.-J.; Clase, C.M.; Deo, R.; A Herzog, C.; E Kasner, S.; Passman, R.S.; Pecoits-Filho, R.; Reinecke, H.; et al. Chronic kidney disease and arrhythmias: Conclusions from a kidney disease: Improving global outcomes (KDIGO) controversies conference. *Eur. Hearth J.* **2018**, *39*, 2314–2325. [CrossRef]
54. Banerjee, D.; Wang, A.Y.-M. Personalizing heart failure management in chronic kidney disease patients. *Nephrol. Dial. Transplant.* **2022**, *37*, 2055–2062. [CrossRef]
55. Bhatt, D.L.; Szarek, M.; Pitt, B.; Cannon, C.P.; Leiter, L.A.; McGuire, D.K.; Lewis, J.B.; Riddle, M.C.; Inzucchi, S.E.; Kosiborod, M.N.; et al. Sotagliflozin in Patients with Diabetes and Chronic Kidney Disease. *N. Engl. J. Med.* **2021**, *384*, 129–139. [CrossRef] [PubMed]
56. Bocchi, E.A.; Salemi, V.M.C. Ivabradine for treatment of heart failure. *Expert Opin. Drug Saf.* **2019**, *18*, 393–402. [CrossRef]
57. Kenny, H.C.; Abel, E.D. Heart Failure in Type 2 Diabetes Mellitus: Impact of Glucose-Lowering Agents, Heart Failure Therapies, and Novel Therapeutic Strategies. *Circ. Res.* **2019**, *124*, 121–141. [CrossRef]

58. Lloyd-Jones, D.M.; Allen, N.B.; Anderson, C.A.; Black, T.; Brewer, L.C.; Foraker, R.E.; Grandner, M.A.; Lavretsky, H.; Perak, A.M.; Sharma, G.; et al. Life's Essential 8: Updating and Enhancing the American Heart Association's Construct of Cardiovascular Health: A Presidential Advisory From the American Heart Association. *Circulation* **2022**, *146*, E18–E43. [CrossRef]
59. Folsom, A.R.; Olson, N.C.; Lutsey, P.L.; Roetker, N.S.; Cushman, M. American Heart Association's Life's Simple 7 and incidence of venous thromboembolism. *Am. J. Hematol.* **2015**, *90*, E92. [CrossRef]
60. O'connor, C.M.; Whellan, D.J.; Lee, K.L.; Keteyian, S.J.; Cooper, L.S.; Ellis, S.J.; Leifer, E.S.; Kraus, W.E.; Kitzman, D.W.; Blumenthal, J.A.; et al. Efficacy and safety of exercise training in patients with chronic heart failure: HF-ACTION randomized controlled trial. *JAMA* **2009**, *301*, 1439–1450. [CrossRef]
61. Osuna, P.M.; Brown, S.J.; Tabatabai, L.S.; Hamilton, D.J. Stage-Based Management of Type 2 Diabetes Mellitus with Heart Failure. *Methodist DeBakey Cardiovasc. J.* **2018**, *14*, 257–265. [CrossRef]
62. Vrhovac, I.; Eror, D.B.; Klessen, D.; Burger, C.; Breljak, D.; Kraus, O.; Radović, N.; Jadrijević, S.; Aleksic, I.; Walles, T.; et al. Localizations of Na(+)-D-glucose cotransporters SGLT1 and SGLT2 in human kidney and of SGLT1 in human small intestine, liver, lung, and heart. *Pflugers Arch. Eur. J. Physiol.* **2015**, *467*, 1881–1898. [CrossRef] [PubMed]
63. Karakasis, P.; Fragakis, N.; Patoulias, D.; Theofilis, P.; Sagris, M.; Koufakis, T.; Vlachakis, P.K.; Rangraze, I.R.; El Tanani, M.; Tsioufis, K.; et al. The Emerging Role of Glucagon-like Peptide-1 Receptor Agonists in the Management of Obesity-Related Heart Failure with Preserved Ejection Fraction: Benefits beyond What Scales Can Measure? *Biomedicines* **2024**, *12*, 2112. [CrossRef]
64. McMurray, J.J.V.; Solomon, S.D.; Inzucchi, S.E.; Køber, L.; Kosiborod, M.N.; Martinez, F.A.; Ponikowski, P.; Sabatine, M.S.; Anand, I.S.; Bělohlávek, J.; et al. Dapagliflozin in Patients with Heart Failure and Reduced Ejection Fraction. *N. Engl. J. Med.* **2019**, *381*, 1995–2008. [CrossRef]
65. Anker, S.D.; Butler, J.; Filippatos, G.; Ferreira, J.P.; Bocchi, E.; Böhm, M.; Brunner–La Rocca, H.-P.; Choi, D.-J.; Chopra, V.; Chuquiure-Valenzuela, E.; et al. Empagliflozin in Heart Failure with a Preserved Ejection Fraction. *N. Engl. J. Med.* **2021**, *385*, 1451–1461. [CrossRef] [PubMed]
66. Piña, I.L.; Jimenez, S.; Lewis, E.F.; Morris, A.A.; Onwuanyi, A.; Tam, E.; Ventura, H.O. Race and ethnicity in heart failure: JACC focus seminar 8/9. *J. Am. Coll. Cardiol.* **2021**, *78*, 2589–2598. [CrossRef] [PubMed]
67. White-Williams, C.; Rossi, L.P.; Bittner, V.A.; Driscoll, A.; Durant, R.W.; Granger, B.B.; Graven, L.J.; Kitko, L.; Newlin, K.; Shirey, M.; et al. Addressing Social Determinants of Health in the Care of Patients with Heart Failure: A Scientific Statement from the American Heart Association. *Circulation* **2020**, *140*, e905–e932. [CrossRef]
68. Rosengren, A.; Smyth, A.; Rangarajan, S.; Ramasundarahettige, C.; Bangdiwala, S.I.; Alhabib, K.F.; Avezum, A.; Boström, K.B.; Chifamba, J.; Gulec, S.; et al. Socioeconomic status and risk of cardiovascular disease in 20 low-income, middle-income, and high-income countries: The Prospective Urban Rural Epidemiologic (PURE) study. *Lancet Glob. Health* **2019**, *7*, e748–e760. [CrossRef]
69. Echouffo-Tcheugui, J.B.; Bishu, K.G.; Fonarow, G.C.; Egede, L.E. Trends in health care expenditure among US adults with heart failure: The Medical Expenditure Panel Survey 2002–2011. *Am. Hearth J.* **2017**, *186*, 63–72. [CrossRef]
70. Wang, S.Y.; Valero-Elizondo, J.; Ali, H.; Pandey, A.; Cainzos-Achirica, M.; Krumholz, H.M.; Nasir, K.; Khera, R. Out-of-pocket annual health expenditures and financial toxicity from healthcare costs in patients with heart failure in the United States. *J. Am. Hearth Assoc.* **2021**, *10*, e022164. [CrossRef]
71. Velazquez, E.J.; Pfeffer, M.A.; McMurray, J.V.; Maggioni, A.P.; Rouleau, J.; Van de Werf, F.; Kober, L.; White, H.D.; Swedberg, K.; Leimberger, J.D.; et al. VALsartan in acute myocardial iNfarcTion (VALIANT) trial: Baseline characteristics in context. *Eur. J. Hearth Fail.* **2003**, *5*, 537–544. [CrossRef]
72. Maddox, T.M.; Januzzi, J.L., Jr.; Allen, L.A.; Breathett, K.; Brouse, S.; Butler, J.; Davis, L.L.; Fonarow, G.C.; Ibrahim, N.E.; Lindenfeld, J.; et al. 2024 ACC Expert Consensus Decision Pathway for Treatment of Heart Failure with Reduced Ejection Fraction: A Report of the American College of Cardiology Solution Set Oversight Committee. *J. Am. Coll. Cardiol.* **2024**, *83*, 1444–1488. [CrossRef]
73. Gaalema, D.E.; Savage, P.D.; O'Neill, S.; Bolívar, H.A.; Denkmann, D.B.; Priest, J.S.; Khadanga, S.; Ades, P.A. The association of patient educational attainment with cardiac rehabilitation adherence and health outcomes. *J. Cardiopulm. Rehabil. Prev.* **2022**, *42*, 227–234. [CrossRef]

Disclaimer/Publisher's Note: The statements, opinions and data contained in all publications are solely those of the individual author(s) and contributor(s) and not of MDPI and/or the editor(s). MDPI and/or the editor(s) disclaim responsibility for any injury to people or property resulting from any ideas, methods, instructions or products referred to in the content.

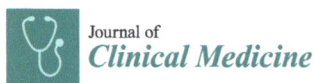 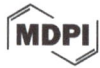

Article

An Observational Study of Evidence-Based Therapies in Older Patients with Heart Failure with Reduced Ejection Fraction: Insights from a Dedicated Heart Failure Clinic

Catarina Silva Araújo [1,†], Irene Marco [2,†], María Alejandra Restrepo-Córdoba [2], Isidre Vila Costa [2], Julián Pérez-Villacastín [2] and Josebe Goirigolzarri-Artaza [2,*]

1. Internal Medicine, Braga Hospital, 4710-243 Braga, Portugal; catarinaaraujo.mi@gmail.com
2. Cardiovascular Institute, Instituto de Investigación Sanitaria, Hospital Clínico San Carlos (IdISSC), C/Prof Martín Lagos S/N, Moncloa-Aravaca, 28040 Madrid, Spain; irene.marco@salud.madrid.org (I.M.)
* Correspondence: josebegoiri@gmail.com; Tel.: +34-913303000
† These authors contributed equally to this work.

Abstract: Background/Objectives: Despite significant advances in the management of heart failure with reduced ejection fraction (HFrEF), data concerning older patients remain limited. The purpose of this study was to evaluate the implementation of guideline-directed medical therapy (GDMT) in older patients with HFrEF along with cardiac events and variation in clinical and echocardiographic parameters during follow-up in a heart failure (HF) clinic. **Methods:** We conducted a retrospective observational analysis of patients with HFrEF aged ≥ 80 years who attended an HF clinic between March 2022 and February 2023. The primary outcome was a composite of the first episode of worsening HF or cardiovascular death. All-cause death was also recorded. **Results:** We included 110 patients (30.9% females; mean age 82.9 years). After a median follow-up of 25.5 months, left ventricular ejection fraction (LVEF) improved (mean difference 12.5% ($p < 0.001$)). New York Heart Association class improved in 37% of patients, and N-terminal pro-B-type natriuretic peptide levels decreased (3091 (158–53354) to 1802 (145–19509), $p < 0.001$). The primary outcome occurred in 34 patients (30.9%). Patients without the primary outcome were more likely to receive sodium-glucose co-transporter-2 inhibitors (SGLT2i) (23.5% versus 67.1%, $p < 0.001$) and angiotensin receptor-neprilysin inhibitors, angiotensin-converting enzyme inhibitors, or angiotensin-receptor blockers (67.6% versus 84.2%, $p < 0.05$). These patients also received a greater number of GDMT medications (2 (0–4) versus 3 (1–4), $p < 0.01$) and demonstrated a higher LVEF at the last visit (41.2 ± 10.2% versus 47.1 ± 9.4%, $p < 0.05$). Survival analysis demonstrated a significant association between LVEF recovery (hazard ratio (HR) 0.35, $p < 0.01$), treatment with two or more GDMT medications (HR 0.29, $p < 0.01$), vasodilator use (HR 0.36, $p < 0.01$), and SGLT2i prescription (HR 0.17, $p < 0.001$) and a reduced risk of the primary endpoint. **Conclusions:** The optimization of HF treatment is achievable in older patients and may be associated with a reduction in cardiac events.

Keywords: heart failure; guideline-directed medical therapies; geriatric cardiology

Citation: Araújo, C.S.; Marco, I.; Restrepo-Córdoba, M.A.; Vila Costa, I.; Pérez-Villacastín, J.; Goirigolzarri-Artaza, J. An Observational Study of Evidence-Based Therapies in Older Patients with Heart Failure with Reduced Ejection Fraction: Insights from a Dedicated Heart Failure Clinic. *J. Clin. Med.* **2024**, *13*, 7171. https://doi.org/10.3390/jcm13237171

Academic Editors: Cristina Tudoran and Larisa Anghel

Received: 30 October 2024
Revised: 18 November 2024
Accepted: 22 November 2024
Published: 26 November 2024

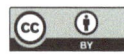

Copyright: © 2024 by the authors. Licensee MDPI, Basel, Switzerland. This article is an open access article distributed under the terms and conditions of the Creative Commons Attribution (CC BY) license (https://creativecommons.org/licenses/by/4.0/).

1. Introduction

Heart failure (HF) is associated with significant morbidity and mortality, and its prevalence exponentially increases with age, reaching 10% in those over 80 years old. This condition has emerged as a significant challenge in the elderly population, representing the leading cause of hospitalization in this age group [1–3]. More than half of those hospitalized for HF are over 75 years old. The prognosis also worsens with age, with 1- and 5-year mortality rates of 19.5% and 54.4% for 80 year olds [4]. While preserved ejection fraction is more prevalent in older individuals with HF, a considerable proportion presents with reduced ejection fraction (HFrEF) [5].

Advances in HFrEF diagnosis and management have shown great reductions in cardiovascular events, hospitalizations, and mortality in clinical trials over the last few decades [6]. In view of these results, international guidelines have endorsed the so-called "4 pillars" for HFrEF treatment: angiotensin receptor-neprilysin inhibitor—ARNI, or angiotensin-converting enzyme inhibitor—ACE-I); beta-blockers; mineralocorticoid receptor antagonist (MRA) and sodium-glucose co-transporter 2 inhibitors (SGLT2i) (dapagliflozin/empagliflozin) [1,7,8]. However, the use of guideline-directed medical therapy (GDMT) can be challenging in this population. There are limited data about HFrEF treatment in older patients as they are underrepresented in major randomized clinical trials [9–11]. In addition, clinical trials aimed at this specific population are marginal [12]. Also, clinicians can be overcautious in the presence of multiple comorbidities and polypharmacy. HF clinics may offer a means of enhancing the quality of care for this population, facilitating close follow-up and meticulous titration of GDMT [13].

This study aimed to evaluate the degree of implementation of HF therapies in an older population with HFrEF, assessing clinical and echocardiographic changes and documenting the occurrence of cardiac events during follow-up within an HF clinic.

2. Materials and Methods

2.1. Patient Selection and Study Design

This study was an observational, single-center retrospective analysis of consecutive elderly patients diagnosed with HFrEF who visited a tertiary hospital heart failure clinic led by cardiologists during one year (from March 2022 to February 2023). The selection of this timeframe ensures a standardized management of HFrEF following the ESC practice guidelines of HF issued in late 2021 [1]. Patients that were 80 years old or older at the time of first visit and were at least 75 years old at the time of HF diagnosis were included. Exclusion criteria included severe primary valvular heart disease requiring intervention, a life expectancy of less than 6 months, and a follow-up period of less than 6 months in the HF clinic. This study was conducted in compliance with the Declaration of Helsinki and reviewed by the Institutional Review Board Ethical Committee of our center (24/720-E).

2.2. Data Collection and Follow-Up

Data from the first and last clinical evaluation were retrospectively collected. Demographic, clinical, laboratory, echocardiographic, and electrocardiographic data were recorded. Echocardiographic parameters registered included left ventricular ejection fraction (LVEF), left ventricular end-diastolic diameter (LVEDD), mitral valve regurgitation, and the presence of right ventricular dysfunction. The New York Heart Association (NYHA) classification was used to assess functional class. Glomerular filtration rate (GFR) was estimated with Chronic Kidney Disease Epidemiology Collaboration (CKD-EPI) equation. LVEF at diagnosis and the suspected etiology of HF were also registered.

A $\geq$10-point increase from diagnosis with a final LVEF of >40% at the last visit was considered improved LVEF, and LVEF recovery was defined as an increase in LVEF of at least 10% to a value $\geq$50%. Primary outcome was defined as the composite of the first episode of worsening HF (HF hospital admission or need for intravenous diuretics in the outpatient clinic) or cardiovascular death. All-cause death was also addressed. HF treatments at the time of the first episode of worsening HF and one month after its occurrence were also registered.

All required information was extracted from the electronic records system and compiled into an anonymized Excel sheet using a standardized extraction procedure, which included validation rules. Medical charts were revised to ensure their reliability and accuracy before data extraction. When multiple sources were available, cross-checking was performed to identify any discrepancies. A single individual conducted data extraction, while a different expert reviewed the extracted data to ensure accuracy prior to analysis.

2.3. Statistical Analysis

The collected data were analyzed using the software IBM SPSS® version 23.0 and GraphPad Prism 10®. Pie charts were designed with Microsoft Excel®. The Kolmogorov–Smirnov test was used to test the existence of a normal distribution in continuous quantitative variables. Continuous variables with a normal distribution were presented as mean and standard deviation. The median, interquartile range, and minimum and maximum values were used for those with a non-normal distribution. Categorical variables were presented as absolute numbers and percentages. Between-group analyses of categorical variables were performed with the chi-square, Fisher's exact, and McNemar tests. The Kruskal–Wallis, Man–Whitney U, Wilcoxon, Spearman, and paired samples t-tests were used for continuous variables. Analysis of binary outcomes such as LVEF recovery was performed with logistic regression, using a backward stepwise approach for multivariate analysis with $p = 0.05$ for inclusion and $p = 0.10$ for exclusion. Time-to-first-event curves were obtained using the Kaplan–Meier method and compared with log-rank test. Hazard ratios (HR) were obtained using univariate Cox regression analysis, including predefined variables (GDMT, LVEF recovery). A 95% confidence interval was considered, with statistical significance at $p < 0.05$.

3. Results

3.1. Sample Description

This study included 110 patients (30.9% females; 80 ± 6 years at HF diagnosis and 82 ± 4 years at first evaluation). Baseline characteristics are described in Table 1. Diabetes was present in 41.8% of patients and chronic kidney disease in 50.9%. Mean LVEF at diagnosis was 32.4%, with the most common cause of HF being non-ischemic dilated cardiomyopathy (37.3%), followed by ischemic cardiomyopathy. Two-thirds of the patients included in this study were referred to the HF clinic after a hospital admission for HF.

Table 1. Sample description.

	n = 110
Female sex	34 (30.9%)
Age at Diagnosis (years) **	80.1 ± 6.1
Age at First Visit (years) *	82.9 ± 4.1
Duration of Follow-up (months) **	25.5 (14–47)
Hypertension	97 (88.2%)
Dyslipidemia	78 (70.9%)
Diabetes	46 (41.8%)
Smoking	
Yes	2 (1.8%)
Ex-smoker	45 (40.9%)
Moderate/severe COPD	5 (4.5%)
Sleep apnea with CPAP	9 (8.2%)
Chronic kidney disease (GFR < 45 mL/min/1.73 m^2)	56 (50.9%)
LVEF at Diagnosis (%) *	32.4 ± 5.4
Etiology of heart failure	
Dilated cardiomyopathy, non-ischemic	41 (37.3%)
Ischemic	36 (32.7%)
Valvular	12 (10.9%)
Mix (valvular + ischemic)	13 (11.8%)
Amyloidosis	2 (1.8%)
Other	6 (5.5%)

Table 1. Cont.

	n = 110
Reason for referral to the HF clinic	
Heart failure admission	67 (60.9%)
Presence of symptoms or signs of HF	33 (30%)
Casual finding on echocardiogram	9 (8.2%)
Sudden cardiac death episode	1 (0.9%)

* Mean ± standard deviation; ** Median (percentiles 25–75) (minimum–maximum); CPAP—continuous positive airway pressure; COPD—chronic obstructive pulmonary disease; GFR—glomerular filtration rate; HF—heart failure; LVEF—left ventricle ejection fraction.

3.2. Follow-Up

The median follow-up time was 25.5 months. Differences between first and last visits are described in Table 2.

Table 2. Differences from first to last visit at the Heart Failure Clinic.

	First Visit	Last Visit	p
NYHA class			
I	19 (17.3%)	30 (27.3%)	
II	66 (60%)	66 (60%)	<0.01
III	25 (22.7%)	13 (11.8%)	
IV	0	1 (0.9%)	
ECG Rhythm			
Sinus rhythm	64 (58.2%)	59 (53.6%)	
Atrial fibrillation	44 (40%)	49 (44.5%)	NS
Auricular pacing	2 (1.8%)	2 (10.8%)	
QRS morphology			
LBBB	29 (26.4%)	32 (29.1%)	
RBBB	13 (11.8%)	17 (15.5%)	NS
IVCD	9 (8.2%)	4 (3.6%)	
Ventricular Pacing	14 (12.7%)	18 (16.4%)	
LVEF (%) ***	32.7 ± 8.4	45.2 ± 10	<0.001
LVEDD (cm) ***	5.6 ± 0.9	5.2 ± 0.9	<0.001
Grade III/IV mitral regurgitation	21 (19.1%)	6 (5.7%)	<0.001
Moderate/severe RV systolic disfunction	10 (9.1%)	12 (11.4%)	NS
NT-proBNP (ng/L) *	3091 (158–53,354)	1802 (145–19,509)	<0.001
Estimated GFR (mL/min/1.73 m^2) ***	54.5 ± 18	47.2 ± 14.8	<0.001
ARNI	27 (24.5%)	66 (60%)	<0.001
ACE-I or ARB	63 (57.3%)	22 (20%)	<0.001
ARNI, ACE-I, or ARB	90 (81.8%)	88 (80%)	NS
Beta-blocker	94 (85.5%)	89 (80.9%)	NS
SGLT2i	26 (23.6%)	71 (64.5%)	<0.001
MRA	61 (55.5%)	59 (53.6%)	NS
Number of drug classes *	3 (0–4) (2–3)	3 (0–4) (2–4)	
0/0 **	3 (2.7%)/7 (6.4%)	4 (3.6%)/5 (4.5%)	
1/1 **	13 (11.8%)/29 (26.4%)	11 (10%)/15 (13.6%)	
2/2 **	35 (31.8%)/49 (44.5%)	20 (18.2%)/25 (22.7%)	<0.05/<0.001
3/3 **	48 (43.6%)/19 (17.3%)	44 (40%)/40 (36.4%)	
4/4 **	11 (10.0%)/6 (5.5%)	31 (28.2%)/25 (22.7%)	

Table 2. *Cont.*

	First Visit	Last Visit	p
ICD			
Primary prevention	9 (8.2%)	9 (8.2%)	NS
Secondary prevention	3 (2.7%)	3 (2.7%)	
CRT	11 (10%)	16 (14.6%)	NS

* Median (percentiles 25–75); ** With ARNI as neurohormonal antagonist; *** Mean ± standard deviation; ACE-I—angiotensin-converting enzyme inhibitor; ARB—angiotensin-receptor blocker; ARNI—angiotensin receptor-neprilysin inhibitor; CRT—cardiac resynchronization therapy; ECG—electrocardiogram; GFR—glomerular filtration rate; ICD—implantable cardioverter-defibrillator; IVCD—intraventricular conduction delay; LBBB—left bundle branch block; LVEDD—left ventricular end-diastolic diameter; LVEF—left ventricular ejection fraction; MRA—mineralocorticoid receptor antagonist; NS—non-significant; NYHA—New York Heart Association; RBBB—right bundle branch block; SGLT2i—sodium-glucose co-transporter 2 inhibitor.

At the initial visit, over half of the patients were in the NYHA class II (60%), while 22.7% were in the NYHA class III and 17.3% in the NYHA class I. A significant improvement in NYHA functional class was observed during follow-up (Figure 1). Specifically, 37% of patients improved to a better functional class, and 27.3% were in the NYHA class I ($p < 0.05$) at the last visit. Atrial fibrillation and left ventricular bundle branch were described at first visit in 40% and 26% of patients, with no significant differences during follow-up. NT-proBNP levels significantly decreased during follow-up (median 3091 vs. 1802, $p < 0.001$), and a significant reduction was also observed in estimated GFR (54.5 ± 18.0 vs. 47.2 ± 14.8, $p < 0.001$).

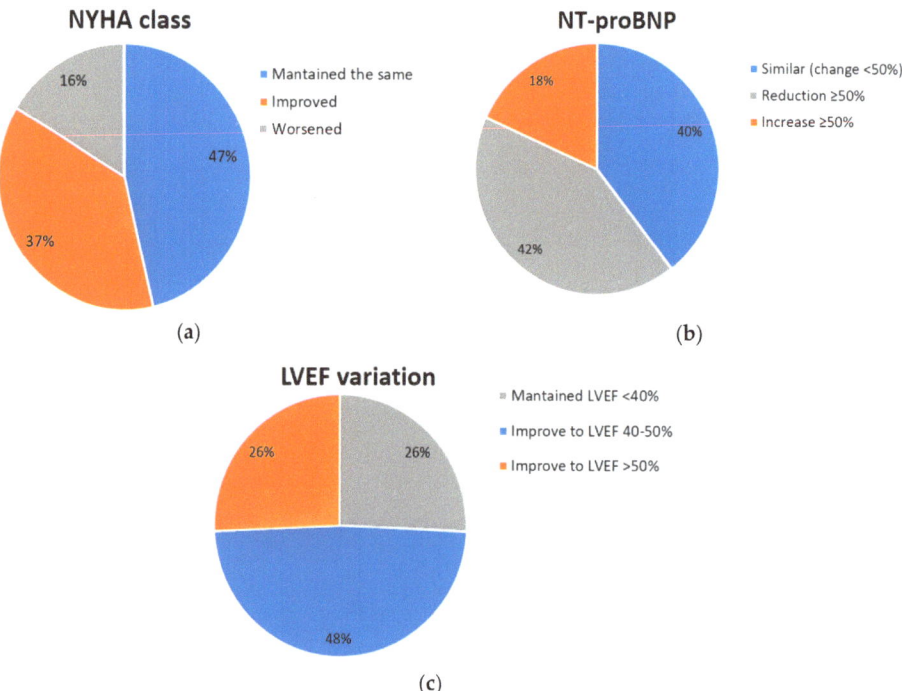

Figure 1. *Cont.*

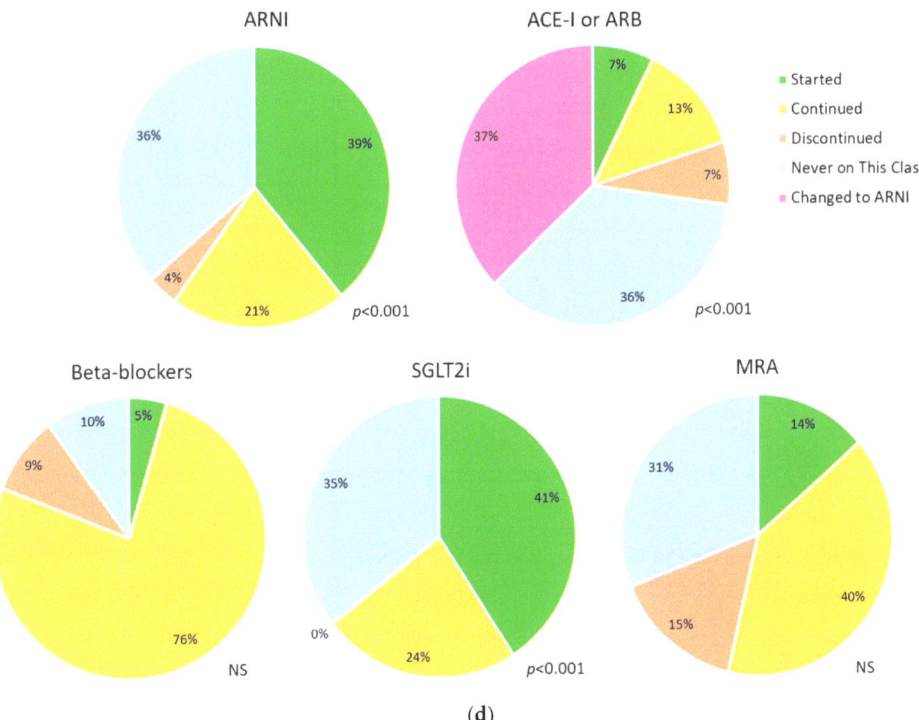

Figure 1. Variation in NYHA class (**a**), NT-proBNP levels (**b**), LVEF (**c**) and medical therapies (**d**) from first to last visit at the Heart Failure Clinic. ACE-I—angiotensin-converting enzyme inhibitor; ARB—angiotensin-receptor blocker; ARNI—angiotensin receptor-neprilysin inhibitor; LVEF—left ventricle ejection fraction; MRA—mineralocorticoid receptor antagonist; NYHA—New York Heart Association; NS—non-significant; SGLT2i—sodium-glucose co-transporter 2 inhibitor.

LVEF significantly improved from first to last visit, with an absolute difference of 12.5% ($p < 0.001$). Improved LVEF was observed in 53% of patients, and 27% showed LVEF recovery. Grade III or IV mitral regurgitation was present in 19.1% of patients at first visit, with a significant reduction to 5.7% at last visit ($p < 0.001$). No significant changes were observed in right ventricular ejection fraction.

At first visit, almost a quarter of patients were already under ARNI treatment, and 57.3% were receiving ACE-I or ARB.

At last follow-up, ARNI and SGLT2i use significantly increased to 60% and 64.5%, respectively ($p < 0.01$). Prescriptions for beta-blockers and mineralocorticoid receptor antagonists (MRA) were 85.5% and 55.5% at the initial visit, respectively, and did not show significant changes at the last visit. Patients with more than two drug classes increased from 53.6% to 68.2% ($p < 0.05$). Figure 1 shows changes in HF therapy between the first and last visit. Eleven patients were treated with cardiac resynchronization therapy (CRT) at the first visit, and five additional patients received this therapy during follow-up. Twelve patients carried an implantable cardiac defibrillator (ICD) at first visit, with no new implants during the time of study.

Multivariate analysis was performed to identify predictors of LVEF recovery. After adjustment, only age was associated with a lower probability of LVEF recovery, with no positive impact of the initiation of three or more HF medical therapies (Table 3).

Table 3. Predictors of LVEF recovery.

	Univariate		Multivariate	
	OR (CI 95%)	p	OR (CI 95%)	p
Age	0.82 (0.71–0.95)	0.009	0.82 (0.71–0.95)	0.010
Female sex	1.5 (0.61–3.69)	0.38		
Chronic kidney disease (GFR < 45 mL/min/1.73 m^2)	0.79 (0.34–1.87)	0.60		
LVEF at diagnosis	1.00 (0.93–1.08)	0.90		
Ischemic cardiomyopathy	0.36 (0.12–1.04)	0.059	0.36 (0.12–1.07)	0.066
3 or more HF therapies	1.29 (0.50–3.31)	0.60		

GFR—glomerular filtration rate; HF—heart failure; LVEF—left ventricle ejection fraction.

3.3. Clinical Outcomes

Thirty-four patients (30.9%) experienced the composite primary outcome during follow-up (Table 4). The majority of these events (94.1%) consisted of the first episode of worsening heart failure. Principio del formularioFinal del formulario

Table 4. Primary outcome and mortality during follow-up.

Primary Outcome (Composite of First HF Hospitalization or CV Death)	34 (30.9%)
HF hospitalization/IV diuretics	32 (94.1%)
CV death	2 (5.9%)
All-cause death	14 (12.7%)
CV Death	6 (42.9%)
Cardiac death secondary to progression of heart failure	2 (14.3%)
Sudden/arrhythmic cardiac death	2 (14.3%)
Cardiac death (not arrhythmic or heart failure related)	2 (14.3%)
Non-cardiac death	7 (50%)
Death of unknown cause	1 (7.1%)

CV—cardiovascular, HF—heart failure, IV—intravenous.

Table 5 compares patients according to the occurrence of the primary outcome. Patients who did not experience the primary outcome were significantly more likely to receive treatment with SGLT2i ($p < 0.001$) and ARNI/ACE-I or ARB ($p < 0.05$) and were prescribed a greater number of disease-modifying HF medications ($p < 0.05$). These patients also exhibited a higher LVEF at the last follow-up visit ($p < 0.05$).

Table 5. Differences in guideline-directed medical therapy and left ventricular ejection fraction according to the occurrence of the primary outcome.

	Primary Outcome		
	YES (n = 34; 30.1%)	NO (n = 76; 69.1%)	p
ARNI	17 (50%)	46 (60.5%)	NS
ACE-I or ARB	6 (17.6%)	18 (10.5%)	NS
ARNI, ACE-I, or ARB	23 (67.6%)	64 (84.2%)	<0.05
Beta-blocker	27 (79.4%)	64 (84.2%)	NS
SGLT2i	8 (23.5%)	51 (67.1%)	<0.001
MRA	16 (47.1%)	41 (53.9%)	NS
Number of drug classes *	2 (0–4) (1–3)	3 (1–4) (2–4)	<0.01

Table 5. *Cont.*

	Primary Outcome		
	YES (n = 34; 30.1%)	NO (n = 76; 69.1%)	p
LVEF at first visit (%) **	33.1 ± 7.7	32.5 ± 8.8	NS
LVEF at last visit (%) **	41.2 ± 10.2	47.1 ± 9.4	<0.05

* Median (percentiles 25–75) (minimum–maximum); ** Mean ± standard deviation; ACE-I—angiotensin-converting enzyme inhibitor; ARB—angiotensin-receptor blocker; ARNI—angiotensin receptor-neprilysin inhibitor; LVEF—left ventricle ejection fraction; MRA—mineralocorticoid receptor antagonist; NS—non-significant; SGLT2i—sodium-glucose co-transporter 2 inhibitor.

Figures 2 and 3 show a graphical representation of survival free from the primary outcome, depending on LVEF recovery, number, and type of HF disease-modifying drugs. Patients who recovered LVEF were at lower risk of the primary outcome (HR 0.35 [95% CI 0.17–0.72] $p < 0.01$). The use of two or more HF drug classes also had a positive effect on survival free from cardiac events (HR 0.29 [95% CI 0.10–0.86], $p < 0.01$). Regarding the implementation of GDMT, Kaplan–Meier curves and log-rank test also showed a benefit for vasodilator therapy (ARNI, ACE-I or ARB) (HR 0.36, $p < 0.01$) and SGLT2i use (HR 0.17 [95% CI 0.15–0.95], $p < 0.001$).

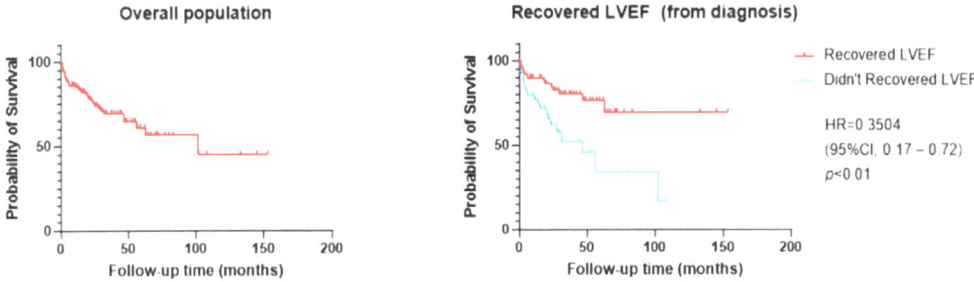

Figure 2. Kaplan–Meier curves for the composite primary outcome of time to cardiovascular death or the first episode of worsening heart failure, presented for the overall population and according to LVEF recovery. LVEF recovery was defined as LVEF increase of at least 10% from LVEF at diagnosis to a value over 50%.

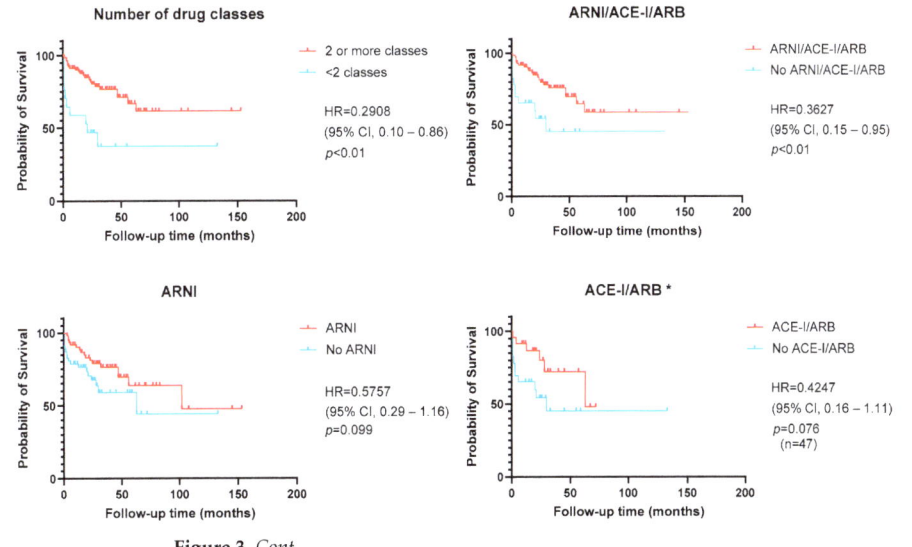

Figure 3. *Cont.*

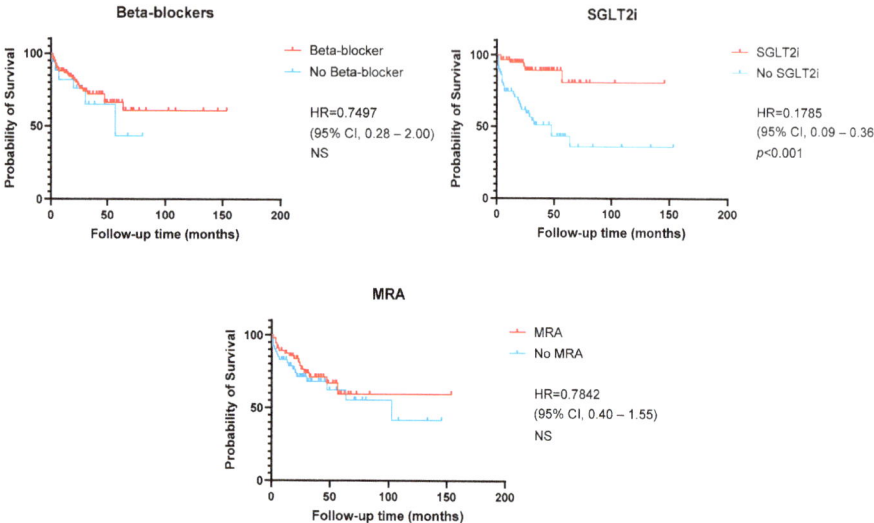

Figure 3. Kaplan–Meier curves for the composite primary outcome of time to cardiovascular death or the first episode of worsening heart failure, according to guideline-directed medical therapy. * Patients with ARNI were excluded. ACE-I—angiotensin-converting enzyme inhibitor; ARB—angiotensin-receptor blocker; ARNI—angiotensin receptor-neprilysin inhibitor; MRA—mineralocorticoid receptor antagonist; NS—non-significant; SGLT2i—sodium-glucose co-transporter 2 inhibitor.

Concerning overall mortality, survival analysis showed a benefit for patients who recovered LVEF (HR = 0.2771 [95% CI 0.10–1.01], $p < 0.05$) but no differences when analyzing each drug class (Figures 4 and 5).

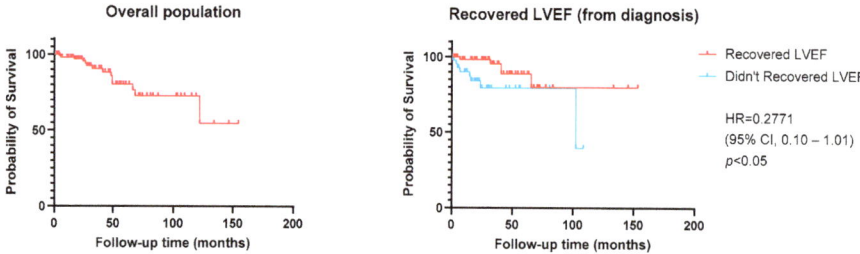

Figure 4. Kaplan–Meier curves for all-cause mortality, presented for the overall population and according to LVEF recovery. LVEF recovery was defined as LVEF increase of at least 10% from LVEF at diagnosis to a value over 50%.

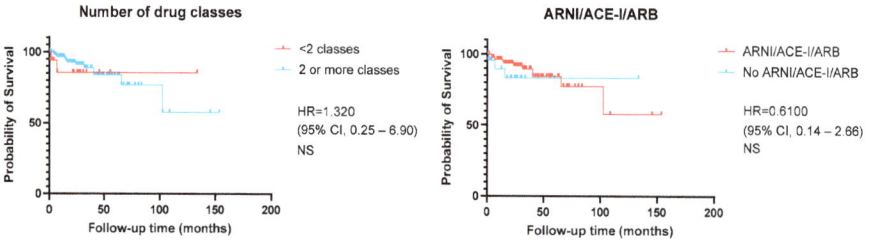

Figure 5. *Cont.*

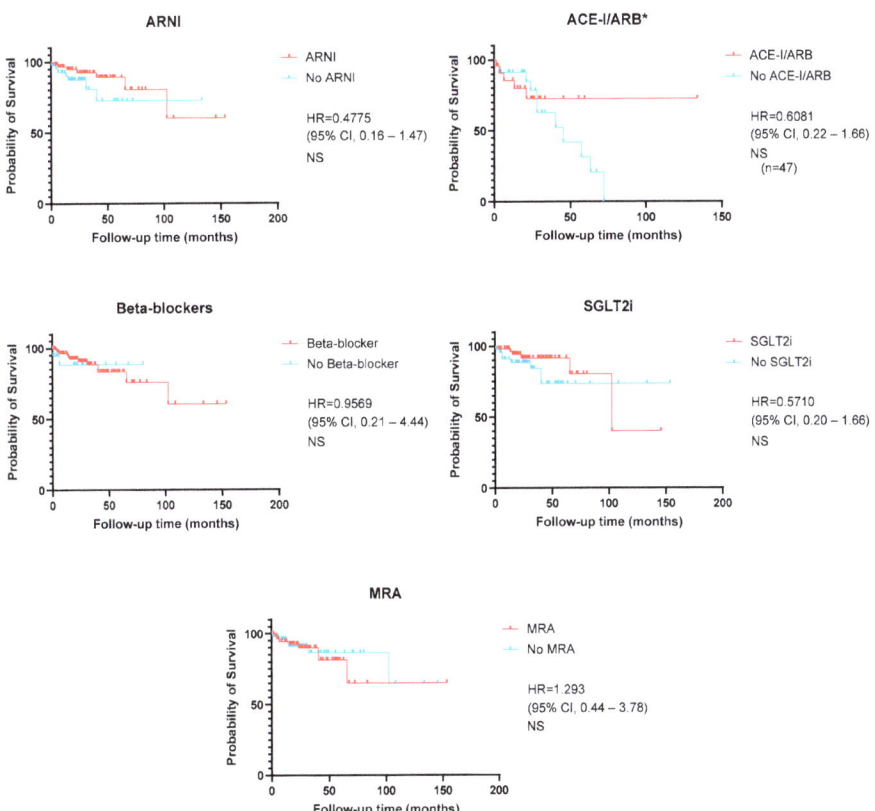

Figure 5. Kaplan–Meier curves for all-cause mortality, according to guideline-directed medical thearpy. * Patients with ARNI were excluded. ACE-I—angiotensin-converting enzyme inhibitor; ARB—angiotensin-receptor blocker; ARNI—angiotensin receptor-neprilysin inhibitor; GDMT: guideline-directed medical therapy; MRA—mineralocorticoid receptor antagonist; NS—non-significant; SGLT2i—sodium-glucose co-transporter 2 inhibitor.

3.4. Treatment Changes After the First Episode of Worsening Heart Failure

No significant differences in HF treatment were observed after the first episode of worsening HF, with no optimization or dropout of drug classes one month after said event. Table 6 compares both time points, and Figure 6 shows the dosage for each individual medical therapy.

Table 6. Changes in guideline-directed medical therapy after the first episode of worsening heart failure.

	Time of Event (n = 32)	One Month After (n = 32)	Change ** (%)	p
ARNI	16 (50%)	14 (43.8%)	−6.2	NS
ACE-I or ARB	5 (15.6%)	8 (25%)	+9.4	NS
ARNI, ACE-I, or ARB	21 (65.6%)	22 (68.8%)	+3.2	NS
Beta-blocker	25 (78.1%)	25 (78.1%)	0	NS
SGLT2i	6 (18.8%)	8 (25%)	+6.2	NS
MRA	16 (50%)	16 (50%)	0	NS
Number of drug classes *	2 (1–3)	2 (1–3)	0 ((−1)–2)	NS

* Median (percentiles 25–75); ** Changes over time ACE-I—angiotensin–converting enzyme inhibitor; ARB—angiotensin–receptor blocker; ARNI—angiotensin receptor-neprilysin inhibitor; MRA—mineralocorticoid receptor antagonist; NS—non-significant; SGLT2i—sodium–glucose co-transporter 2 inhibitor.

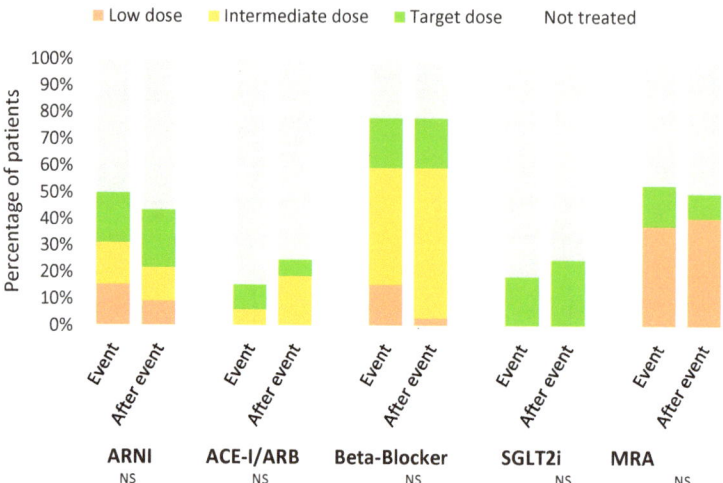

Figure 6. Changes in GDMT dosage after the first episode of worsening HF. ACE-I—angiotensin-converting enzyme inhibitor; ARB—angiotensin-receptor blocker; ARNI—angiotensin receptor-neprilysin inhibitor; LVEF—left ventricle ejection fraction; MRA—mineralocorticoid receptor antagonist; NS—non-significant; SGLT2i—sodium-glucose co-transporter 2 inhibitor.

4. Discussion

This study reports the clinical and echocardiographic characteristics, treatment, and cardiac outcomes of a cohort of adults over 80 years with HFrEF. A high level of implementation of GDMT in older populations is feasible. LVEF recovery, a greater number of HF medical therapies, and treatment with a vasodilator agent or SGLT2i were associated with a reduction in the combined primary outcome of the first episode of worsening HF and cardiovascular death.

In this cohort, elderly patients with HFrEF who initiated a structured follow-up at the HF clinic received three or more HF drug classes in more than two-thirds of cases, with ARNI prescription in 60% and SLGT2i in 64.5% of patients at the last visit. The implementation of GDMT was higher than previously described in observational cohorts [14–19]. Real-world data usually show an underusage of HF therapies in the elderly in comparison to younger patients [20]. Also, recent registries such as CHECK-HF registry and EORP demonstrate an implementation of HF medical therapies significantly higher in patients aged less than 60 years and a decline in the use of GDMT with advanced age [14,16]. Available data about ARNI and SGLTi use in the elderly are very limited. In a recent prospective study of patients with a mean age of 83.3 years, only 14.3% of those with a theoretical indication for ARNI therapy were receiving the medication [18]. Similarly, in another recent registry of 364 octogenarians with HFrEF, only 15.1% were treated with SGLT2i and 26.4% with ARNIs [19].

Initiation and up-titration of HF medical therapies in older patients can be challenging. Elderly people with HF frequently present other major illnesses, with a high prevalence of chronic kidney disease, high cardiovascular risk, and frailty, which can interfere with drug efficacy and tolerability [5,21,22]. Comorbidities were frequent in our study, with more than half of the patients presenting chronic kidney disease. Indeed, chronic kidney disease is one of the main reasons for suboptimal use or non-up-titration of GDMT [23,24]. Also, polypharmacy increases the risk of adverse drug reactions and is associated with a higher treatment burden, which may be another potential explanation for the lower implementation of GDMT in the elderly [25,26]. Healthcare system characteristics and reimbursement policies of HF therapies can also have an impact on GDMT implementation [20]. The Spanish healthcare system usually covers the full price of prescription costs in the elderly, which may have favored GDMT prescription in our cohort. Follow-up at a dedicated HF clinic led by cardiologists may help explain the high rates of GDMT prescription in our cohort. First, older patients attending Cardiology HF clinics may be a selected, less frail group compared to the broader population of octogenarians. Second, cardiologists may be more attuned to the importance of GDMT implementation than geriatricians or general practitioners. Finally, dedicated HF clinics facilitate frequent consultations, offering a unique opportunity for careful up-titration of GDMT [13], which might not be possible in other settings. The application of our findings may, therefore, be limited outside this context; however, it does not invalidate the fact that GMDT is achievable with the proper resources. Also, our findings highlight the importance of referring older patients with HFrEF to dedicated HF clinics independently of their biological age if frailty is not a major concern.

Despite the complexities of GDMT implementation in older adults, its use was associated with a reduction in the primary outcome in our cohort. The implementation of two or more drug classes, or the prescription of any vasodilator agent (ACE-I/ARB/ARNI) or SGLT2i, was associated with a significant prognostic benefit. In line with our results, a growing body of evidence suggests that HF medical therapies are safe and benefit the elderly similarly to younger patients. Sacubitril/valsartan has proven to be superior to enalapril across the spectrum of age in a post hoc analysis of the PARADIGM-HF trial [9], and its use has been associated with a significant reduction in mortality in patients over 75 years [18]. Regarding ACE-I/ARB, post hoc analysis of major studies and meta-analysis has not found age-related heterogeneity [27–29], and no higher risk has been observed of syncope-related hospitalization when compared to younger patients [30]. SGLT2i constitutes the latest addition to the arsenal of HF therapies, so evidence concerning their use in the elderly is minimal. Prespecified subgroup analysis of major clinical trials did not show significant age-related heterogeneity [10,31]. Our study showed a notable protective effect of SLGT2i, which should be confirmed in further studies. The pleiotropic effects of this drug class may confer additional benefits in elderly patients by influencing other comorbidities such as reducing kidney disease progression [32] or atrial fibrillation risk [33]. In this cohort, beta-blockers or MRA administration was not associated with a risk reduction. Noteworthily, the prescription of both medications did not increase from the first to last visit in the HF clinic, although beta-blocker prescription was already high at first visit. It is well known that physicians have more concerns about beta-blockers and MRA adverse effects in the elderly population. The SENIORS trial, one of the few randomized clinical trials in an older population, showed that nebivolol was well tolerated and effective in reducing mortality and morbidity in patients of age >70 years with HF, regardless of the initial LVEF [34]. In this line, a subgroup analysis of the MERIT-HF trial described that metoprolol improved survival, reduced hospitalizations, and was safe and well tolerated in patients over 65 years [35]. An explanation for our different findings could be that patients in our study were older than those in the SENIORS trial (mean age 83 years versus 76 years). Indeed, some studies and meta-analyses have raised concerns about beta-blocker tolerability in very elderly patients, where difficulties in achieving target doses may diminish their impact [36]. In that sense, our cohort may not have been of large enough size to demonstrate an already attenuated effect. The small sample size of our cohort may also explain the absence of a positive impact of MRA administration. A meta-analysis of RALES, EMPHASIS-HF and TOPCAT did find a beneficial effect in mortality and morbidity in patients over 75 years [37]. However, studies display significant inter-study heterogeneity concerning mortality in patients with HFrEF over 75 years, suggesting that MRA's effect may depend on the patient baseline characteristics [38]. Impaired renal function or the risk of hyperkaliemia may limit the use of MRA in frail, comorbid older patients. However, age alone should not be a barrier to prescribing MRA, as it often is currently [39]. Rather, a careful, individualized approach should guide ARM implementation. Our study suggests that there may be room for improvement concerning MRA prescription in the elderly, warranting close monitoring of renal function and potassium levels. Regarding concerns about worsening kidney function under GDMT, our study did observe a significant reduction in estimated GFR from the first to last visit, although it may be explained by age being included in the CKD-EPI creatinine equation [40].

Overall mortality analysis was limited by a relatively low mortality rate (fourteen deaths in more than two years of median follow-up), despite the mean age at first visit being very similar to the Spanish life expectancy [41]. As expected, half of the deaths were not secondary to cardiac causes [42]. This finding highlights the critical importance of comorbidities in this subset of patients and their associated competitive risks. Additionally, it underscores that the management of older patients with HFrEF and efforts to improve their quality of life should include strategies to address non-cardiac comorbidities.

Concerning implantable devices, CRT was not underused in our cohort when compared to the rates of CRT observed in recent major clinical trials including younger populations [10,43]. This strategy aligns with several retrospective studies, suggesting that older patients benefit similarly in terms of resynchronization response and reductions in HF-related hospitalizations [44–47]. In opposition, ICD implantation was infrequent in our cohort. ICD benefits are more controversial in the elderly, as the risk of arrhythmic death is lower with a higher competing risk of non-arrhythmic death, including non-cardiac deaths [48]. More studies are needed to assess ICD survival benefits in contemporary elderly people treated with GDMT.

During follow-up, most patients improved their functional class, LVEF, LVEDD, and degree of mitral regurgitation. A decrease in NT-proBNP levels was also observed, which is expected to be associated with a better prognosis [49,50]. It is noteworthy that only age demonstrated a negative impact on LVEF recovery, a finding consistent with previous reports [51]. This association may have attenuated GDMT's effect on LVEF recovery in our cohort. However, this finding emphasizes GDMT's effect on prognosis independently of LVEF recovery.

Recent guidelines suggest that a cardiac event, particularly a heart failure admission, is an opportunity for evidence-based treatment optimization [1]. Different than expected, no significant changes were observed when analyzing GDMT use before and after a first episode of worsening HF. Worse kidney function, hypotension, and higher frailty after admission could hinder this opportunity in the elderly.

Our study presented some limitations, mostly those inherent to a retrospective analysis, which only enables hypotheses generation. The small sample size may have prevented us from extracting further conclusions from data analysis. Also, lower-than-expected mortality in our cohort prevented a further analysis of the treatment effect on mortality. Frequent cardiology consultations may have impacted outcomes, such as worsening heart failure, which might have been more frequent in a less controlled environment. Also, follow-up in an HF clinic led by cardiologists may have introduced a selection bias towards more robust elderly patients, with frailer patients being followed at geriatric outpatient clinics. This may explain the high level of implementation of GDMT and low mortality rates. In this sense, data concerning frailty or comorbidity scores such as the Charlson comorbidity index could have provided valuable information. However, this finding does not undermine the fact that chronological age by itself should not be a limitation for GDMT use. In this sense, future studies should focus on the impact of frailty rather than age on GDMT's effect. On the other hand, comparing with a younger matched control group could have strengthened our analysis by providing further insight into the specific effects of GDMT in the elderly. Future studies could use this approach to enhance our understanding of the matter. Ultimately, the relative importance of non-cardiac deaths highlights the differential features of this patient subset. Randomized clinical trials involving older patients are essential, with primary outcomes focusing on quality-of-life measures rather than overall mortality.

5. Conclusions

The optimization of HF treatment is achievable in older patients and may be associated with a reduction in cardiac events. Although further studies are needed, these results should encourage us to pursue a higher level of GDMT prescription in our seniors as it may benefit them significantly.

Author Contributions: Conceptualization, C.S.A., J.G.-A. and M.A.R.-C.; methodology, C.S.A., J.G.-A. and M.A.R.-C.; formal analysis, C.S.A. and I.M.; investigation, C.S.A.; resources, C.S.A.; data curation, C.S.A. and I.M.; writing—original draft preparation, C.S.A. and I.M.; writing—review and editing, I.M., J.G.-A. and M.A.R.-C.; visualization, C.S.A. and I.M.; supervision, J.G.-A., J.P.-V. and I.V.C.; project administration, C.S.A., I.M., J.G.-A., M.A.R.-C., J.P.-V. and I.V.C. All authors have read and agreed to the published version of the manuscript.

Funding: This research received no external funding.

Institutional Review Board Statement: This study was conducted in accordance with the Declaration of Helsinki and reviewed by the Institutional Review Board of Hospital Clínico San Carlos (reference: 24/720-E; date: 23 October 2024).

Informed Consent Statement: Patient consent was waived due to the retrospective design of this study.

Data Availability Statement: The raw data supporting the conclusions of this article will be made available by the authors on request.

Conflicts of Interest: The authors declare no conflicts of interest.

References

1. McDonagh, T.A.; Metra, M.; Adamo, M.; Baumbach, A.; Böhm, M.; Burri, H.; Čelutkiene, J.; Chioncel, O.; Cleland, J.G.F.; Coats, A.J.S.; et al. 2021 ESC Guidelines for the Diagnosis and Treatment of Acute and Chronic Heart Failure. *Eur. Heart J.* **2021**, *42*, 3599–3726. [CrossRef] [PubMed]
2. Murphy, S.P.; Ibrahim, N.E.; Januzzi, J.L. Heart Failure with Reduced Ejection Fraction: A Review. *JAMA J. Am. Med. Assoc.* **2020**, *324*, 488–504. [CrossRef] [PubMed]
3. Bozkurt, B.; Ahmad, T.; Alexander, K.M.; Baker, W.L.; Bosak, K.; Breathett, K.; Fonarow, G.C.; Heidenreich, P.; Ho, J.E.; Hsich, E.; et al. Heart Failure Epidemiology and Outcomes Statistics: A Report of the Heart Failure Society of America. *J. Card. Fail.* **2023**, *29*, 1412–1451. [CrossRef]
4. Dharmarajan, K.; Rich, M.W. Epidemiology, Pathophysiology, and Prognosis of Heart Failure in Older Adults. *Heart Fail. Clin.* **2017**, *13*, 417–426. [CrossRef]
5. Hamada, T.; Kubo, T.; Kawai, K.; Nakaoka, Y.; Yabe, T.; Furuno, T.; Yamada, E.; Kitaoka, H. Clinical Characteristics and Frailty Status in Heart Failure with Preserved vs. Reduced Ejection Fraction. *ESC Heart Fail.* **2022**, *9*, 1853–1863. [CrossRef] [PubMed]
6. Mozzini, C.; Pagani, M. The Heart Failure Knights. *Curr. Probl. Cardiol.* **2023**, *48*, 101834. [CrossRef]
7. McDonagh, T.A.; Metra, M.; Adamo, M.; Gardner, R.S.; Baumbach, A.; Böhm, M.; Burri, H.; Butler, J.; Celutkiene, J.; Chioncel, O.; et al. 2023 Focused Update of the 2021 ESC Guidelines for the Diagnosis and Treatment of Acute and Chronic Heart Failure Developed by the Task Force for the Diagnosis and Treatment of Acute and Chronic Heart Failure of the European Society of Cardiology (ESC) With the Special Contribution of the Heart Failure Association (HFA) of the ESC. *Eur. Heart J.* **2023**, *44*, 3627–3639. [CrossRef]
8. Heidenreich, P.A.; Bozkurt, B.; Aguilar, D.; Allen, L.A.; Byun, J.J.; Colvin, M.M.; Deswal, A.; Drazner, M.H.; Dunlay, S.M.; Evers, L.R.; et al. 2022 AHA/ACC/HFSA Guideline for the Management of Heart Failure: A Report of the American College of Cardiology/American Heart Association Joint Committee on Clinical Practice Guidelines. *Circulation* **2022**, *145*, E895–E1032. [CrossRef]
9. Jhund, P.S.; Fu, M.; Bayram, E.; Chen, C.H.; Negrusz-Kawecka, M.; Rosenthal, A.; Desai, A.S.; Lefkowitz, M.P.; Rizkala, A.R.; Rouleau, J.L.; et al. Efficacy and Safety of LCZ696 (Sacubitril-Valsartan) According to Age: Insights from PARADIGM-HF. *Eur. Heart J.* **2015**, *36*, 2576–2584. [CrossRef]
10. Martinez, F.A.; Serenelli, M.; Nicolau, J.C.; Petrie, M.C.; Chiang, C.E.; Tereshchenko, S.; Solomon, S.D.; Inzucchi, S.E.; Køber, L.; Kosiborod, M.N.; et al. Efficacy and Safety of Dapagliflozin in Heart Failure with Reduced Ejection Fraction According to Age: Insights from DAPA-HF. *Circulation* **2020**, *141*, 100–111. [CrossRef]
11. Tahhan, A.S.; Vaduganathan, M.; Greene, S.J.; Fonarow, G.C.; Fiuzat, M.; Jessup, M.; Lindenfeld, J.; O'Connor, C.M.; Butler, J. Enrollment of Older Patients, Women, and Racial and Ethnic Minorities in Contemporary Heart Failure Clinical Trials: A Systematic Review. *JAMA Cardiol.* **2018**, *3*, 1011–1019. [CrossRef] [PubMed]
12. McMurray, J. Making Sense of SENIORS. *Eur. Heart J.* **2005**, *26*, 203–206. [CrossRef] [PubMed]
13. Seferović, P.M.; Piepoli, M.F.; Lopatin, Y.; Jankowska, E.; Polovina, M.; Anguita-Sanchez, M.; Störk, S.; Lainščak, M.; Miličić, D.; Milinković, I.; et al. Heart Failure Association of the European Society of Cardiology Quality of Care Centres Programme: Design and Accreditation Document. *Eur. J. Heart Fail.* **2020**, *22*, 763–774. [CrossRef] [PubMed]
14. Veenis, J.F.; Brunner-La Rocca, H.P.; Linssen, G.C.M.; Geerlings, P.R.; Van Gent, M.W.F.; Aksoy, I.; Oosterom, L.; Moons, A.H.M.; Hoes, A.W.; Brugts, J.J. Age Differences in Contemporary Treatment of Patients with Chronic Heart Failure and Reduced Ejection Fraction. *Eur. J. Prev. Cardiol.* **2019**, *26*, 1399–1407. [CrossRef] [PubMed]

15. Forman, D.E.; Cannon, C.P.; Hernandez, A.F.; Liang, L.; Yancy, C.; Fonarow, G.C. Influence of Age on the Management of Heart Failure: Findings from Get with the Guidelines-Heart Failure (GWTG-HF). *Am. Heart J.* **2009**, *157*, 1010–1017. [CrossRef]
16. Lainščak, M.; Milinkovic, I.; Polovina, M.; Crespo-Leiro, M.G.; Lund, L.H.; Anker, S.; Laroche, C.; Ferrari, R.; Coats, A.J.S.; McDonagh, T.; et al. Sex- and Age-Related Differences in the Management and Outcomes of Chronic Heart Failure: An Analysis of Patients from the ESC HFA EORP Heart Failure Long-Term Registry. *Eur. J. Heart Fail.* **2020**, *22*, 92–102. [CrossRef]
17. Fonarow, G.C.; Abraham, W.T.; Albert, N.M.; Stough, W.G.; Gheorghiade, M.; Greenberg, B.H.; O'Connor, C.M.; Sun, J.L.; Yancy, C.; Young, J.B. Age- and Gender-Related Differences in Quality of Care and Outcomes of Patients Hospitalized with Heart Failure (from OPTIMIZE-HF). *Am. J. Cardiol.* **2009**, *104*, 107–115. [CrossRef]
18. Roca, L.N.; García, M.C.; Germán, J.B.; Becerra, A.J.B.; Otero, J.M.R.; Chapel, J.A.E.; López, C.R.; Lázaro, A.M.P.; Urquía, M.T.; Tuñón, J. Use and Benefit of Sacubitril/Valsartan in Elderly Patients with Heart Failure with Reduced Ejection Fraction. *J. Clin. Med.* **2024**, *13*, 4772. [CrossRef]
19. Balaguer Germán, J.; Cortés García, M.; Rodríguez López, C.; Romero Otero, J.M.; Esteban Chapel, J.A.; Bollas Becerra, A.J.; Nieto Roca, L.; Taibo Urquía, M.; Pello Lázaro, A.M.; Tuñón Fernández, J. Impact of SGLT2 Inhibitors on Very Elderly Population with Heart Failure with Reduce Ejection Fraction: Real Life Data. *Biomedicines* **2024**, *12*, 1507. [CrossRef]
20. Milinković, I.; Polovina, M.; Coats, A.J.S.; Rosano, G.M.C.; Seferović, P.M. Medical Treatment of Heart Failure with Reduced Ejection Fraction in the Elderly. *Card. Fail. Rev.* **2022**, *8*, e17. [CrossRef]
21. Rich, M.W. Pharmacotherapy of Heart Failure in the Elderly: Adverse Events. *Heart Fail. Rev.* **2012**, *17*, 589–595. [CrossRef] [PubMed]
22. Díez-Villanueva, P.; Jiménez-Méndez, C.; Alfonso, F. Heart Failure in the Elderly. *J. Geriatr. Cardiol.* **2021**, *18*, 219–232. [CrossRef] [PubMed]
23. Greene, S.J.; Butler, J.; Albert, N.M.; DeVore, A.D.; Sharma, P.P.; Duffy, C.I.; Hill, C.L.; McCague, K.; Mi, X.; Patterson, J.H.; et al. Medical Therapy for Heart Failure with Reduced Ejection Fraction: The CHAMP-HF Registry. *J. Am. Coll. Cardiol.* **2018**, *72*, 351–366. [CrossRef]
24. Ouwerkerk, W.; Voors, A.A.; Anker, S.D.; Cleland, J.G.; Dickstein, K.; Filippatos, G.; Van Der Harst, P.; Hillege, H.L.; Lang, C.C.; Ter Maaten, J.M.; et al. Determinants and Clinical Outcome of Uptitration of ACE-Inhibitors and Beta-Blockers in Patients with Heart Failure: A Prospective European Study. *Eur. Heart J.* **2017**, *38*, 1883–1890. [CrossRef]
25. Stefil, M.; Dixon, M.; Bahar, J.; Saied, S.; Mashida, K.; Heron, O.; Shantsila, E.; Walker, L.; Akpan, A.; Lip, G.Y.H.; et al. Polypharmacy in Older People with Heart Failure: Roles of the Geriatrician and Pharmacist. *Card. Fail. Rev.* **2022**, *8*, e34. [CrossRef] [PubMed]
26. Unlu, O.; Levitan, E.B.; Reshetnyak, E.; Kneifati-Hayek, J.; Diaz, I.; Archambault, A.; Chen, L.; Hanlon, J.T.; Maurer, M.S.; Safford, M.M.; et al. Polypharmacy in Older Adults Hospitalized for Heart Failure. *Circ. Heart Fail.* **2020**, *13*, E006977. [CrossRef]
27. Flather, M.D.; Yusuf, S.; Køber, L.; Pfeffer, M.; Hall, A.; Murray, G.; Torp-Pedersen, C.; Ball, S.; Pogue, J.; Moyé, L.; et al. Long-Term ACE-Inhibitor Therapy in Patients with Heart Failure or left-Ventricular Dysfunction: A Systematic Overview of Data from individual Patients. *Lancet* **2000**, *355*, 1575–1581. [CrossRef]
28. Baruch, L.; Glazer, R.D.; Aknay, N.; Vanhaecke, J.; Thomas Heywood, J.; Anand, I.; Krum, H.; Hester, A.; Cohn, J.N. Morbidity, Mortality, Physiologic and Functional Parameters in Elderly and Non-Elderly Patients in the Valsartan Heart Failure Trial (Val-HeFT). *Am. Heart J.* **2004**, *148*, 951–957. [CrossRef]
29. Pfeffer, M.A.; Swedberg, K.; Granger, C.B.; Held, P.; McMurray, J.J.; Michelson, E.L.; Olofsson, B.; Östergren, J.; Yusuf, S.; CHARM Investigators and Committees. Effects of Candesartan on Mortality and Morbidity in patients with Chronic Heart Failure: The CHARM-Overall Programme. *Lancet* **2003**, *362*, 759–766. [CrossRef]
30. Savarese, G.; Dahlstrom, U.; Vasko, P.; Pitt, B.; Lund, L.H. Association between Renin–Angiotensin System Inhibitor Use and Mortality/Morbidity in Elderly Patients with Heart Failure with Reduced Ejection Fraction: A Prospective Propensity Score-Matched Cohort Study. *Eur. Heart J.* **2018**, *39*, 4257–4265. [CrossRef]
31. Packer, M.; Anker, S.D.; Butler, J.; Filippatos, G.; Pocock, S.J.; Carson, P.; Januzzi, J.; Verma, S.; Tsutsui, H.; Brueckmann, M.; et al. Cardiovascular and Renal Outcomes with Empagliflozin in Heart Failure. *N. Engl. J. Med.* **2020**, *383*, 1413–1424. [CrossRef] [PubMed]
32. Kitaoka, K.; Yano, Y.; Nagasu, H.; Kanegae, H.; Chishima, N.; Akiyama, H.; Tamura, K.; Kashihara, N. Kidney Outcomes of SGLT2 Inhibitors among Older Patients with Diabetic Kidney Disease in Real-World Clinical Practice: The Japan Chronic Kidney Disease Database Ex. *BMJ Open Diabetes Res. Care* **2024**, *12*, e004115. [CrossRef] [PubMed]
33. Mariani, M.V.; Manzi, G.; Pierucci, N.; Laviola, D.; Piro, A.; D'Amato, A.; Filomena, D.; Matteucci, A.; Severino, P.; Miraldi, F.; et al. SGLT2i effect on atrial fibrillation: A network meta-analysis of randomized controlled trials. *J. Cardiovasc. Electrophysiol.* **2024**, *35*, 1754–1765. [CrossRef] [PubMed]
34. Flather, M.D.; Shibata, M.C.; Coats, A.J.; Van Veldhuisen, D.J.; Parkhomenko, A.; Borbola, J.; Cohen-Solal, A.; Dumitrascu, D.; Ferrari, R.; Lechat, P.; et al. Randomized Trial to Determine the Effect of Nebivolol on Mortality and Cardiovascular Hospital Admission in Elderly Patients with Heart Failure (SENIORS). *Eur. Heart J.* **2005**, *26*, 215–225. [CrossRef]
35. Deedwania, P.C.; Gottlieb, S.; Ghali, J.K.; Waagstein, F.; Wikstrand, J.C.M. Efficacy, Safety and Tolerability of β-Adrenergic Blockade with Metoprolol CR/XL in Elderly Patients with Heart Failure. *Eur. Heart J.* **2004**, *25*, 1300–1309. [CrossRef]
36. Parrini, I.; Lucà, F.; Rao, C.M.; Cacciatore, S.; Riccio, C.; Grimaldi, M.; Gulizia, M.M.; Oliva, F.; Andreotti, F. How to Manage Beta-Blockade in Older Heart Failure Patients: A Scoping Review. *J. Clin. Med.* **2024**, *13*, 2119. [CrossRef]

37. Ferreira, J.P.; Rossello, X.; Eschalier, R.; McMurray, J.J.; Pocock, S.; Girerd, N.; Rossignol, P.; Pitt, B.; Zannad, F. MRAs in elderly HF Patients: Individual patient-data meta-analysis of RALES, EMPHASIS-HF, and TOPCAT. *JACC Heart Fail.* **2019**, *7*, 1012–1021. [CrossRef]
38. Japp, D.; Shah, A.; Fisken, S.; Denvir, M.; Shenkin, S.; Japp, A. Mineralocorticoid receptor antagonists in elderly patients with heart failure: A systematic review and meta-analysis. *Age Ageing* **2017**, *46*, 18–25. [CrossRef]
39. Savarese, G.; Savarese, G.; Carrero, J.; Carrero, J.; Pitt, B.; Pitt, B.; Anker, S.D.; Anker, S.D.; Rosano, G.M.; Rosano, G.M.; et al. Factors associated with underuse of mineralocorticoid receptor antagonists in heart failure with reduced ejection fraction: An analysis of 11 215 patients from the Swedish Heart Failure Registry. *Eur. J. Heart Fail.* **2018**, *20*, 1326–1334. [CrossRef]
40. Levey, A.S.; Stevens, L.A.; Schmid, C.H.; Zhang, Y.; Castro III, A.F.; Feldman, H.I.; Kusek, J.W.; Eggers, P.; Van Lente, F.; Greene, T.; et al. A New Equation to Estimate Glomerular Filtration Rate. *Ann. Intern. Med.* **2009**, *150*, 604–612. [CrossRef]
41. Health Data Overview for the Kingdom of Spain. Available online: https://data.who.int/countries/724 (accessed on 28 October 2024).
42. Conrad, N.; Judge, A.; Canoy, D.; Tran, J.; Pinho-Gomes, A.-C.; Millett, E.R.C.; Salimi-Khorshidi, G.; Cleland, J.G.; McMurray, J.J.V.; Rahimi, K. Temporal Trends and Patterns in Mortality After Incident Heart Failure: A Longitudinal Analysis of 86,000 Individuals. *JAMA Cardiol.* **2019**, *4*, 1102–1111. [CrossRef] [PubMed]
43. Armstrong, P.W.; Pieske, B.; Anstrom, K.J.; Ezekowitz, J.; Hernandez, A.F.; Butler, J.; Lam, C.S.; Ponikowski, P.; Voors, A.A.; Jia, G.; et al. Vericiguat in Patients with Heart Failure and Reduced Ejection Fraction. *N. Engl. J. Med.* **2020**, *382*, 1883–1893. [CrossRef]
44. Camanho, L.E.M.; Saad, E.B.; Slater, C.; Inacio, L.A.O.; Vignoli, G.; Dias, L.C.; de Mello Spineti, P.P.; Mourilhe-Rocha, R. Clinical Outcomes and Mortality in Old and Very Old Patients Undergoing Cardiac Resynchronization Therapy. *PLoS ONE* **2019**, *14*, e0225612. [CrossRef]
45. Yokoyama, H.; Shishido, K.; Tobita, K.; Moriyama, N.; Murakami, M.; Saito, S. Impact of Age on Mid-Term Clinical Outcomes and Left Ventricular Reverse Remodeling after Cardiac Resynchronization Therapy. *J. Cardiol.* **2021**, *77*, 254–262. [CrossRef] [PubMed]
46. Behon, A.; Merkel, E.D.; Schwertner, W.R.; Kuthi, L.K.; Veres, B.; Masszi, R.; Kovács, A.; Lakatos, B.K.; Zima, E.; Gellér, L.; et al. Long-Term Outcome of Cardiac Resynchronization Therapy Patients in the Elderly. *Geroscience* **2023**, *45*, 2289–2301. [CrossRef]
47. Verbrugge, F.H.; Dupont, M.; De Vusser, P.; Rivero-Ayerza, M.; Van Herendael, H.; Vercammen, J.; Jacobs, L.; Verhaert, D.; Vandervoort, P.; Tang, W.H.W.; et al. Response to Cardiac Resynchronization Therapy in Elderly Patients (≥70 Years) and Octogenarians. *Eur. J. Heart Fail.* **2013**, *15*, 203–210. [CrossRef]
48. Fernandes, G.C.; Heist, E.K. Primary Prevention Defibrillators in Elderly Persons: How Old Is Too Old? *JACC Clin. Electrophysiol.* **2023**, *9*, 989–991. [CrossRef]
49. Ma, B.; Zhao, M.; Guo, Z.; Zhao, Z. Research on the Correlation between Plasma BNP and the Condition and Prognosis of Chronic Heart Failure. *Cell Mol. Biol.* **2022**, *67*, 274–280. [CrossRef] [PubMed]
50. Daubert, M.A.; Adams, K.; Yow, E.; Barnhart, H.X.; Douglas, P.S.; Rimmer, S.; Norris, C.; Cooper, L.; Leifer, E.; Desvigne-Nickens, P.; et al. NT-ProBNP Goal Achievement Is Associated with Significant Reverse Remodeling and Improved Clinical Outcomes in HFrEF. *JACC Heart Fail.* **2019**, *7*, 158–168. [CrossRef]
51. Goh, Z.M.; Javed, W.; Shabi, M.; Klassen, J.R.L.; Saunderson, C.E.D.; Farley, J.; Spurr, M.; Dall'armellina, E.; Levelt, E.; Greenwood, J.; et al. Early Prediction of Left Ventricular Function Improvement in Patients with New-Onset Heart Failure and Presumed Non-Ischaemic Aetiology. *Open Heart* **2023**, *10*, e002429. [CrossRef]

Disclaimer/Publisher's Note: The statements, opinions and data contained in all publications are solely those of the individual author(s) and contributor(s) and not of MDPI and/or the editor(s). MDPI and/or the editor(s) disclaim responsibility for any injury to people or property resulting from any ideas, methods, instructions or products referred to in the content.

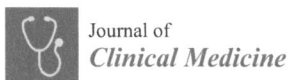

Article

Use and Benefit of Sacubitril/Valsartan in Elderly Patients with Heart Failure with Reduced Ejection Fraction

Luis Nieto Roca [1,†], Marcelino Cortés García [2,*,†], Jorge Balaguer Germán [2], Antonio José Bollas Becerra [2,*], José María Romero Otero [2], José Antonio Esteban Chapel [2], Carlos Rodríguez López [2], Ana María Pello Lázaro [2], Mikel Taibo Urquía [2] and José Tuñón [2]

[1] Cardiology Department, Son Espases University Hospital, 07120 Balearic Islands, Spain; luis.nietor@quironsalud.es
[2] Cardiology Department, Fundación Jiménez Díaz University Hospital, 28040 Madrid, Spain; jtunon@quironsalud.es (J.T.)
* Correspondence: mcortesg@quironsalud.es (M.C.G.); antonio.bollas@quironsalud.es (A.J.B.B.)
† These authors contributed equally to this work.

Abstract: Background: Heart failure (HF) is a highly prevalent syndrome in elderly subjects. Currently, multiple drugs have shown clinical benefits in patients with HF and reduced ejection fraction (HFrEF). However, evidence is scarce in elderly patients (beyond 75 years old), even more so for the latest drugs, such as angiotensin receptor-neprilysin inhibitors (ARNIs). This study aims to evaluate the use and benefits of ARNIs in elderly patients with HFrEF. **Methods**: A prospective observational cohort study was designed. Patients with left ventricular systolic dysfunction (defined by left ventricular ejection fraction [LVEF] < 40%) and age $\geq$ 75 years from January 2016 to December 2020 were prospectively included. Patients with an indication for ARNIs at inclusion or throughout follow-up were selected. Clinical, electrocardiographic and echocardiographic variables were collected. **Results**: A total of 616 patients were included, 34.4% of them female, with a mean age of 83.3 years, mean LVEF of 28.5% and ischemic etiology in 53.9% of patients. Only 14.3% of patients were taking ARNIs. After a mean follow-up of 34 months, 50.2% of patients died, and 62.2% had a cardiac event (total mortality or hospital admission due to HF). Multivariate Cox regression analysis showed that the use of ARNIs was independently and significantly associated with lower rates of mortality [HR 0.36 (95% CI 0.21–0.61)], with similar results in relation to all-cause mortality in a propensity-score-matched analysis [HR 0.33 (95% CI 0.19–0.57)]. **Conclusions**: We observed an important underuse of ARNIs in a cohort of elderly HFrEF patients, in which treatment with ARNIs was associated with a significant reduction in mortality. Greater implementation of clinical practice guidelines in this group of patients could improve their prognosis.

Keywords: HFrEF; elderly; ARNI; propensity score

1. Introduction

Heart failure (HF) is a highly prevalent syndrome among the elderly. The incidence of HF progressively increases with age, reaching around 20% among people over 75 years old [1]. Nowadays, many pharmacological and non-pharmacological therapies have been shown to reduce all-cause mortality and hospitalizations [2]. Clinical trials, however, usually exclude elderly patients or under-represent them, raising concerns about the external validity of their results [3]. Angiotensin-converting enzyme inhibitors (ACEIs), angiotensin receptor blockers (ARBs), beta-blockers (BBs) and mineralocorticoid receptor antagonists (MRAs) are drugs with a longer run in the field of heart failure, which have demonstrated their role in reducing morbimortality and improving left ventricular ejection fraction (LVEF) in elder populations [4–9]. Additionally, in the last few years, angiotensin receptor-neprilysin inhibitors (ARNIs) and sodium-glucose transport protein 2 inhibitors (SGLT2i) have become an important therapeutic group for heart failure with reduced ejection fraction (HFrEF). Although we know that neprilysin inhibition in patients with reduced LVEF through ARNIs is associated with significantly improved survival, hospitalizations and quality of life results [10], the evidence in the elderly subpopulation is very scarce. There are no clinical trials focused on ARNIs in this subgroup of patients. We only have sub-analyses of the main ARNI trials (which show clinical benefit in elderly patients) [10–12]. On the other hand, even though small observational studies reflect more disparate results, most of them seem to favor the use of ARNIs in terms of safety and clinical efficacy [13–16]. Nonetheless, the number of publications relating to this concrete subject is relatively small; many of them are subgroup analyses of greater populations, with age intervals far under the clinical practice ones and with significantly smaller populations.

Both ARNIs and SGLT2i appear to suffer from this paucity of evidence. However, there are some observational studies for SGLT2i in elderly patients with HFrEF that look at clinically relevant endpoints like mortality and hospitalization [17], unlike with ARNIs. Thus, the aim of our study is to evaluate the role of ARNI therapy in a population of very elderly patients with HFrEF.

2. Materials and Methods

2.1. Patient Selection and Study Design

We carried out a single-center, prospective, observational cohort study. We consecutively enlisted 891 patients 75 years of age or older with an LVEF lower than or equal to 40% as measured by 2-dimensional echocardiography from January 2016 to December 2020. A specific database compiled in the cardiac imaging department of our center was used to screen for patients meeting the criteria. We selected patients with a clinical indication for the use of ARNIs at the time of inclusion or throughout follow-up. Ultimately, 616 patients were included in our study. All patients received regular medical supervision according to their symptoms and the indications of their physicians (cardiologists or general practitioners) to optimize treatment. The study design and protocol have been revised and approved by the clinical research ethics committee of our institution (Ref. EO093-18 FJD). This investigation was carried out in accordance with the principles outlined in the Declaration of Helsinki.

2.2. Data Collection

All data, including clinical events and death during follow-up, were collected from patients' electronic health records or, if not available, from telephone interviews with patients or relatives. At the beginning of follow-up, variables recorded included baseline clinical characteristics, cardiovascular risk factors, comorbidities, the glomerular filtration rate (GFR) calculated by the Chronic Kidney Disease Epidemiology Collaboration (CKD-EPI) equation, electrocardiographic (rhythm, heart rate and QRS complex width) and echocardiographic findings, New York Heart Association (NYHA) functional class and the type and dose of cardiovascular drugs. At the end of follow-up, data regarding HF treatment, LVEF and NYHA functional class were gathered.

2.3. Outcomes and Follow-Up

The outcomes analyzed in our study were the rate of all-cause mortality and major cardiovascular events. Major cardiovascular events were defined as either death from any cause or admission due to heart failure (HF). HF admission was defined as admission to a healthcare facility lasting > 24 h due to the worsening of HF symptoms and followed by specific treatment for HF (regardless of the cause of decompensation).

2.4. Statistical Analysis

Data were subjected to descriptive statistical analysis via frequency measurements (absolute frequencies and percentages) for qualitative variables and using mean and standard deviation for quantitative variables. The magnitude of the effects of the variables was expressed in the form of hazard ratios (HRs) and 95% confidence intervals (CIs). Univariate analysis of the quantitative variables was performed using Student's t-test when the variables were normally distributed and the Mann–Whitney U-test when the distribution was not normal. Qualitative variables were analyzed using χ^2 or Fisher's exact test. Because observational studies do not allow for randomization, we planned two different approaches to avoid potential confounding factors: multivariate Cox proportional hazard and propensity score (PS)-matched analysis. These two analyses were used to determine significant predictors of cardiovascular events and mortality.

First, we performed a multivariate analysis with Cox (backward stepwise) regression. Of all of the baseline variables collected, we selected those with the potential to act as confounding factors. The selection criteria were as follows: first, clinical and biological plausibility and, second, the statistical criterion of Mickey, excluding all of those variables that returned a p value > 0.20 on univariate analysis. Multivariate Cox regression analyses were performed for all-cause mortality and cardiovascular events, including clinical variables [age, frailty, NYHA class, previous HF admissions and comorbidities, such as diabetes mellitus, hypertension, chronic lung disease (asthma, chronic obstructive pulmonary disease or sleep apnea/hypopnea syndrome) and peripheral vascular disease (demonstrated atherosclerotic disease in all arteries other than coronary arteries and aorta)], GFR, electrocardiographic variables (presence of sinus rhythm and of a wide QRS complex), LVEF at baseline and follow-up and variables related to therapy [use of ARNIs, ACEI/ARB, BB, MRA, SGLT2i, diuretics and cardiac resynchronization therapy (CRT) or implantable cardioverter-defibrillator (ICD)].

Second, we performed a PS-matched analysis. The PS was calculated with an ordered logistic regression model, taking the ARNI group as the dependent variable and adopting a parsimonious approach. In the first step, all of the following variables were included in the univariate analysis: age, gender, diabetes mellitus, hypertension, GFR, chronic lung disease, peripheral vascular disease, cerebrovascular disease, any degree of cognitive impairment, any degree of functional disability, the ischemic origin of reduced ejection fraction [defined as evidence of significant disease of a major coronary vessel (at least 70% stenosis or, in the case of the left main coronary artery, 50% stenosis) as evidenced by coronary angiography or coronary CT scan, regardless of whether the significant lesion has been revascularized or not], previous HF admission, LVEF and NYHA class I or II (vs. III, IV or not available) at the onset of follow-up. All variables with a p value < 0.2 were entered into a multivariate binary logistic regression model, which served to estimate the PS of every patient. Patient matching was performed at a 2:1 ratio with the nearest neighbor method (caliper = 0.2 × standard deviation (SD) [logitPs]). Results are expressed as HR and 95% CIs. Statistical analyses were performed with SPSS version 22.0 (SPSS, Inc, Chicago, IL, USA).

3. Results

3.1. Baseline Characteristics

During the study period, 616 consecutive patients with an LVEF ≤ 40% were assessed for eligibility. Table 1 shows the baseline characteristics of our population (total population and propensity score-selected population). In terms of sex, 65.6% were male, and the mean age was 83.3 ± 5.1 years. According to cardiovascular risk factors, 81.2% were hypertensive, 35.4% were diabetic, and 57.1% were dyslipidemic. Regarding comorbidities, 53.6% had been diagnosed with chronic kidney disease (GFR < 60 mL/m/m^2) and 17.7% with chronic lung disease, with chronic obstructive pulmonary disease being the most frequent entity. Ischemic etiology was found in 53.9% of the cases. The mean LVEF was 28.5 ± 7.8%. Further, 86.8% presented with NYHA class I-II, and 58.7% of the subjects were at sinus rhythm at inclusion.

At the end of follow-up, the percentage of patients taking ARNIs was 14.3% of the total cohort. BBs were used by 76.9% of patients, ACEIs/ARBs by 55.5%, MRAs by 40.4% and SGLT2 inhibitors (SGLT2i) by 4.2%. Ivabradine was received by 4.4% of the cohort, and 71.8% of patients underwent diuretic treatment.

Table 1. Baseline characteristics of the study population.

	Total Population (N = 616)	ARNI (after Propensity Score Matching) (N = 258)		
		Yes (N = 86)	No (N = 172)	p-Value
Age, years ± SD	83.3 ± 5.1	80.6 ± 3.8	80.9 ± 4.3	NS
Male, n (%)	404 (65.6)	60 (69.8)	115 (66.9)	NS
High blood pressure, n (%)	500 (81.2)	67 (77.9)	139 (80.8)	NS
Diabetes mellitus, n (%)	218 (35.4)	29 (33.7)	62 (36.0)	NS
Hyperlipidemia, n (%)	352 (57.1)	48 (55.8)	93 (54.1)	NS
Current smoker, n (%)	253 (41.1)	41 (47.7)	71 (41.3)	NS
BMI > 30kg/m^2, n (%)	66 (10.7)	9 (10.5)	28 (16.3)	NS
Chronic lung disease, n (%)	109 (17.7)	16 (18.6)	37 (21.5)	NS
Stroke/TIA, n (%)	100 (16.2)	9 (10.5)	13 (7.6)	NS
Peripheral artery disease, n (%)	78 (12.7)	11 (12.8)	17 (9.9)	NS
Chronic liver disease, n (%)	14 (2.3)	1 (1.2)	3 (1.7)	NS
Chronic kidney disease, n (%)	330 (53.6)	42 (48.8)	74 (43.0)	NS
Cognitive impairment, n (%)	75 (12.1)	0 (0)	11 (8.2)	NS
Functional disability, n (%)	94 (15.3)	8 (9.3)	11 (6.4)	NS
LVEF, % ± SD	28.5 ± 7.8	28.6 ± 7.5	28.4 ± 8.0	NS
Ischemic LV dysfunction, n (%)	287 (53.9)	50 (59.5)	79 (51)	NS
Previous HF admission, n (%)	269 (43.7)	34 (39.5)	78 (45.3)	NS
QRS > 120 ms, n (%)	155 (60.3)	56 (65.9)	99 (57.6)	NS
Sinus rhythm, n (%)	361 (58.7)	50 (41.2)	101 (41.3)	NS
GFR, mL/min/1.73 m^2, ± SD	56.9 ± 18.4	60.8 ± 14.8	60.4 ± 17.8	NS
Hemodialysis, n (%)	13 (2.1)	0 (0)	5 (2.9)	NS
NYHA class				
I–II, n (%)	519 (86.8)	73 (90.1)	149 (87.1)	NS
III–IV, n (%)	79 (13.2)	8 (9.9)	22 (12.9)	NS
Beta-blockers, n (%)	474 (76.9)	78 (90.7)	139 (80.8)	NS
ACEi/ARB, n (%)	342 (55.5)	–	114 (66.3)	–
MRA, n (%)	249 (40.4)	50 (58.1)	78 (45.3)	NS
SGLT2i, n (%)	26 (4.2)	15 (17.4)	7 (4.1)	0.001
Diuretics, n (%)	442 (71.8)	67 (77.7)	123 (71.5)	NS
Digoxin, n (%)	60 (9.7)	4 (4.7)	15 (8.7)	NS
Ivabradine, n (%)	27 (4.4)	7 (8.1)	7 (4.1)	NS
Amiodarone, n (%)	68 (11.0)	10 (11.6)	20 (11.6)	NS
Anticoagulation, n (%)	296 (48.1)	47 (54.7)	88 (51.2)	NS
ICD/CRT, n (%)	65 (16.6)	19 (22.1)	20 (11.6)	NS

ACEi: angiotensin-converting enzyme inhibitor, ARB: angiotensin receptor blocker, BMI: body mass index, CRT: cardiac resynchronization therapy, GFR: glomerular filtration rate, HF: heart failure, ICD: implantable cardioverter defibrillator, LV: left ventricle, LVEF: left ventricular ejection fraction, MRA: mineralocorticoid receptor antagonist, SGLT2i: sodium-glucose cotransporter 2 inhibitors, NS: not significant, NYHA: New York Heart Association, SD: standard deviation, TIA: transient ischemic attack.

We also analyzed the reasons for not using ARNIs in those patients who did not receive this drug by means of a thorough examination of the possible causes throughout the available medical records. Among those patients not receiving ARNIs, 85.8% of the patients did not have a clear contraindication for ARNIs. Within the remaining 14.2%, the main cause for not being treated with ARNIs was impaired renal function (7.2%), followed by drug-induced hypotension (4.7%) and hyperkalemia (0.8%).

3.2. Outcomes

After a follow-up of 34 ± 21 months, 309 patients (50.2%) had died, and 383 patients (62.2%) had developed a major cardiovascular event (death or hospitalization for HF). Of the patients who died, the cause of death was cardiovascular in 72 cases (23.3%), and non-cardiovascular causes accounted for 188 deaths (60.8%). We were unable to determine the cause of death in 49 patients (15.8%).

We performed a multivariate Cox regression analysis of our study population to identify significant predictors of total mortality, following the methodology described above. Table 2 shows the results of univariate and multivariate analyses of overall mortality. A multivariate Cox regression analysis revealed that the use of ARNIs was independently associated with lower rates of mortality (HR 0.36 [95% CI 0.21–0.61]) as compared with those who were not receiving sacubitril/valsartan. Similarly, we found a clear relationship between BB intake and reduction in mortality [multivariate Cox regression analysis HR 0.62 (0.48–0.80)]. SGLT2i showed a significant association between its use and reduction in mortality but only for the univariate analysis [HR 0.12 (0.03–0.5)]. On the other hand, neither ACEIs/ARBs nor MRAs were associated with a significant improvement in mortality.

A similar analysis was performed to evaluate potential predictors for total cardiovascular events. ARNI was independently associated with a significant reduction in cardiovascular events [HR 0.69 (0.49–0.99)]. The use of BBs and ACEIs/ARBs was also associated with a significant reduction in events (Table 3).

Table 2. Univariate and multivariate analyses for overall mortality.

	Univariate Analysis		Multivariate Analysis	
	HR	95% CI	HR	95% CI
Age	1.09	1.07–1.12	1.05	1.02–1.08
Sex	0.97	0.77–1.37		
High blood pressure	1.02	0.76–1.77		
Diabetes mellitus	1.27	1.01–1.60	1.36	1.07–1.72
Hyperlipidemia	1.10	0.87–1.38		
Chronic lung disease	1.30	0.98–1.71		
Stroke/TIA	1.17	0.87–1.57		
GFR	0.99	0.98–0.99	0.99	0.98–0.99
Functional disability	0.40	0.26–0.61	1.28	1.04–1.58
Ischemic LV dysfunction	1.35	1.05–1.73		
Previous HF admission	1.32	1.06–1.66		
QRS > 120 ms	0.84	0.64–1.11		
No sinus rhythm	1.22	0.98–1.54	1.33	1.06–1.68
LVEF	0.99	0.98–1.00		
LVEF improvement	0.48	0.36–0.62	0.49	0.37–0.64
NYHA class III–IV	1.26	0.92–1.74		
Beta-blockers	0.53	0.41–0.67	0.62	0.48–0.80
ARNI	0.27	0.16–0.44	0.36	0.21–0.61
ACEi/ARB	0.88	0.70–1.10		

Table 2. Cont.

	Univariate Analysis		Multivariate Analysis	
	HR	95% CI	HR	95% CI
MRA	1.09	0.83–1.44		
SGLT2i	**0.12**	**0.03–0.50**		
ICD/CRT	**0.53**	**0.35–0.82**		

Included variables in the multivariate analysis: age, GFR, diabetes, previous HF, sinus rhythm, QRS duration, functional disability, ACEi/ARBs, beta-blocker, MRA, ARNI, SGLT2i, digoxin, anticoagulation, LVEF improvement and ICD/CRT. ACEi: angiotensin-converting enzyme inhibitor, ARB: angiotensin receptor blocker, CRT: cardiac resynchronization therapy, GFR: glomerular filtration rate, HF: heart failure, ICD: implantable cardioverter defibrillator, LV: left ventricle, LVEF: left ventricular ejection fraction, MRA: mineralocorticoid receptor antagonist, SGLT2i: sodium-glucose cotransporter 2 inhibitors, NYHA: New York Heart Association, TIA: transient ischemic attack. Statistically significant variables are indicated in **bold**.

Table 3. Univariate and multivariate analyses for cardiovascular events.

	Univariate Analysis		Multivariate Analysis	
	HR	95% CI	HR	95% CI
Age	**1.06**	**1.04–1.08**	**1.04**	**1.02–1.07**
Sex	0.99	0.80–1.22		
High blood pressure	1.16	0.89–1.52		
Diabetes mellitus	**1.23**	**1.00–1.51**	**1.32**	**1.07–1.63**
Hyperlipidemia	1.10	0.90–1.35		
Chronic lung disease	1.29	1.00–1.66		
Stroke/TIA	1.15	0.88–1.49		
GFR	**0.99**	**0.98–0.99**	0.99	0.98–1.00
Ischemic LV dysfunction	1.14	0.92–1.42		
Previous HF admission	**1.43**	**1.17–1.75**	**1.36**	**1.1–1.68**
QRS > 120 ms	1.09	0.89–1.35		
Non-sinus rhythm	**1.28**	**1.05–1.57**	**1.32**	**1.07–1.62**
LVEF	0.99	0.98–1.00		
LVEF improvement	**0.67**	**0.53–0.83**	**0.72**	**0.57–0.90**
NYHA class III–IV	1.09	0.81–1.46		
Beta-blockers	**0.64**	**0.51–0.79**	**0.70**	**0.49–0.88**
ARNI	**0.27**	**0.16–0.44**	**0.69**	**0.49–0.99**
ACEi/ARB	**0.72**	**0.59–0.88**	**0.68**	**0.54–0.85**
MRA	1.01	0.82–1.24		
SGLT2i	**0.43**	**0.22–0.83**		
ICD/CRT	0.79	0.56–1.11		

Included variables in the multivariate analysis: age, GFR, diabetes, previous HF, sinus rhythm, QRS duration, functional disability, ACEi/ARBs, beta-blocker, MRA, ARNI, SGLT2i, digoxin, anticoagulation, LVEF improvement and ICD/CRT. ACEi: angiotensin-converting enzyme inhibitor, ARB: angiotensin receptor blocker, CRT: cardiac resynchronization therapy, GFR: glomerular filtration rate, HF: heart failure, ICD: implantable cardioverter defibrillator, LV: left ventricle, LVEF: left ventricular ejection fraction, MRA: mineralocorticoid receptor antagonist, SGLT2i: sodium-glucose cotransporter 2 inhibitors, NYHA: New York Heart Association, TIA: transient ischemic attack. Statistically significant variables are indicated in **bold**.

Finally, a statistical analysis was performed through PS matching, specifically aimed at analyzing the effect of ARNIs in our population. Table 1 shows the baseline characteristics of the selected groups according to the aforementioned methodology with and without ARNI. No significant differences were described between the two groups with respect to age, sex, comorbidities or HF treatments except for the use of SGLT2i (greater in the ARNI group). The PS-matching analysis showed again that the use of ARNIs was associated with a significant reduction in mortality [HR 0.33 (95% CI 0.19–0.57)].

Kaplan–Meier curves for mortality in the overall population and in the PS-matching population comparing those under treatment with ARNIs to those not treated with ARNIs are shown in Figure 1.

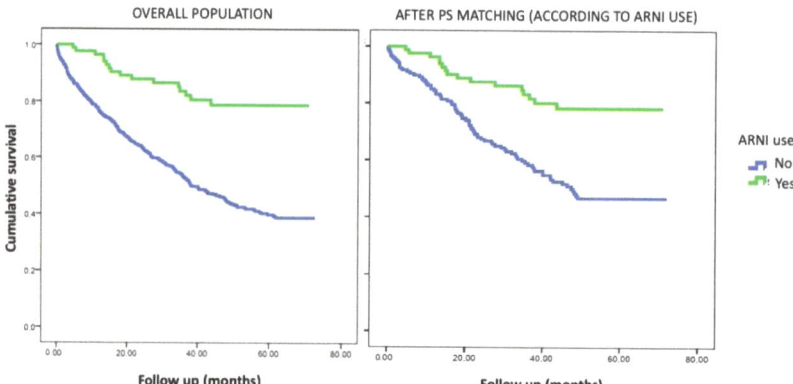

Figure 1. Kaplan–Meier curves for mortality, first showing results for the overall population and then after PS (propensity score) matching according to ARNI use. ARNIs: angiotensin receptor-neprilysin inhibitors.

4. Discussion

Our study highlights that the use of ARNIs in a cohort of elderly patients (>75 years old) with HFrEF (LVEF $\leq$ 40%) was associated with increased survival and an improvement in long-term prognosis despite a significant underuse. These results are consistent with those shown in the main trials focused on the general HFrEF population. Nevertheless, our results represent a novel contribution to the body of evidence of ARNI treatment in that it directly evaluates mortality and cardiovascular events in a very elderly cohort instead of relegating them to subgroup or post hoc analyses.

PARADIGM-HF was a guideline-changing trial. It introduced sacubitril/valsartan to the heart failure drug repertoire after showing significant and safe improvements in LVEF, NT-proBNP levels and morbimortality in patients with HFrEF [10]. Additional benefits of ARNIs included an improvement in symptoms, an improvement in quality of life, a reduction in the incidence of diabetes requiring insulin treatment [18], a reduction in the decline of GFR [19] and a reduced rate of hyperkalemia [20]. In this trial, almost 50% were over 65 years old; nevertheless, the proportion of patients > 75 years was just 18.6% (7% > 80 years and 1.44% > 85 years).

Of the overall population included in the PIONEER-HF trial (which demonstrated the efficacy and safety of sacubitril/valsartan in acute decompensated HF), only 36.5% were >65 years old [11]. The median age in the TRANSITION study (showing the feasibility of early initiation of sacubitril/valsartan after acute decompensated HF) was 68 years old, with no specific information regarding the proportion of patients older than 75 years [12].

Most patients in these pivotal trials belong to these "younger elders" between 65 and 75 years of age. The "real" elders are clearly underrepresented (a mere 18.6% versus almost 30% between 65 and 75 in PARADIGM-HF). In addition, current evidence regarding the use of ARNIs in patients > 75 years old and with HFrEF is mostly supported by post hoc or subgroup analysis. In one of them, where patients of the PARADIGM-HF trial were analyzed according to age, a persistent benefit was described beyond 65 years old. However, this was mainly driven by those between 65 and 74 years old, and, even though the results in terms of mortality were relatively stable across the age range, they did not reach statistical significance in the > 75-year-old group. Sacubitril/valsartan was demonstrated to be safe with no greater rate of adverse events; moreover, there was a possible clinical benefit in these patients despite lower doses [21]. On the other hand, the few trials that have directly focused on elderly patients either consider surrogate clinical endpoints or have a very short follow-up period [22].

Considering the lack of elderly-focused trials and the aforementioned underrepresentation in the main HF trials [23,24], real-world registries have shed some more light on the use of ARNIs in the "real elders". In a real-world series including 205 patients beyond 70 years of age, sacubitril/valsartan was, first, safe, with no significant rate of adverse events compared to the younger group; in addition, its withdrawal was linked with poorer prognosis [25]. A more recent trial based on the FDA adverse events reporting system database showed similar rates of adverse events in patients over 75 years of age when compared with younger peers. [26]. In addition, in a recent large cohort study comparing elderly patients with HFrEF treated with ARNIs versus those receiving ACEIs/ARBs in the UK, the use of ARNIs was associated with a lower risk of hospitalization for HF and all-cause mortality (mainly driven by those patients who previously received a renin-angiotensin system blocker and switched to ARNIs) [27]. Clinical assumptions can also be made regarding our current knowledge of natriuretic peptides and the effects of this inhibition. Along this line, it is well known that they have similar effects in old patients when compared with younger populations [28,29]. Hence, we could expect similar hemodynamic and clinical benefits in this subgroup of patients. Therefore, even though all available data seem to support the use of ARNIs in patients with HFrEF and >75 years old, there is still no solid evidence of their clinical benefit in this population.

On the other hand, HF is a very relevant entity in the elderly. It is well known that the prevalence of HF reaches up to 20% among people over 75 years old [1,2]. Most patients with HF are elderly, constituting up to 80% of patients suffering from this disease with both the incidence and prevalence of the condition increasing with age [30]. Age has been associated with a greater risk of cardiovascular events and mortality, especially in patients with HF [31]. We must consider that elderly patients have different clinical profiles than younger ones, characterized by complex comorbidities and frailty. The latter is an independent predictor of adverse outcomes, and it is associated with poorer prognosis in terms of quality of life, hospitalization and mortality [32]. As a matter of fact, we must point out that despite comorbidities and polypharmacy, age does not seem to be associated with lower adherence to medical treatment [33]. In this regard, efforts to maintain strict compliance and improve clinical results are essential.

Although guidelines proclaim that pharmacotherapy and other treatments of HFrEF in elderly patients are recommended to be the same as for younger patients [2,34], in the real world, the use of guideline-directed medical therapy is notoriously lower in older patients despite its potential benefits [2,23,35–37]. As an example of this, Euro Heart Failure Survey II reported that the use of ACEi/ARBs in patients over age 80 with HFrEF is approximately 60% at admission due to HF, with this rate rising to 75% at discharge [38]. This percentage is relatively low given that these drugs have been proven to protect against mortality. The use of these drugs is frequently limited by the already mentioned presence of different comorbidities, adverse events and polypharmacy [38]. Elders are also less frequently referred to a cardiologist [39,40]. Altogether, these factors contribute to the lower rate of appropriate HF treatment and may result in lower adherence to current clinical guidelines among elderly patients. In addition, optimal doses are frequently not achieved in these patients despite their positive impact on prognosis [41,42]. Therefore, elderly patients with HF also very often do not benefit from an optimized medical regimen. This underuse is concerning given the growing evidence for each HF-specific drug in this subgroup of patients. Despite the small number of trials that have targeted older HF patients (such as the SENIORS trial [43] or the CIBIS-ELD trial [44]), these trials have reinforced the idea of the clinical benefit and safety of using anti-remodeling drugs and opened the door toward the use of HF-specific drugs in elderly patients with HFrEF. Nevertheless, most of the current data regarding the use of HF drugs in the elderly still come from sub-analyses and observational studies. Some of them have proven to be useful in bringing some light to the use of ACEi/ARBs and BBs in elderly patients, even in the context of frequent clinical situations and comorbidities (such as CKD) [37,45–48]. Therefore, we still have a real gap in evidence regarding the use of guideline-directed medical therapy in elderly HF patients.

The use of ARNIs is no exception to this situation. Insights from the CHAMP trial show that among patients with HF and > 65 years old, only 12.9% were taking ARNIs [36]. In line with these results, just 14.3% of our patients were taking any dose of sacubitril/valsartan at the end of the follow-up. Moreover, almost 86% of our patients did not have a clear clinical reason for not being on ARNIs. It is quite significant that even with the growing evidence regarding the safe use of ARNIs in this population since 2018, the proportion of patients remains almost the same in different but comparable cohorts [36]. Our study also highlights the reasons for not starting or withdrawing sacubitril/valsartan, with impaired renal function and symptomatic hypotension being the two main ones. Nonetheless, in more than 80% of patients, there was no clear reason for not initiating ARNIs. This could be explained by the lower rate of adherence to clinical guidelines in this subgroup of patients, probably due to the already mentioned factors (polypharmacy, comorbidities, relatively fewer referrals to the cardiologist, etc.).

In our study, we found a significant reduction in cardiovascular events and total mortality associated with the use of ARNIs in our population of very elderly patients with HFrEF. This is even more interesting in the context of low rates of use of sacubitril/valsartan. Another important fact is that our study included a significant population of 616 patients with HFrEF and older than 75 years old. There are few studies directly focused on and with such a cohort size in this range of age [49]. In addition, our cohort comes directly from real-world clinical practice, with a mean age (83 years old) much higher than those from the pivotal trials [10–12,21].

Our research presents some limitations. Firstly, it is an observational study, with the subsequent risk of biases. Secondly, it is a single-center study, explaining the relatively small sample size, which may affect the statistical results provided. Another limitation is that we could not ascertain the cause of death in almost 16% of our population because it was not available (we do not have access to the complete history of other centers).

Despite the limitations of our study, it appears unlikely that future randomized trials regarding the use of ARNIs in the elderly will be conducted, especially if we consider the small number of them carried out in the cardiovascular field in the last decade [43,44,49]. Our study addresses clinically relevant endpoints, with a long follow-up period, in a cohort with scarce clinical evidence. As such, the results of this paper are both innovative and potentially applicable to daily clinical practice, regardless of the observational nature of the registry. Further research using real-world data could help to design larger studies and generate more research for this "forgotten" population.

5. Conclusions

Based on the findings of our study, treatment with ARNIs in elderly patients presenting with HFrEF was associated with a significant reduction in mortality and cardiovascular events. However, a significant underuse in this population was observed. Those patients not being treated with sacubitril/valsartan did not have a clear contraindication in most of the cases. Our data support that an increased use of ARNIs in this subgroup of patients would probably lead to a significant improvement in prognosis. Nevertheless, more studies focused on this subgroup are needed to confirm these findings.

Author Contributions: Conceptualization, L.N.R., J.B.G. and M.C.G.; methodology, M.C.G.; validation, M.T.U., A.M.P.L. and J.T.; formal analysis, M.C.G.; investigation, L.N.R. and J.B.G.; data curation, C.R.L., J.M.R.O., J.A.E.C. and L.N.R.; writing—original draft preparation, L.N.R.; writing—review and editing, M.C.G. and A.J.B.B.; supervision, M.T.U., A.M.P.L. and J.T. All authors have read and agreed to the published version of the manuscript.

Funding: This research received no external funding.

Institutional Review Board Statement: The study was conducted according to the guidelines of the Declaration of Helsinki and approved by the Clinical Research Ethics Committee of Hospital Universitario Fundación Jiménez Díaz (Ref. EO093-18 FJD) on 31 July 2018.

Informed Consent Statement: Patient consent was waived due to only using anonymized data from the medical records of patients seen at our center.

Data Availability Statement: The data presented in this study are available from the corresponding authors upon reasonable request.

Conflicts of Interest: The authors declare no conflicts of interest.

References

1. Díez-Villanueva, P.; Jiménez-Méndez, C.; Alfonso, F. Heart failure in the elderly. *J. Geriatr. Cardiol.* **2021**, *18*, 219–232. [CrossRef]
2. McDonagh, T.A.; Metra, M.; Adamo, M.; Gardner, R.S.; Baumbach, A.; Böhm, M.; Burri, H.; Butler, J.; Čelutkienė, J.; Chioncel, O.; et al. 2021 ESC Guidelines for the diagnosis and treatment of acute and chronic heart failure. *Eur. J. Heart Fail.* **2021**, *42*, 3599–3726. [CrossRef]
3. Cherubini, A.; Oristrell, J.; Pla, X.; Ruggiero, C.; Ferretti, R.; Diestre, G.; Clarfield, A.M.; Crome, P.; Hertogh, C.; Lesauskaite, V.; et al. The persistent exclusion of older patients from ongoing clinical trials regarding heart failure. *Arch. Intern. Med.* **2011**, *171*, 550–556. [CrossRef]
4. CONSENSUS Trial Study Group. Effects of enalapril on mortality in severe congestive heart failure. Results of the Cooperative North Scandinavian Enalapril Survival Study (CONSENSUS). *N. Engl. J. Med.* **1987**, *316*, 1429–1435. [CrossRef]
5. Cleland, J.G.F.; Tendera, M.; Adamus, J.; Freemantle, N.; Gray, C.S.; Lye, M.; O'Mahony, D.; Polonski, L.; Taylor, J.; on behalf of the PEP investigators. The perindopril in elderly people with chronic heart failure (PEP-CHF) study. *Eur. Heart J.* **2006**, *27*, 2338–2345. [CrossRef]
6. Cohen-Solal, A.; McMurray, J.J.; Swedberg, K.; Pfeffer, M.A.; Puu, M.; Solomon, S.D.; Michelson, E.L.; Yusuf, S.; Granger, C.B.; for the CHARM Investigators. Benefits and safety of candesartan treatment in heart failure are independent of age: Insights from the Candesartan in Heart failure—Assessment of Reduction in Mortality and Morbidity Programme. *Eur. Heart J.* **2008**, *29*, 3022–3028. [CrossRef]
7. Kotecha, D.; Manzano, L.; Krum, H.; Rosano, G.; Holmes, J.; Altman, D.G.; Collins, P.D.; Packer, M.; Wikstrand, J.; Coats, A.J.S.; et al. Effect of age and sex on efficacy and tolerability of β blockers in patients with heart failure with reduced ejection fraction: Individual patient data meta-analysis. *BMJ* **2016**, *353*, i1855. [CrossRef]
8. Ferreira, J.P.; Rossello, X.; Eschalier, R.; McMurray, J.J.; Pocock, S.; Girerd, N.; Rossignol, P.; Pitt, B.; Zannad, F. MRAs in elderly HF Patients: Individual patient-data meta-analysis of RALES, EMPHASIS-HF, and TOPCAT. *JACC Heart Fail.* **2019**, *7*, 1012–1021. [CrossRef]
9. Japp, D.; Shah, A.; Fisken, S.; Denvir, M.; Shenkin, S.; Japp, A. Mineralocorticoid receptor antagonists in elderly patients with heart failure: A systematic review and meta-analysis. *Age Ageing* **2017**, *46*, 18–25. [CrossRef] [PubMed]
10. Mcmurray, J.J.V.; Packer, M.; Desai, A.S.; Gong, J.; Lefkowitz, M.P.; Rizkala, A.R.; Rouleau, J.L.; Shi, V.C.; Solomon, S.D.; Swedberg, K.; et al. Angiotensin-neprilysin inhibition versus enalapril in heart failure. *N. Engl. J. Med.* **2014**, *371*, 993–1004. [CrossRef]
11. Velazquez, E.J.; Morrow, D.A.; DeVore, A.D.; Duffy, C.I.; Ambrosy, A.P.; McCague, K.; Rocha, R.; Braunwald, E. Angiotensin–Neprilysin inhibition in acute decompensated heart failure. *N. Engl. J. Med.* **2019**, *380*, 539–548. [CrossRef] [PubMed]
12. Wachter, R.; Senni, M.; Belohlavek, J.; Straburzynska-Migaj, E.; Witte, K.K.; Kobalava, Z.; Fonseca, C.; Goncalvesova, E.; Cavusoglu, Y.; Fernandez, A.; et al. Initiation of sacubitril/valsartan in haemodynamically stabilised heart failure patients in hospital or early after discharge: Primary results of the randomised TRANSITION study. *Eur. J. Heart Fail.* **2019**, *21*, 998–1007. [CrossRef]
13. Cofiño, J.B.; Fernández, Á.Á.; Rodríguez, M.F. ICyFA-010—Empleo anecdótico de sacubitrilo/valsartan en paciente anciano hospitalizado. In Proceedings of the XXXVIII Congreso Nacional de la SEMI/XV Congreso de la SOMIMACA, Madrid, Spain, 22–24 November 2017. Available online: https://www.revclinesp.es/es-congresos-xxxviii-congreso-nacional-sociedad-espanola-54-sesion-insuficiencia-cardiaca-fibrilacion-auricular-3553-empleo-anecdotico-de-sacubitrilo-valsartan-en-41820 (accessed on 24 April 2022).
14. Camafort, M.; Formiga, F. Sacubitrilo-valsartán también debe ser la primera elección a valorar en el paciente mayor con insuficiencia cardiaca con fracción de eyección reducida. *Rev. Esp. Geriatría Gerontol.* **2021**, *56*, 67–68. [CrossRef] [PubMed]
15. Martín, P.M.; Lorite, I.R.; Escobar, M.M.; Ronda, M.V.; Rangel, L.S.; Moreno, M. ICyFA-054—Eficacia y seguridad de sacubitril/valsartan en un programa de insuficiencia cardiaca de Medicina Interna. In Proceedings of the XXXVIII Congreso Nacional de la SEMI/XV Congreso de la SOMIMACA, Madrid, Spain, 22–24 November 2017. Available online: https://www.revclinesp.es/es-congresos-xxxviii-congreso-nacional-sociedad-espanola-54-sesion-insuficiencia-cardiaca-fibrilacion-auricular-3553-eficacia-y-seguridad-de-sacubitril-valsartan-41830 (accessed on 24 April 2022).
16. Vicent, L.; Esteban-Fernández, A.; Gómez-Bueno, M.; De-Juan, J.; Díez-Villanueva, P.; Iniesta, M.; Ayesta, A.; González-Saldívar, H.; Rojas-González, A.; Bover-Freire, R.; et al. Clinical profile of a nonselected population treated with sacubitril/valsartan is different from PARADIGM-HF trial. *J. Cardiovasc. Pharmacol.* **2018**, *72*, 112–116. [CrossRef] [PubMed]

17. Germán, J.B.; García, M.C.; López, C.R.; Otero, J.M.R.; Chapel, J.A.E.; Becerra, A.J.B.; Roca, L.N.; Urquía, M.T.; Lázaro, A.M.P.; Fernández, J.T. Impact of SGLT2 Inhibitors on Very Elderly Population with Heart Failure with Reduce Ejection Fraction: Real Life Data. *Biomedicines* **2024**, *12*, 1507. [CrossRef] [PubMed]
18. Seferovic, J.P.; Claggett, B.; Seidelmann, S.B.; Seely, E.W.; Packer, M.; Zile, M.R.; Rouleau, J.L.; Swedberg, K.; Lefkowitz, M.; Shi, V.C.; et al. Effect of sacubitril/valsartan versus enalapril on glycaemic control in patients with heart failure and diabetes: A post-hoc analysis from the PARADIGM-HF trial. *Lancet Diabetes Endocrinol.* **2017**, *5*, 333–340. [CrossRef] [PubMed]
19. Damman, K.; Gori, M.; Claggett, B.; Jhund, P.S.; Senni, M.; Lefkowitz, M.P.; Prescott, M.F.; Shi, V.C.; Rouleau, J.L.; Swedberg, K.; et al. Renal effects and associated outcomes during angiotensin-neprilysin inhibition in heart failure. *JACC Heart Fail.* **2018**, *6*, 489–498. [CrossRef] [PubMed]
20. Desai, A.S.; Vardeny, O.; Claggett, B.; McMurray, J.J.V.; Packer, M.; Swedberg, K.; Rouleau, J.L.; Zile, M.R.; Lefkowitz, M.; Shi, V.; et al. Reduced risk of hyperkalemia during treatment of heart failure with mineralocorticoid receptor antagonists by use of sacubitril/valsartan compared with enalapril: A secondary analysis of the PARADIGM-HF trial. *JAMA Cardiol.* **2017**, *2*, 79. [CrossRef]
21. Jhund, P.S.; Fu, M.; Bayram, E.; Chen, C.-H.; Negrusz-Kawecka, M.; Rosenthal, A.; Desai, A.S.; Lefkowitz, M.P.; Rizkala, A.R.; Rouleau, J.L.; et al. Efficacy and safety of LCZ696 (sacubitril-valsartan) according to age: Insights from PARADIGM-HF. *Eur. Heart J.* **2015**, *36*, 2576–2584. [CrossRef]
22. Armentaro, G.; Condoleo, V.; Pelaia, C.; Cassano, V.; Miceli, S.; Maio, R.; Salzano, A.; Pelle, M.C.; Perticone, M.; Succurro, E.; et al. Short term effect of sacubitril/valsartan on comprehensive geriatric assessment in chronic heart failure: A real life analysis. *Intern. Emerg. Med.* **2023**, *18*, 113–125. [CrossRef]
23. Reddy, K.P.; Faggioni, M.; Eberly, L.A.; Halaby, R.; Sanghavi, M.; Lewey, J.; Mehran, R.; Coylewright, M.; Herrmann, H.C.; Giri, J.; et al. Enrollment of older patients, women, and racial and ethnic minorities in contemporary heart failure clinical trials: A systematic review. *JAMA Cardiol.* **2018**, *3*, 1011. [CrossRef]
24. Greene, S.J.; DeVore, A.D.; Sheng, S.; Fonarow, G.C.; Butler, J.; Califf, R.M.; Hernandez, A.F.; Matsouaka, R.A.; Tahhan, A.S.; Thomas, K.L.; et al. Representativeness of a heart failure trial by race and sex: Results from ASCEND-HF and GWTG-HF. *JACC Heart Fail.* **2019**, *7*, 980–992. [CrossRef]
25. Esteban-Fernández, A.; Díez-Villanueva, P.; Vicent, L.; Bover, R.; Gómez-Bueno, M.; De Juan, J.; Iniesta, M.; García-Aguado, M.; Martínez-Sellés, M. Sacubitril/Valsartan is useful and safe in elderly people with heart failure and reduced ejection fraction. Data from a real-word cohort. *Rev. Espanola Geriatr. Gerontol.* **2020**, *55*, 65–69. [CrossRef]
26. Lerman, T.T.; Greenberg, N.; Fishman, B.; Goldman, A.; Talmor-Barkan, Y.; Bauer, M.; Goldberg, I.; Goldberg, E.; Kornowski, R.; Krause, I.; et al. The real-world safety of sacubitril / valsartan among older adults (≥75): A pharmacovigilance study from the FDA data. *Int. J. Cardiol.* **2024**, *397*, 131613. [CrossRef] [PubMed]
27. Desai, R.J.; Patorno, E.; Vaduganathan, M.; Mahesri, M.; Chin, K.; Levin, R.; Solomon, S.D.; Schneeweiss, S. Effectiveness of angiotensin-neprilysin inhibitor treatment versus renin-angiotensin system blockade in older adults with heart failure in clinical care. *Heart* **2021**, *107*, 1407–1416. [CrossRef]
28. Mulkerrin, E.; Brain, A.; Hampton, D.; Penney, M.D.; Sykes, D.; Williams, J.; Coles, G.; Woodhouse, K. Reduced renal hemodynamic response to atrial natriuretic peptide in elderly volunteers. *Am. J. Kidney Dis.* **1993**, *22*, 538–544. [CrossRef]
29. Hausdorff, J.M.; Clark, B.A.; Shannon, R.P.; Elahi, D.; Wei, J.Y. Hypotensive response to atrial natriuretic peptide administration is enhanced with age. *J. Gerontol. A Biol. Sci. Med. Sci.* **1995**, *50*, M169–M172. [CrossRef]
30. Go, A.S.; Mozaffarian, D.; Roger, V.L.; Benjamin, E.J.; Berry, J.D.; Borden, W.B.; Bravata, D.M.; Dai, S.; Ford, E.S.; Fox, C.S.; et al. Executive summary: Heart disease and stroke statistics—2013 update: A report from the American Heart Association. *Circulation* **2013**, *127*, 143–152. [CrossRef]
31. Metra, M.; Cotter, G.; El-Khorazaty, J.; Davison, B.A.; Milo, O.; Carubelli, V.; Bourge, R.C.; Cleland, J.G.; Jondeau, G.; Krum, H.; et al. Acute heart failure in the elderly: Differences in clinical characteristics, outcomes, and prognostic factors in the VERITAS study. *J. Card. Fail.* **2015**, *21*, 179–188. [CrossRef]
32. Uchmanowicz, I.; Gobbens, R.J. The relationship between frailty, anxiety and depression, and health-related quality of life in elderly patients with heart failure. *Clin. Interv. Aging* **2015**, *10*, 1595–1600. [CrossRef]
33. Krueger, K.; Botermann, L.; Schorr, S.G.; Griese-Mammen, N.; Laufs, U.; Schulz, M. Age-related medication adherence in patients with chronic heart failure: A systematic literature review. *Int. J. Cardiol.* **2015**, *184*, 728–735. [CrossRef] [PubMed]
34. Heidenreich, P.A.; Bozkurt, B.; Aguilar, D.; Allen, L.A.; Byun, J.J.; Colvin, M.M.; Deswal, A.; Drazner, M.H.; Dunlay, S.M.; Evers, L.R.; et al. 2022 AHA/ACC/HFSA guideline for the management of heart failure: A report of the American College of Cardiology/American Heart Association Joint Committee on Clinical Practice Guidelines. *Circulation* **2022**, *145*, e895–e1032. [CrossRef]
35. Seo, W.-W.; Park, J.J.; Park, H.A.; Cho, H.-J.; Lee, H.-Y.; Kim, K.H.; Yoo, B.-S.; Kang, S.-M.; Baek, S.H.; Jeon, E.-S.; et al. Guideline-directed medical therapy in elderly patients with heart failure with reduced ejection fraction: A cohort study. *BMJ Open.* **2020**, *10*, e030514. [CrossRef]
36. Peri-Okonny, P.A.; Mi, X.; Khariton, Y.; Patel, K.K.; Thomas, L.; Fonarow, G.C.; Sharma, P.P.; Duffy, C.I.; Albert, N.M.; Butler, J.; et al. Target doses of heart failure medical therapy and blood pressure: Insights from the CHAMP-HF registry. *JACC Heart Fail.* **2019**, *7*, 350–358. [CrossRef] [PubMed]

37. Martínez-Milla, J.; García, M.C.; Urquía, M.T.; Castillo, M.L.; Arbiol, A.D.; Monteagudo, A.L.R.; Mariscal, M.L.M.; Figuero, S.B.; Franco-Pelaéz, J.A.; Tuñón, J. Blockade of renin-angiotensin-aldosterone system in elderly patients with heart failure and chronic kidney disease: Results of a single-center, observational cohort study. *Drugs Aging* **2019**, *36*, 1123–1131. [CrossRef] [PubMed]
38. Komajda, M.; Hanon, O.; Hochadel, M.; Follath, F.; Swedberg, K.; Gitt, A.; Cleland, J.G. Management of octogenarians hospitalized for heart failure in Euro Heart Failure Survey I. *Eur. Heart J.* **2007**, *28*, 1310–1318. [CrossRef] [PubMed]
39. Rutten, F.H.; Grobbee, D.E.; Hoes, A.W. Differences between general practitioners and cardiologists in diagnosis and management of heart failure: A survey in every-day practice. *Eur. J. Heart Fail.* **2003**, *5*, 337–344. [CrossRef]
40. Johansson, S.; Wallander, M.A.; Ruigómez, A.; García Rodríguez, L.A. Incidence of newly diagnosed heart failure in UK general practice. *Eur. J. Heart Fail.* **2001**, *3*, 225–231. [CrossRef]
41. Yancy, C.W.; Fonarow, G.C.; Albert, N.M.; Curtis, A.B.; Stough, W.G.; Gheorghiade, M.; Heywood, J.T.; McBride, M.L.; Mehra, M.R.; O'Connor, C.M.; et al. Influence of patient age and sex on delivery of guideline-recommended heart failure care in the outpatient cardiology practice setting: Findings from IMPROVE HF. *Am. Heart J.* **2009**, *157*, 754–762.e2. [CrossRef]
42. Pulignano, G.; Del Sindaco, D.; Tavazzi, L.; Lucci, D.; Gorini, M.; Leggio, F.; Porcu, M.; Scherillo, M.; Opasich, C.; Di Lenarda, A.; et al. Clinical features and outcomes of elderly outpatients with heart failure followed up in hospital cardiology units: Data from a large nationwide cardiology database (IN-CHF Registry). *Am. Heart J.* **2002**, *143*, 45–55. [CrossRef]
43. Flather, M.D.; Shibata, M.C.; Coats, A.J.; Van Veldhuisen, D.J.; Parkhomenko, A.; Borbola, J.; Cohen-Solal, A.; Dumitrascu, D.; Ferrari, R.; Lechat, P.; et al. Randomized trial to determine the effect of nebivolol on mortality and cardiovascular hospital admission in elderly patients with heart failure (SENIORS). *Eur. Heart J.* **2005**, *26*, 215–225. [CrossRef]
44. Düngen, H.-D.; Apostolović, S.; Inkrot, S.; Tahirović, E.; Töpper, A.; Mehrhof, F.; Prettin, C.; Putniković, B.; Neskovic, A.N.; Krotin, M.; et al. Titration to target dose of bisoprolol vs. carvedilol in elderly patients with heart failure: The CIBIS-ELD trial. *Eur. J. Heart Fail.* **2011**, *13*, 670–680. [CrossRef] [PubMed]
45. Martínez-Milla, J.; Cortés-García, M.; Palfy, J.A.; Taibo-Urquía, M.; López-Castillo, M.; Devesa-Arbiol, A.; Monteagudo, A.L.R.; Mariscal, M.L.M.; Jiménez-Varas, I.; Figuero, S.B.; et al. Beta-blocker therapy in elderly patients with renal dysfunction and heart failure. *J. Geriatr. Cardiol.* **2021**, *18*, 20. [CrossRef] [PubMed]
46. Peláez, J.A.F.; García, M.C.; Daza, A.M.R.; Mariscal, M.L.M.; Ropero, G.; Castillo, M.L.; Palfy, J.A.; Lázaro, A.M.P.; Urquía, M.T.; Figuero, S.B.; et al. Relationship between different doses of beta-blockers and prognosis in elderly patients with reduced ejection fraction. *Int. J. Cardiol.* **2016**, *220*, 219–225. [CrossRef] [PubMed]
47. Damman, K.; Tang, W.W.; Felker, G.M.; Lassus, J.; Zannad, F.; Krum, H.; McMurray, J.J. Current evidence on treatment of patients with chronic systolic heart failure and renal insufficiency: Practical considerations from published data. *J. Am. Coll. Cardiol.* **2014**, *63*, 853–871. [CrossRef] [PubMed]
48. Fernandez, A.F.; Hammill, B.G.; O'Connor, C.M.; Schulman, K.A.; Curtis, L.H.; Fonarow, G.C. Clinical effectiveness of beta-blockers in heart failure: Findings from the OPTIMIZE-HF (Organized Program to Initiate Lifesaving Treatment in Hospitalized Patients with Heart Failure) registry. *J. Am. Coll. Cardiol.* **2019**, *53*, 184–192. [CrossRef] [PubMed]
49. Broekhuizen, K.; Pothof, A.; de Craen, A.J.M.; Mooijaart, S.P. Characteristics of randomized controlled trials designed for elderly: A systematic review. *PLoS ONE* **2015**, *10*, e0126709. [CrossRef] [PubMed]

Disclaimer/Publisher's Note: The statements, opinions and data contained in all publications are solely those of the individual author(s) and contributor(s) and not of MDPI and/or the editor(s). MDPI and/or the editor(s) disclaim responsibility for any injury to people or property resulting from any ideas, methods, instructions or products referred to in the content.

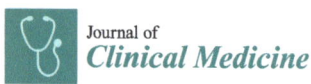 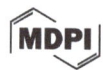

Perspective

The Five Pillars of Acute Right Ventricular Heart Failure Therapy: Can We Keep the Pediment in Balance?

Antoniu Octavian Petriș [1,2], Călin Pop [3,*] and Diana Carmen Cimpoeșu [1,4]

1. Cardiology Clinic, "Grigore T. Popa" University of Medicine and Pharmacy, 700115 Iași, Romania; antoniu.petris@yahoo.ro (A.O.P.); dcimpoiesu@yahoo.com (D.C.C.)
2. "Sf. Spiridon" Clinical County Emergency Hospital, 700111 Iași, Romania
3. Faculty of Medicine, West "Vasile Goldiș" University, 310025 Arad, Romania
4. Emergency Department, "Grigore T. Popa" University of Medicine and Pharmacy, 700115 Iași, Romania
* Correspondence: medicbm@yahoo.com

Abstract: Acute right ventricular heart failure (aRHF), a long-neglected aspect of heart disease, has recently gained attention due to an improved understanding of its pathophysiology and the development of tailored therapeutic strategies. The therapeutic approach is now built on several pillars that aim to support the stable clinical condition of the patient, starting with the central pillar of etiological or specific therapy and extending to various aspects related to hemodynamic support, ventilation support, fluid optimization, and, when necessary, advanced resources such as right ventricular assist devices (e.g., extracorporeal membrane oxygenation—ECMO, Impella RP, or ProtekDuo). This five-pillar approach summarizes the different facets of contemporary treatment for aRHF, although some aspects related to their use are still being clarified.

Keywords: right heart failure; pulmonary embolism; cor pulmonale; pillar; ECMO

Citation: Petriș, A.O.; Pop, C.; Cimpoeșu, D.C. The Five Pillars of Acute Right Ventricular Heart Failure Therapy: Can We Keep the Pediment in Balance? *J. Clin. Med.* **2024**, *13*, 6949. https://doi.org/10.3390/jcm13226949

Academic Editor: Carlos Escobar

Received: 16 October 2024
Revised: 11 November 2024
Accepted: 15 November 2024
Published: 18 November 2024

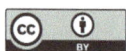

Copyright: © 2024 by the authors. Licensee MDPI, Basel, Switzerland. This article is an open access article distributed under the terms and conditions of the Creative Commons Attribution (CC BY) license (https://creativecommons.org/licenses/by/4.0/).

1. Introduction

Long considered the "weak ventricle", "a passive conduit", "the Cinderella side of the heart", or "a forgotten ventricle", the right ventricle (RV) has recently demonstrated its importance, prompting contemporary investigations and re-evaluations that emphasize its role in maintaining normal heart function.

The RV was not only "forgotten" but also minimized regarding its role in ensuring a normal hemodynamic after early experiments (Starr et al. 1943), which promoted the idea that "a normal, contractile right ventricular wall is not necessary for the maintenance of a normal circulation", a concept that determined the complete exclusion of the RV in Fontan operations (1971) [1]. It can be said that cardiologists have become more and more "LV-centric". The end-diastolic volume of the RV is greater than that of the left ventricle/LV (49–101 mL/m^2 vs. 44–89 mL/m^2), its ejection fraction (45–60%) is less than that of the LV (50–70%) and its elastance (1.30 ± 0.84 mmHg/mL) is also more reduced than that of the LV (5.48 ± 1.23 mmHg/mL) [2]. More recently, the important prognostic role of RV dysfunction was proved in congenital heart disease (CHD), pulmonary hypertension (PH), and left heart failure (LHF). LV contraction generates up to 40% of "weak" RV contractile force, but this is sufficient to pump systemic venous return into the low-pressure system of pulmonary circulation. One of the greatest vulnerabilities of the RV is its greater sensitivity to changes in afterload [3].

Acute right heart failure (aRHF) can be isolated (characterized by increased RV and atrial pressure with systemic congestion) or may be associated with LV damage and reduced systemic cardiac output (due to ventricular interdependence, highlighting the importance of maintaining the transseptal gradient) [4].

Consequently, the etiology of aRHF primarily includes acute pulmonary embolism (aPE), acute cor pulmonale (in previously healthy individuals, high-risk aPE is the most common cause of acute RV failure) [5], acute right myocardial infarction (aRMI, in which the right coronary artery perfuses the RV free wall and the posterior part of the interventricular septum during both systole and diastole activity, making the RV more vulnerable to increases in wall tension and drops in systemic blood pressure) [6], acute respiratory distress syndrome (ARDS, with 20–30% of moderate to severe aRDS cases developing aRHF), acute-to-chronic cor pulmonale (a/cCP) [6], and aRHF post-cardiac surgery (pcsRHF) (in 0.1% of patients after cardiotomy, 2–3% after heart transplantation, and in 10–20% of cases in LV assisted device insertion) [7]. Pericardial pathology is not addressed in this work, although the pericardium participates in maintaining ventricular interdependence and does not readily accommodate acute changes in RV size in response to afterload variations [8].

The management of aRHF typically begins in emergency settings, such as emergency departments and intensive cardiovascular care units, involving a multidisciplinary approach (emergency medicine, cardiology, pneumology, internal medicine, intensivists, and thoracic surgery) [5]. Since the *primum movens* in any emergency approach is its organization, in this work, we propose and verify the consistency of references regarding the establishment of some pillars on which such a therapeutic approach must be built, following the model recently used in LV heart failure (Figure 1). A major pathophysiological specificity of the RV is its heightened sensitivity to increases in afterload, regardless of origin. Accordingly, therapeutic approaches aimed at decreasing excessive RV afterload should be prioritized, while treatment of the underlying cause of RVF can be addressed subsequently. However, identifying the etiology and addressing it is the "gold" solution to interrupt the downward spiral of the patient's clinical condition, with various symptomatic supports used merely to buy time until the main etiology is identified and removed. Of course, specific differences in management strategies may depend on the resources available in different countries and local diagnostic capabilities. Currently, much of what we know about pharmacological or interventional support in aRHF comes from various animal models (canine, porcine, rabbit, and rat), which exhibit differences among models and in local availability, thereby generating variability in the results [9], as well as from case reports, small cohorts, or meta-analysis. The need for randomized, controlled, multicenter studies is obvious. The pillars/columns of aRHF management are part of the therapeutic architecture by which the modern treatment of chronic heart failure, CKD, atrial fibrillation, etc. has recently been constructed. This seems to be an efficient way to highlight the structures that more robustly or more precariously support the condition of stability of the respective patient, allowing for personalized treatment. These management pillars follow the concept of some physiopathological pillars that the optimal approach to aRHF must take into account: primary etiology that must be removed as quickly and as completely as possible, contractility that must be enhanced, preload (volume) that will have to be optimized, post-load (pressure) that will have to be reduced, and secondary organ damage that will have to be prevented. It is important to note the fact that some therapeutic resources support several pillars at the same time or in sequence.

There are a series of therapeutic peculiarities in the case of patients who are older, pregnant, oncologic, etc., but their approach is beyond the scope of our paper.

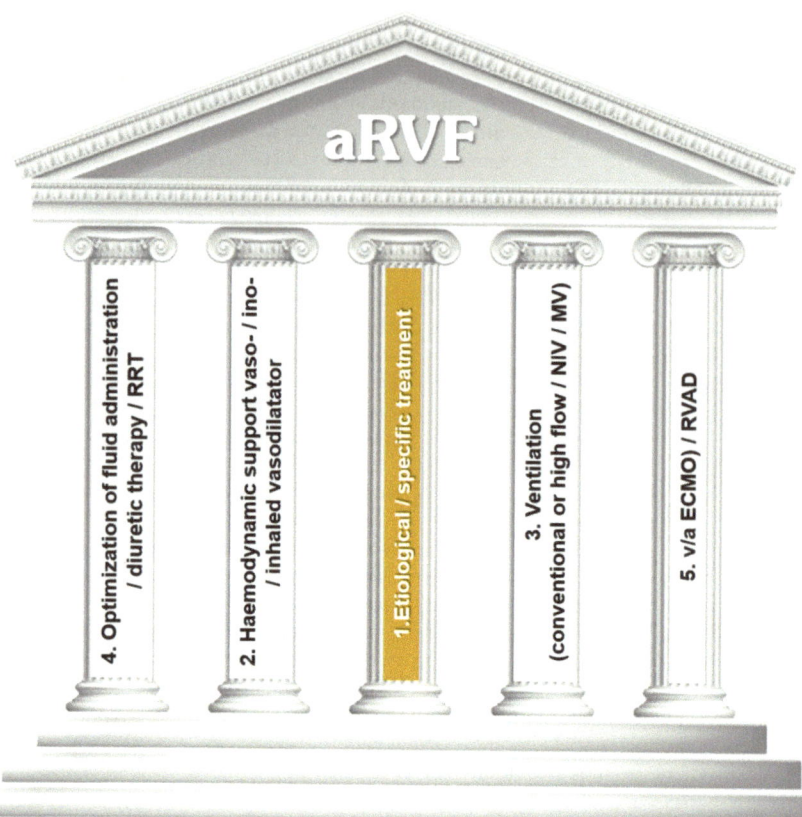

Figure 1. The five-pillar approach for the treatment of aRHF: (1) etiological/specific treatment; (2) hemodynamic support (vaso-/ino-/inhaled vasodilator); (3) ventilation (conventional or high flow/NIV/MV); (4) optimization of fluid administration/diuretic therapy/RRT; and (5) v/a ECMO)/RVAD. NIV—non-invasive ventilation. MV—mechanical ventilation; RRT—renal replacement therapy; v/a—ECMO veno/arterial extracorporeal membrane oxygenation; RVAD—right ventricular assist device; aRHF—acute right heart failure.

2. The First Pillar

Since a decision-making hierarchy could improve the applicability of this framework, especially in emergency conditions, we believe that the first pillar, which is also the central pillar that can ensure stable support, should consist of the etiological/specific treatment, representing an essential target of the management of aRHF. The other pillars intended to support the pediment are added gradually, taking into account the advantages and limitations that each one has. This pillar is best supported by data from clinical trials of varying sizes (e.g., anticoagulation/systemic thrombolysis/percutaneous catheter-directed treatment/surgical pulmonary embolectomy in aPE, PCI/thrombolysis in aRMI, etc.) [10].

Frequently encountered challenges in emergency situations mainly relate to the availability of diagnostic and therapeutic resources because the therapeutic intervention will have to be applied as quickly as possible and must be adapted to the etiology. Sometimes it is challenging to discern if the RV dysfunction is secondary to left-sided cardiac dysfunction, a pulmonary pathology (airway, parenchymal, or vascular disease), an isolated right ventricle aRMI or pulmonary circulation failure (aPE), or a combination of these etiologies.

For the early and appropriate treatment of the underlying causes of aRHF (before RV dysfunction passes the point-of-no-return), diagnostic resources must be available in emergency settings, including a fast and focused clinical assessment, electrocardiography, biomarkers (D-dimers, natriuretic peptides, troponin, and blood lactate), echocardiography (at least a point-of-care ultrasound or POCUS), and other emergency imaging techniques. No specific biomarker has been identified for the early diagnosis of aRVF, but natriuretic peptides and cardiac troponin levels do have prognostic value. In acute pulmonary embolism, for example, levels of NT-proBNP $\geq$ 600 ng/L, heart-type fatty acid binding protein (H-FABP) $\geq$ 6 ng/mL, or copeptin $\geq$ 24 pmol/L may provide additional prognostic information, but these biomarkers have not yet been validated to guide treatment decisions [10]. Echocardiographic evaluation is the most frequently used technique in daily practice and several valuable parameters for an imaging diagnosis of aRVF have been identified: fractional area change (FAC), tricuspid annular plane systolic excursion (TAPSE), the Doppler tissue imaging-derived systolic S' velocity of the tricuspid annulus, or the RV index of myocardial performance (RIMP), and, by using strain echocardiography, RV global and regional longitudinal shortening may be estimated [3].

Invasive hemodynamic parameters indicating the presence of aRVF include elevated central venous pressure (CVP > 15 mmHg), discordant right-to-left filling pressures (the right atrial pressure to pulmonary capillary wedge pressure ratio or RAP/PCWP of > 0.8), a low pulmonary artery pulsatility index (PAPi $\leq$ 1.85, which should be interpreted cautiously in severe tricuspid regurgitation), and a low RV stroke work index (<0.25–0.30 mmHg·L/m^2) [4]. The RAP/PCWP (right atrial pressure to pulmonary capillary wedge pressure) ratio shows that lowering PCWP increases pulmonary artery compliance more than would be anticipated from a fall in pulmonary vascular resistance (PVR) alone [11]. A low PAPi (pulmonary artery pulsatility index) value, derived noninvasively by transthoracic echocardiography, is associated with the markers of right heart failure, RV dysfunction, and worse survival rates [11].

In a previously healthy individual, the most common cause of acute RV failure is suspected to be a high-risk aPE [5], but we must not ignore the possibility of an aRMI involving the RV, whether it is in association with an inferior myocardial infarction (10–50%) or possibly also with the anterior one (13%, according to necroptic studies) [12].

The recommendations from the latest ESC guidelines for the treatment of aPE [10] specify the sequence, recommendation classes, and level of evidence for each therapeutic method. It is recommended that anticoagulation treatment with unfractioned heparin (UHF), including a weight-adjusted bolus injection, should be initiated without delay in patients with high-risk PE (class of recommendation I; level of evidence C). Systemic thrombolytic therapy is recommended for high-risk PE (I, B), while surgical pulmonary embolectomy or percutaneous catheter-directed treatment (such as catheter-directed thrombolysis (CDT), ultrasound-assisted CDT (USCDT), pharmacomechanical CDT, and aspiration thrombectomy) is recommended for patients with high-risk PE, in whom thrombolysis is contraindicated or has failed (I, C). The inferior vena cava filter should only be used in patients with a clear contraindication for anticoagulation (IIa, C); in these cases, the filter should be removed as soon as possible, due to the significant risk of subsequent deep vein thrombosis [5,10]. The routine use of IVC filters is not recommended (III, A).

The management of aRMI, as stated in the latest version of the ESC guidelines on this subject, includes early reperfusion (PCI/thrombolysis), which can lead to rapid hemodynamic improvement, the avoidance of reducing right ventricular preload (i.e., nitrates and diuretics and opioid medications), and the correction of atrio-ventricular (AV) dyssynchrony and/or AV block, with rhythm sequencing if necessary [13].

In the 2021 ESC guidelines regarding the management of patients with isolated aRHF, only two therapeutic indications have the recommendation class and level of evidence mentioned: loop diuretics (Class I) and vasopressors and/or inotropes (Class IIb) [4].

3. The Second Pillar

The second pillar focuses on hemodynamic support (vasopressors, inotropes/lusitropes, or inhaled vasodilators). The rationale for using vasopressors as first-line therapy is driven by the need to maintain right coronary perfusion pressure. The presence of biventricular dysfunction may indicate the use of inotropes. It should be noted that in cardiogenic shock from the right, as opposed to cardiogenic shock that mainly involves the left ventricle, a "double hit phenomenon" has been described. The "double hit phenomenon", described by Hrymak et al., refers to severely reduced organ perfusion (liver, renal, gut, etc.) in a right ventricular shock because of the high CVP associated with low systolic blood pressure, in contrast to what happens during a shock that mainly affects the LV, where the organ perfusion is maintained, because both the central venous pressure (CVP) and the systolic blood pressure are both low [2]. The clinical significance of this phenomenon is that after the "first hit", represented by the damage to the RV (an acute increase in RV afterload or volume results in increased wall tension, septal shift due to transseptal gradient reduction, and tricuspid regurgitation), multiple intra-abdominal organ failure occurs ("double hit"), which must be constantly considered and treated appropriately [2].

Norepinephrine (0.1–0.5 mcg/kg/min) is a reasonable first choice [8], improving systemic hemodynamics (as a potent α1-receptor agonist with weaker β-receptor activity, noradrenaline increases systemic arterial vascular resistance and increases cardiac output through the optimization of cardiac preload and direct inotropism, and also increases systemic blood pressure and coronary artery perfusion) with minimal effect on pulmonary vascular resistance [14]. Vasopressin (0.03 units/min) and vasopressin analogs may be useful as adjunct vasopressors if hypotension persists [10]. Inotropes can be used alone in cases of hypoperfusion without hypotension [4]. Inodilators (inotropes with vasodilatory properties) such as dobutamine, levosimendan, and phosphodiesterase-III inhibitors can reduce cardiac filling pressures, enhance ventriculo-atrial coupling by increasing RV contractility, and restore cardiac output, reducing afterload due to PA vasodilation; however, as inotropic agents may exacerbate arterial hypotension, they may be combined with norepinephrine if necessary [4,10]. Sympathomimetics, including norepinephrine and phenylephrine (the second is not as beneficial in studies on humans compared to those performed on animals), have a direct vasoconstrictive effect on the pulmonary artery, a property not shared by vasopressin [8].

In a/cCP, inotropic-vasoactive drugs and inhaled vasodilators have been proposed during awake intubation following the nebulization of local anesthesia. The simplest pulmonary vasodilator is supplemental oxygen [10], but the addition of inhaled nitric oxide (iNO, iloprost, or epoprostenol) is reasonable as a rescue therapy in patients with ongoing RV dysfunction despite hemodynamic support, appropriate volume status, and supplemental oxygen administration [5,10]. These therapies remain off-label and can increase ventilation/perfusion mismatch or shunting, worsening oxygenation [5]. Some experts argue that pulmonary vasodilators should not be classified as "hemodynamic support" but rather as strategies to decrease RV afterload.

4. The Third Pillar

The third pillar consists of ventilation support using oxygen therapy (either conventionally or via a high-flow nasal cannula, targeting an oxygen saturation of > 90%) [10], non-invasive ventilation (NIV), or mechanical ventilation (MV). Supplemental oxygen should be considered even without hypoxemia [8]. However, while MV may occasionally be required in the management of patients with aRHF (e.g., severe hypoxemia, impaired mentation, or the facilitation of procedures), it should ideally be avoided, particularly in the case of positive pressure ventilation, due to potential hemodynamic consequences, MV being associated with a three-fold higher risk of mortality in high-risk PE or a/cCP [15]. Pulmonary vascular resistance and intrathoracic pressures may increase, and venous return and RV preload may decrease during positive pressure ventilation; furthermore, the option to use positive end-expiratory pressure (PEEP) extends these effects throughout the respiratory cycle, further reducing venous return and RV preload [5]. Therefore, ventilation support in patients with aRVF may worsen the clinical situation and should be avoided in this clinical setting; when necessary, it should be used with caution (ultraprotective settings). Caution is advised regarding the risk of peri-intubation hemodynamic collapse (e.g., with propofol) and pulmonary vasoconstriction (worsening hypoxemia and hypercarbia during induction), with etomidate considered the most hemodynamically neutral induction agent [10]. Hypercarbia may not only occur after induction but can also be present depending on the severity of lung disease when RVF is associated with respiratory compromise. If MV is necessary, it should be approached cautiously with positive end-expiratory pressure and low to moderate tidal volumes; however, correcting hypoxemia may not always be feasible without simultaneous pulmonary reperfusion in high-risk aPE [10]. Early prone positioning is one of the best maneuvers for unloading the RV in aRDS [16].

5. The Fourth Pillar

The fourth pillar relates to the optimization of intravenous fluid (IVF) administration [5], the use of diuretic therapy (the potential benefits of IVF versus fluid removal depend on the baseline status of the patient with aRHF, with loop diuretics remaining the first option in cases of venous congestion; assessing volume responsiveness may be useful) [4,10] or, in some cases, the use of renal replacement therapy (RRT) [4]. A randomized open-label study comparing diuresis with a 0.5-L saline infusion reported a more rapid decrease in natriuretic peptide levels after diuretics, without any difference in RV function or clinical outcomes [17]. Thus, in most cases, IVF administration may be harmful (over-distending the right heart and subsequently increasing wall tension, impairing LV filling, aggravating tricuspid regurgitation, worsening ventricular interdependence, and, consequently, reducing cardiac output) [5]. Although the presentation of fluid optimization with diuretic therapy can be somewhat confusing, the evidence suggests that patients with aRVF usually do not require fluid supplementation, as this may exacerbate the associated systemic venous congestion, sometimes necessitating the removal of excess fluid. Recent contributions emphasize the possibility of false positive indices of fluid responsiveness, such as pulse pressure variation [18]. We need to be careful with volume loading that is guided by central venous pressure (CVP) monitoring, but a CVP of less than 10 mm Hg can almost rule out RV dysfunction with congestion [3]. In patients with ARDS, fluid responsiveness can be predicted, but different thresholds should be used [19]. IV loop diuretic administration should be considered, particularly if evidence exists of RV dysfunction or volume overload [10]. The challenge lies in detecting hypovolemia, which could be prognostic, while avoiding worsening tissue hypoperfusion in patients with systemic venous congestion. This remains an important and complex dilemma.

6. The Fifth Pillar

The fifth pillar represents the most modern approach: the use of veno/arterial extracorporeal membrane oxygenation (v/aECMO) and right ventricular assist devices (RVAD). Where both pulmonary and cardiac support are necessary, v/aECMO is the preferred approach [20]; for pulmonary insufficiency, v/vECMO can be considered (even in the absence of MV) as a bridge to an intervention in cases of progressive RV failure, but not in aPE, as it returns blood to the venous system and does not decrease RV preload [21]. When only cardiac support is needed, options such as Impella RP or ProtekDuo support (but not an intra-aortic balloon pump for isolated aRHF) should be considered. The choice of device depends on the estimated duration of mechanical RV support: short-term (10 to 15 days) devices include ECMO, Impella RP, and PROTEK Duo, while for more than 15 days, surgically implanted devices (Levitronix CentriMag) should be chosen, and, for an assisted VD in which recovery is not expected, the possibility of accessing a heart or heart-lung transplant should be assessed [22]. The association of therapeutic options is also crucial: in 39 studies (n = 6409) involving ECMO for aPE, patients treated with ECMO and catheter-directed therapy had significantly lower mortality compared to those treated with ECMO and systemic thrombolysis [23]. ECMO in high-risk PE and aRVF (refractory cardiac shock or cardiac arrest) cases, in combination with surgical embolectomy or catheter-directed treatment, represents a promising approach. It must be taken into account, as a warning, that ECMO might also induce adverse effects such as a reduction in bronchial arterial blood flow, a reduction in pulmonary blood flow/transpulmonary gradient, and the worsening of lung ischemia [24]. Based on the data currently available, we can state that the potential contraindications and procedural risks of right ventricular assist devices for Impella RP are the lack of an intrinsic oxygenator and a higher risk of hemolysis, for Protek Duo, they are the long insertion time and the high transfusion rate, and for v/a ECMO, they are LV distension and vascular complications [20]. Cost, accessibility, and training requirements remain a continuing challenge for the development of these forms of advanced mechanical support.

7. Conclusions

Acute *cor pulmonale* is a life-threatening entity in which many organs are affected; therefore, it requires a multidisciplinary approach [5]. The therapeutic arsenal for patients with aRHF, like the treatment of heart failure in general, has recently been enriched by a combination of established, newly developed, and re-evaluated drugs, as well as new support devices for the RV. We propose a new architectural framework for a therapeutic approach to aRHF therapy based on five pillars, which would simplify the selection of options in emergency situations and would make sure that none are overlooked. Of course, these five pillars vary in robustness and importance and are based on statistical arguments of varying strengths. This architectural approach prompts the identification of the most appropriate therapeutic resources, adapted to each patient. The wise use of widely available therapeutic resources will have to be supported by increasing availability and access to modern therapeutic resources, as selected by a Heart Team that can be activated in critical moments (e.g., PERT in pulmonary embolism, etc.). If the identification of the etiology is the basis of specific assurances of the functionality of the first pillar, starting from the second pillar (hemodynamic support), there are often antagonistic therapeutic features (the use of vasopressors, inotropes/lusitropes, or, in some situations, inhaled vasodilators); the cautious use of positive end-expiratory pressure with the option of low to moderate tidal volumes (third pillar), the cautious administration of fluids but also recourse to diuretic therapy (fourth pillar), and recourse to ECMO should be made as early as possible, but, depending on the need for cardiac support, Impella RP and PROTEK Duo may prove much more useful. The motto of this pediment-supporting effort might be "*Nec plus ultra*"—nothing further beyond.

8. Future Directions

In the future, *Artificial intelligence* (AI)-enhanced diagnostic and therapeutic strategies may improve the assessment of aRHF and provide optimal management in this acute setting. Progress can be achieved through early diagnosis with the identification of the underlying etiology (specific biomarkers for RV failure, which are commonly used in the current practice of molecular imaging, as well as the identification and use of new hemodynamic indices) and early treatment, even borrowing some effective drugs for LV heart failure (e.g., dapagliflozin for structural RV remodeling and antiarrhythmic effects), or reducing device implantation delays [22]. SGLT2i may improve RV function, based on TAPSE, PAP, and FAC values recorded in HF patients assessed with the CardioMEMS sensor, which showed that empagliflozin caused rapid decreases in PAP, independent of the loop diuretic effect [25,26].

Author Contributions: A.O.P., C.P. and D.C.C. wrote the first draft of the manuscript. A.O.P. conceived and drafted the figure. A.O.P., C.P. and D.C.C. contributed to the critical revision of the manuscript for important intellectual content and confirmed the integrity of the work. All authors have read and agreed to the published version of the manuscript.

Funding: This research received no external funding.

Institutional Review Board Statement: Not applicable.

Informed Consent Statement: Not applicable.

Data Availability Statement: Data sharing is not applicable to this article as no datasets were generated or analyzed during the current outline of advances in our field of expertise.

Conflicts of Interest: The authors declare no conflicts of interest.

References

1. Sanz, J.; Sánchez-Quintana, D.; Bossone, E.; Bogaard, H.J.; Naeije, R. Anatomy, function, and dysfunction of the right ventricle: JACC State-of-the-Art Review. *J. Am. Coll. Cardiol.* **2019**, *73*, 1463–1482. [CrossRef] [PubMed]
2. Hrymak, C.; Strumpher, J.; Jacobsohn, E. Acute right ventricle failure in the Intensive Care Unit: Assessment and management. *Can. J. Cardiol.* **2017**, *33*, 61–71. [CrossRef] [PubMed]
3. Harjola, V.-P.; Mebazaa, A.; Čelutkienė, J.; Bettex, D.; Bueno, H.; Chioncel, O.; Crespo-Leiro, M.G.; Falk, V.; Filippatos, G.; Gibbs, S.; et al. Contemporary management of acute right ventricular failure: A statement from the Heart Failure Association and the Working Group on Pulmonary Circulation and Right Ventricular Function of the European Society of Cardiology. *Eur. J. Heart Fail.* **2016**, *18*, 226–241. [CrossRef] [PubMed]
4. McDonagh, T.A.; Metra, M.; Adamo, M.; Gardner, R.S.; Baumbach, A.; Böhm, M.; Burri, H.; Butler, J.; Čelutkienė, J.; Chioncel, O.; et al. 2021 ESC Guidelines for the diagnosis and treatment of acute and chronic heart failure. *Eur. Heart. J.* **2021**, *42*, 3599–3726. [CrossRef]
5. Arrigo, M.; Price, S.; Harjola, V.-P.; Huber, L.C.; Schaubroeck, H.A.I.; Vieillard-Baron, A.; Mebazaa, A.; Masip, J. Diagnosis and treatment of right ventricular failure secondary to acutely increased right ventricular afterload (acute cor pulmonale). A clinical consensus statement of the Association for Acute CardioVascular Care (ACVC) of the ESC. *Eur. Heart J. Acute Cardiovasc. Care.* **2024**, *13*, 304–312. [CrossRef]
6. Houston, B.A.; Brittain, E.L.; Tedford, R.J. Right ventricular failure. *N. Engl. J. Med.* **2023**, *388*, 1111–1125. [CrossRef]
7. Kaul, T.; Fields, B.L. Postoperative acute refractory right ventricular failure: Incidence, pathogenesis, management and prognosis. *Cardiovasc. Surg.* **2000**, *8*, 1–9. [CrossRef]
8. McGuire, W.C.; Sullivan, L.; Odish, M.F.; Desai, B.; Morris, T.A.; Fernandes, T.M. Management strategies for acute pulmonary embolism in the ICU. *Chest* **2024**, in press. [CrossRef]
9. Andersen, A.; van der Feen, D.E.; Andersen, S.; Schultz, J.G.; Hansmann, G.; Bogaard, H.J. Animal models of right heart failure. *Cardiovasc. Diagn. Ther.* **2020**, *10*, 1561–1579. [CrossRef]
10. Konstantinides, S.V.; Meyer, G.; Becattini, C.; Bueno, H.; Geersing, G.-J.; Harjola, V.-P.; Huisman, M.V.; Humbert, M.; Jennings, C.S.; Jiménez, D.; et al. 2019 ESC guidelines for the diagnosis and management of acute pulmonary embolism developed in collaboration with the European Respiratory Society (ERS). *Eur. Heart J.* **2020**, *41*, 543–603. [CrossRef]
11. Konstam, M.A.; Kiernan, M.S.; Bernstein, D.; Bozkurt, B.; Jacob, M.; Kapur, K.; Kociol, R.D.; Lewis, E.F.; Mehra, M.R.; Pagani, F.D.; et al. Evaluation and management of right-sided heart failure. A scientific statement from the American Heart Association. *Circulation* **2018**, *137*, e578–e622. [CrossRef] [PubMed]
12. Femia, G.; French, J.K.; Juergens, C.; Leung, D.; Lo, S. Right ventricular myocardial infarction: Pathophysiology, clinical implications and management. *Rev. Cardiovasc. Med.* **2021**, *22*, 1229–1240. [CrossRef] [PubMed]
13. Steg, P.G.; James, S.K.; Atar, D.; Badano, L.P.; Blömstrom-Lundqvist, C.; Borger, M.A.; Di Mario, C.; Dickstein, K.; Ducrocq, G.; Fernandez-Aviles, F.; et al. Task Force on the management of ST-segment elevation acute myocardial infarction of the European Society of Cardiology (ESC). ESC Guidelines for the management of acute myocardial infarction in patients presenting with ST-segment elevation. *Eur. Heart J.* **2012**, *33*, 2569–2619. [CrossRef] [PubMed]
14. Legrand, M.; Zarbock, A. Ten tips to optimize vasopressors use in the critically ill patient with hypotension. *Intensive Care Med.* **2022**, *48*, 736–739. [CrossRef]
15. Disselkamp, M.; Adkins, D.; Pandey, S.; Yataco, A.O.C. Physiologic approach to mechanical ventilation in right ventricular failure. *Ann. Am. Thorac. Soc.* **2018**, *15*, 383–389. [CrossRef]
16. Guerin, C.; Beuret, P.; Constantin, J.M.; Bellani, G.; Garcia-Olivares, P.; Roca, O.; Meertens, J.H.; Maia, P.A.; Becher, T.; Peterson, J.; et al. A prospective international observational prevalence study on prone positioning of ARDS patients: The APRONET (ARDS Prone Position Network) study. *Intensive Care Med.* **2018**, *44*, 22–37. [CrossRef]
17. Ferrari, E.; Sartre, B.; Labbaoui, M.; Heme, N.; Asarisi, F.; Redjimi, N.; Fourrier, E.; Squara, F.; Bun, S.; Berkane, N.; et al. Diuretics versus volume expansion in the initial management of acute intermediate high-risk pulmonary embolism. *Lung* **2022**, *200*, 179–185. [CrossRef]
18. Vieillard-Baron, A.; Prigent, A.; Repessé, X.; Goudelin, M.; Prat, G.; Evrard, B.; Charron, C.; Vignon, P.; Geri, G. Right ventricular failure in septic shock: Characterization, incidence and impact on fluid responsiveness. *Crit. Care.* **2020**, *24*, 630. [CrossRef]
19. Joseph, A.; Evrard, B.; Petit, M.; Prat, G.; Slama, M.; Charron, C.; Vignon, P.; Goudelin, M.; Vieillard-Baron, A. Fluid responsiveness in acute respiratory distress syndrome patients: A post hoc analysis of the HEMOPRED study. *Intensive Care Med.* **2024**, *50*, 1850–1860. [CrossRef]
20. Kadri, A.N.; Alrawashdeh, R.; Soufi, M.K.; Elder, A.J.; Elder, Z.; Mohamad, T.; Gnall, E.; Elder, M. Mechanical support in high-risk pulmonary embolism: Review article. *J. Clin. Med.* **2024**, *13*, 2468. [CrossRef]

21. Götzinger, F.; Lauder, L.; Sharp, A.S.P.; Lang, I.M.; Rosenkranz, S.; Konstantinides, S.; Edelman, E.R.; Böhm, M.; Jaber, W.; Mahfoud, F. Interventional therapies for pulmonary embolism. *Nat. Rev. Cardiol.* **2023**, *20*, 670–684. [CrossRef] [PubMed]
22. Monteagudo-Vela, M.; Tindale, A.; Monguió Santín, E.; Reyes-Copa, G.; Panoulas, V. Right ventricular failure: Current strategies and future development. *Front. Cardiovasc. Med.* **2023**, *10*, 998382. [CrossRef] [PubMed]
23. Boey, J.J.E.; Dhundi, U.; Ling, R.R.; Chiew, J.K.; Fong, N.C.-J.; Chen, Y.; Hobohm, L.; Nair, P.; Lorusso, R.; MacLaren, G.; et al. Extracorporeal membrane oxygenation for pulmonary embolism: A systematic review and meta-analysis. *J. Clin. Med.* **2024**, *13*, 64. [CrossRef] [PubMed]
24. Helms, J.; Carrier, M.; Klok, F.A. High-risk pulmonary embolism in the intensive care unit. *Intensive Care Med.* **2023**, *49*, 579–582. [CrossRef]
25. Mariani, M.V.; Manzi, G.; Pierucci, N.; Laviola, D.; Piro, A.; D'Amato, A.; Filomena, D.; Matteucci, A.; Severino, P.; Miraldi, F.; et al. SGLT2i effect on atrial fibrillation: A network meta-analysis of randomized controlled trials. *J. Cardiovasc. Electrophysiol.* **2024**, *35*, 1754–1765. [CrossRef]
26. Tufan Cinar, T.; Saylik, F.; Cicek, V.; Pay, L.; Khachatryan, A.; Alejandro, J.; Erdem, A.; Hayiroglu, M.I. Effects of SGLT2 inhibitors on right ventricular function in heart failure patients: Updated meta-analysis of the current literature. *Kardiol. Pol.* **2024**, *82*, 416–422. [CrossRef]

Disclaimer/Publisher's Note: The statements, opinions and data contained in all publications are solely those of the individual author(s) and contributor(s) and not of MDPI and/or the editor(s). MDPI and/or the editor(s) disclaim responsibility for any injury to people or property resulting from any ideas, methods, instructions or products referred to in the content.

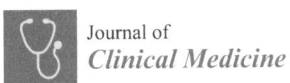

Article

Pulsatile Left Ventricular Assistance in High-Risk Percutaneous Coronary Interventions: Short-Term Outcomes

Josko Bulum [1,†], Marcelo B. Bastos [2,*,†], Ota Hlinomaz [3], Oren Malkin [4], Tomasz Pawlowski [5], Milan Dragula [6] and Robert Gil [7]

1. Department of Internal Medicine, University Hospital Center Zagreb, 10000 Zagreb, Croatia; jbulum@kbc-zagreb.hr
2. Thoraxcentrum, Erasmus Medical Center, 3015 GD Rotterdam, The Netherlands
3. Department of Cardiology, International Clinical Research Center, St. Anne University Hospital and Masaryk, University School of Medicine, 656 91 Brno, Czech Republic
4. PulseCath BV, 6811 KS Arnhem, The Netherlands
5. Department of Cardiology, National Institute of Medicine, 02-507 Warsaw, Poland
6. Department of Cardiology, University Hospital in Martin, 036 01 Martin, Slovakia
7. Department of Cardiology, National Medical Institute of the Internal Affairs and Administration Ministry, 02-005 Warsaw, Poland
* Correspondence: m.barrosbastos@erasmusmc.nl; Tel.: +31-10-7035260
† These authors contributed equally to this work as first authorship.

Abstract: Objectives: To document the real-world experience with the use of pneumatic pulsatile mechanical circulatory support (MCS) with the PulseCath iVAC2L during high-risk percutaneous coronary interventions (HR-PCIs). **Background**: The use of MCS in HR-PCIs may reduce the rate of major adverse cardiovascular events (MACEs) at 90 days. The PulseCath iVAC2L is a short-term pulsatile transaortic left ventricular (LV) assist device that has been in use since 2014. The iVAC2L Registry tracks its safety and efficacy in a variety of hospitals worldwide. **Methods**: The iVAC2L Registry is a multicenter, observational registry that aggregates clinical data from patients treated with the iVAC2L worldwide. A total of 293 consecutive cases were retrospectively collected and analyzed. Estimated rates of in-hospital clinical endpoints were described. All-cause mortality was used as the primary endpoint and other outcomes of interest were used as secondary endpoints. The rates obtained were reported and contextualized. **Results**: The in-hospital rate of all-cause mortality was 1.0%, MACE was 3.1%. Severe hypotension occurred in 8.9% of patients. Major bleeding and major vascular complications occurred in 1.0 and 2.1%, respectively. Acute myocardial infarction occurred in 0.7% of patients. Cerebrovascular events occurred in 1.4% of patients. Cardiac arrest occurred in 1.7% of patients. A statistically significant improvement in blood pressure was observed with iVAC2L activation. **Conclusions**: The results of the present study suggest that the iVAC2L is capable of improving hemodynamics with a low rate of adverse events. However, confirmatory studies are needed to validate these findings.

Keywords: registry; mechanical circulatory support; PulseCath; iVAC2L; pulsatile; high-risk; percutaneous coronary intervention; real world; LV assist device; coronary disease; heart failure; cardiogenic shock; ACS/NSTE-ACS; depressed LV function; mitral regurgitation dilated non-ischemic cardiomyopathy; ischemic cardiomyopathy

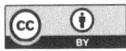

1. Introduction

Due to the recent advances in cardiovascular therapeutics, the growing use of short-term mechanical circulatory support (MCS) devices is now an established trend. MCS is available in a variety of support modalities, each with the common goal of improving prognosis after high-risk invasive interventions.

The intra-aortic balloon pump (IABP) is the most commonly utilized modality; however, its use tends to decrease in favor of new and more powerful ones, which now have class IIb recommendation for prophylactic use in high-risk percutaneous coronary interventions (HR-PCIs) [1–3]. Despite evidence favoring pulsatile flow [4,5], all current short-term MCS devices are continuous-flow devices (CFDs), with PulseCath iVAC2L (PulseCath BV, Arnhem, The Netherlands) being the only exception. Numerous large-scale studies have examined the utilization of short-term MCS in a real-world context. Nevertheless, to date, no reports have addressed the use of pulsatile flow (PF) in a real-world setting.

Three single-center prospective studies have already demonstrated the safety and efficacy of the iVAC2L [5]. The iVAC2L Registry is an open, multicenter registry that collects data on the real-world use of the iVAC2L on a global scale. This report presents the initial findings from the iVAC2L Registry.

2. Methods

Description of the iVAC2L. The iVAC2L comprises a membrane pump connected to a nitinol-reinforced polyurethane bi-directional flow catheter. The catheter has a length of 92 cm, with an outer diameter of 17 French (Fr). It features a stainless steel inlet tip and a patented two-way valve, illustrated in Supplementary Figure S1. The chamber is subdivided by a flexible membrane into a blood chamber and a helium chamber. The catheter is then inserted into the femoral artery and positioned with the inlet tip inside the LV, where it operates in synchrony with the cardiac cycle. During diastole, the helium chamber receives helium from the IABP driver, resulting in the ejection of blood back into the ascending aorta with a stroke volume of around 21 mL. During systole, the helium chamber undergoes a deflation, which is accompanied by a refill of the blood chamber. The pump typically produces an additional flow of 1.5 to 1.8 L/min, though it has the capacity to reach up to 2.5 L/min (data not yet published). The optimal performance of the device is achieved at rates between 70 and 90 beats per minute (bpm).

Study population and data collection: The iVAC2L Registry is a multicenter, international registry that retrospectively collects data on the utilization of iVAC2L in a range of indications. Participation is entirely voluntary. In order to guarantee strict adherence to the Declaration of Helsinki, it is recommended that operators seek verbal consent from patients regarding their willingness to have their data utilized for research purposes and to provide data only upon confirmation.

To ensure the highest degree of completeness and accuracy, data were collected via the use of a standardized Clinical Report Form (CRF). Furthermore, all information was completed at the site with the assistance of the clinical team. The data sources included medical records, ancillary diagnostic tests, specialist reports, and communications from treating physicians. Subsequently, the CRFs were subjected to a review by a medical specialist for coherence, completeness, and accuracy.

The present analysis encompasses individuals aged 18 years and above who underwent iVAC2L during HR-PCIs for coronary artery disease, and excludes procedures driven by indications other than HR-PCIs, as well as cases of acute extra-cardiac disease. The data were anonymized at the time of collection and remained anonymous throughout the analysis. HR-PCI was defined as any percutaneous intervention for coronary disease involving an unusually high risk of periprocedural circulatory collapse, as determined by the treating physician.

Clinical Endpoints. The data were collected retrospectively. The adjudication of events was conducted by the attending physicians in accordance with the prevailing standards of practice at the local level. The primary endpoint was all-cause in-hospital mortality. Secondary endpoints included major adverse cardiovascular events (MACEs), major vascular complications, major bleeding, acute kidney injury (AKI), and the occurrence of severe hypotension while on circulatory support. The composite endpoint of MACE was defined as the occurrence of in-hospital all-cause mortality, cerebrovascular event, acute myocardial infarction (AMI), and repeat revascularization. Severe hypotension was defined as a mean arterial pressure (MAP) of less than 60 mmHg for a minimum of 10 min or the presence of shock of any etiology. A major vascular complication was defined as a clinically significant vascular injury, bleeding, or limb ischemia. All other endpoints were adjudicated at the local level by local teams using local standards of practice and definitions.

Statistical Analysis. Continuous data are presented as either mean ± SD or median (25th–75th quartiles), as appropriate. Categorical data are presented as frequencies and percentages. The results of the study include a description of the subjects' baseline characteristics, procedural data, and clinical endpoints. Baseline and procedural data are presented for descriptive purposes, and no statistical tests were performed. The hemodynamic data were analyzed utilizing either Student's *t*-test for paired samples or the Wilcoxon signed-rank test for paired samples, depending on the statistical distribution. The Bonferroni correction was employed to account for multiplicity. To investigate the major factors associated with severe hypotension and in-hospital MACE, uni- and multivariate logistic regressions were conducted. For the multivariate analyses, stepwise backward and forward selections were employed. The data were collected and stored using Microsoft Excel 2019 (Microsoft Corporation, Redmond, WA, USA), and the analysis was performed using the R v4.0.2 statistical package. All statistical tests were based on a two-tailed significance level of 5%.

3. Results

A total of 302 consecutive patients received iVAC2L during high-risk cardiovascular procedures in 37 countries between November 2013 and October 2023 (Figures 1 and 2). Of the aforementioned patients, seven were excluded from the analysis due to indications other than HR-PCI, and one due to the lack of clinical outcomes. In-hospital outcomes were ascertainable in 99.7% of cases ($n = 293$).

The baseline demographic and procedural characteristics are presented in Table 1; Table 2, respectively. The median age was 71 years (range: 64–77 years), and 85% of the participants were male. The ejection fraction (EF) was 30% (25–40%), and the SYNTAX score was 33 (28–40). The majority of patients exhibited moderate to severe symptoms of heart failure, with 71% classified as NYHA class III or IV. Additionally, 50% of the cohort was deemed ineligible for CABG. A history of acute myocardial infarction (AMI) was present in 53% of the cohort, while renal insufficiency, previous cerebrovascular events, and peripheral arterial disease were also common.

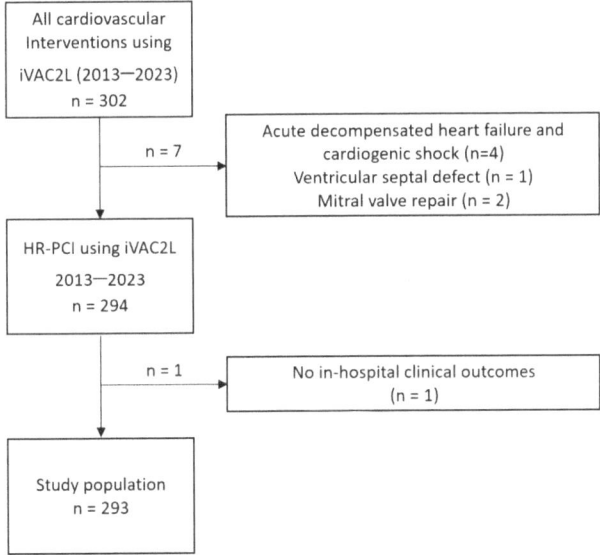

Figure 1. Study flowchart. HR-PCI: high-risk percutaneous coronary intervention.

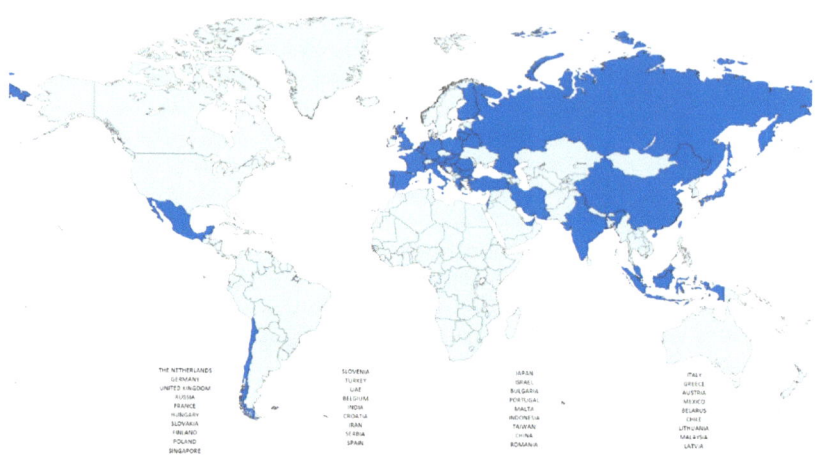

Figure 2. Countries whose centers provided data to the iVAC2L Registry until 2023 (in blue).

Table 1. Baseline demographics, n = 293. Data are presented as mean $\pm$ SD or median (25th to 75th quartiles) as appropriate. Count data are presented as percentages (no. of available observations).

Baseline Characteristics	
Age (years)	71 (64 to 77)
SYNTAX	33 (28 to 40)
EF (%)	30 (25 to 40)
Gender (male) (%)	84.8 (264)
NYHA classification III/IV (%)	71.3 (174)
EF < 40% (%)	69.2 (273)
Hypertension (%)	76.4 (216)
Type II Diabetes (%)	38.5 (218)
Previous Stroke (%)	9.3 (205)
Previous Myocardial Infarction (%)	52.5 (217)
Peripheral Artery Disease (%)	13.9 (216)
Renal Insufficiency (%)	23.3 (219)
Cancer (%)	4.5 (176)
Not surgical candidate (%)	50 (224)
Previous PCI (%)	38.5 (208)
Previous CABG (%)	33.7 (208)
Three-vessel Disease (%)	56.1 (278)
Unprotected Left Main (%)	35.1 (228)
Multivessel Disease (%)	72.3 (285)

Procedural characteristics. Lesions in the left main coronary artery or the left anterior descending artery and its branches were treated in 59% and 71% of cases, respectively. The median duration of the procedure was 67 (45–100) minutes. Rotational atherectomy was employed in 19% of cases. Data on the maximum flow produced by the iVAC2L were available in 63% of cases and were estimated to be 1.6 (1.4–1.7) L/min, with a range of (1.0–2.5) L/min. The MAP at baseline was 80 $\pm$ 17 mmHg, with a systolic blood pressure (SBP) of 117 $\pm$ 24 mmHg.

Table 2. Procedural characteristics, $n = 293$. Data are presented as mean ± SD or median (25th to 75th quartiles) as appropriate. Count data are presented as percentages (no. available observations).

Procedural Characteristics	
Stented LM (%)	59.1 (274)
Stented LAD and branches (%)	70 (249)
Stented LCX and branches (%)	50.8 (252)
Stented RCA and branches (%)	31.9 (254)
Heart Rate (bpm)	71 (63.8 to 80)
SBP (mmHg)	117.3 ± 23.7
DBP (mmHg)	61.3 ± 16.3
MAP (mmHg)	80 ± 16.8
CPO (Watt)	0.75 ± 0.27
CO (L/min)	4.47 ± 1.27
Pump flow (L/min)	1.6 (1.4 to 1.7)
Rotational Atherectomy (%)	19 (183)
Support time (min)	67 (45 to 100)

Clinical Endpoints. A summary of the clinical endpoints is provided in Figures 3 and 4. The incidence of all-cause mortality, cardiovascular events (CVEs), and acute myocardial infarction (AMI) was 1.0%, 1.4%, and 0.7%, respectively. A total of 3.1% of cases resulted in a MACE. Major vascular complications were observed in 2.1% of cases, none of which necessitated urgent cardiac or vascular surgery. Major bleeding was observed in 1.0% of cases. One patient presented with a major bleeding complication that required surgical intervention but succumbed before surgery could be performed. Dislodgement of the iVAC2L occurred in 5% of cases, while the necessity for removal of the iVAC2L (including escalation to alternative devices) was observed in 1.0% of instances. Endotracheal intubation was required in 3.7% of cases. Severe hypotension occurred in 8.9% of cases. Cardio-pulmonary resuscitation (CPR) was necessary in 1.6% of cases. When only elective or semi-elective procedures were selected ($n = 174$), these rates were 3.5% and 1.7%, respectively.

Hemodynamic effects. Findings are shown in Figure 5 and in Supplementary Table S1. Data on heart rate, blood pressure, cardiac output and mPCWP were available in 78%, 76%, 17%, and 17% of all cases, respectively.

Relative to the pre-support state (i.e., baseline), measurements taken with iVAC2L activated showed significant increases in both SBP (117.3, 95%CI: [114.2–120.4] vs. 121.2, 95%CI: [118.2–124.2] mmHg, $p < 0.01$) and DBP (61.3, 95%CI: [59.2–63.5] vs. 63.8, 95%CI: [61.9–65.8] mmHg, $p < 0.01$). The heart rate remained constant (73.4, 95% CI: [71.4–75.4] vs. 74.6, 95% CI: [72.7–76.4] bpm, $p = 0.26$). There was a significant increase in CO (4.47, 95% CI: [4.13–4.81] vs. 4.78, 95% CI: [4.42–5.14] L/min, $p < 0.05$) and CPO (0.74, 95% CI: [0.67–0.82] vs. 0.84, 95% CI: [0.76–0.92] Watts, $p < 0.01$). No alterations were observed in the mPCWP (15.8, 95% CI: [13.6–18.1] vs. 17.1, 95% CI: [14.7–19.6] mmHg, $p = 0.14$) when assessed in the entire cohort.

In patients who received inotropes and/or vasopressors at any point ($n = 27, 9.2\%$), cardiac output (CO), blood pressure, and heart rate remained unaltered. However, CPO increased numerically in this subgroup from 0.75 (95% CI: [0.52, 0.99]) vs. 0.9 (95% CI: [0.68, 1.13]) Watts, $p = 0.37$. Additionally, mPCWP demonstrated a non-significant trend toward a decrease from 28.8 (95% CI: [24.4, 33.1]) vs. 20.3 (95% CI: 16.4, 24.3) mmHg, $p = 0.08$.

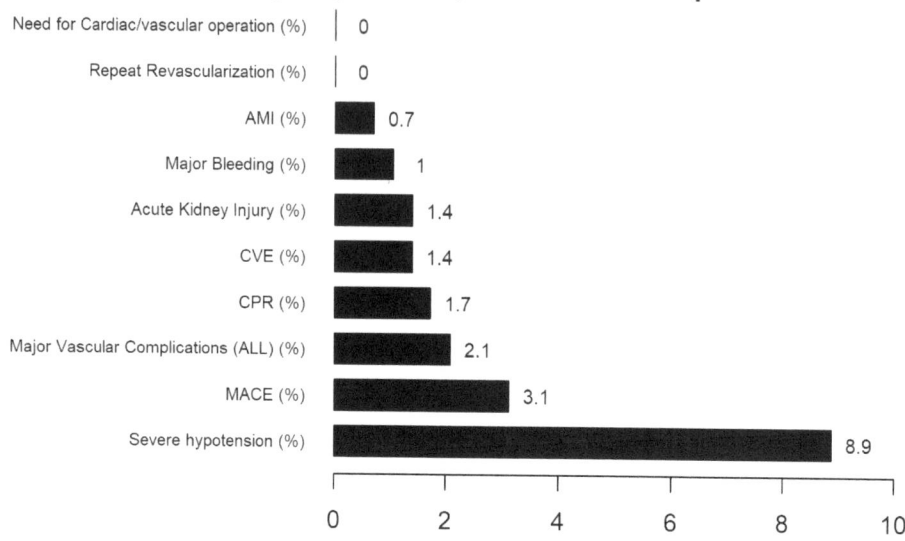

Figure 3. In-hospital clinical outcomes from the iVAC2L Registry. MACE: Major Adverse Cardiovascular Event. AMI: Acute Myocardial Infarction. CVE: Cerebrovascular Event. CPR: Cardiopulmonary Resuscitation.

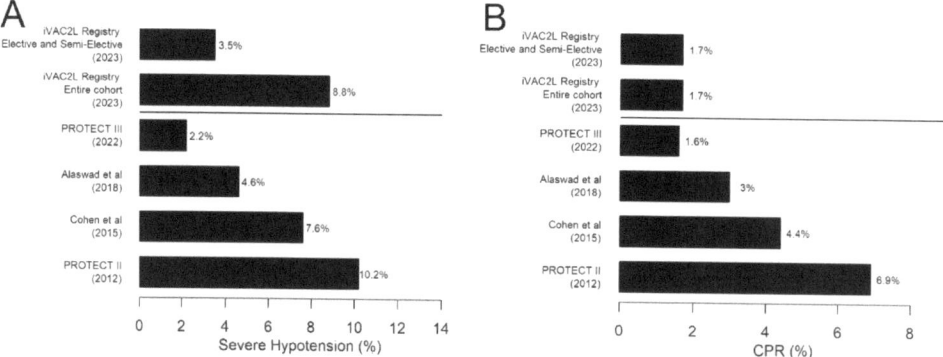

Figure 4. (**A**) Rates of severe hypotension found in the most relevant studies on the use of short-term mechanical circulatory support in high-risk PCI. (**B**) Rates of CPR found in the most relevant studies on the use of short-term mechanical circulatory support in high-risk PCI [3,6,7]. CPR: Cardiopulmonary Resuscitation.

Independent predictors of severe hypotension were Emergent Case and Endotracheal Intubation. Previous MI and a pre-procedural SBP > 100 mmHg were non-significantly related (AUC: 0.80). Independent predictors of in-hospital MACE were Multivessel PCI, Male Gender, Pre-support MAP > 80 mmHg, Hypertension, and Vasoactive Drugs, AUC = 0.89 (Figure 6).

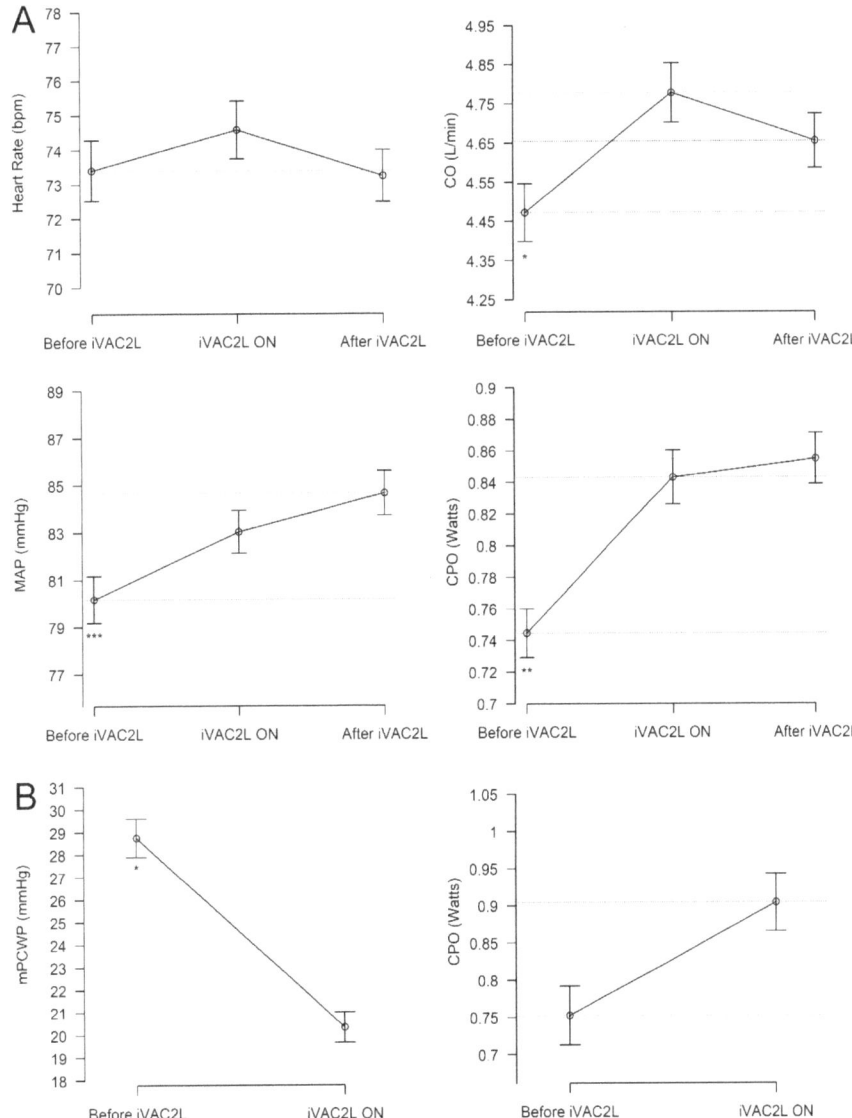

Figure 5. (**A**) Hemodynamic changes obtained with the activation of iVAC2L showing improvements in blood pressure, CO, and CPO. (**B**) Hemodynamic measurements taken before implementation of iVAC2L and during support. Data are presented as mean ± SE. p-values derive from t-tests or Wilcoxon's test for paired samples. * $p < 0.05$; ** $p < 0.01$; *** $p < 0.01$ compared to "iVAC 2L ON". CO: cardiac output. MAP: mean arterial pressure. CPO: cardiac power output. mPCWP: mean pulmonary capillary wedge pressure.

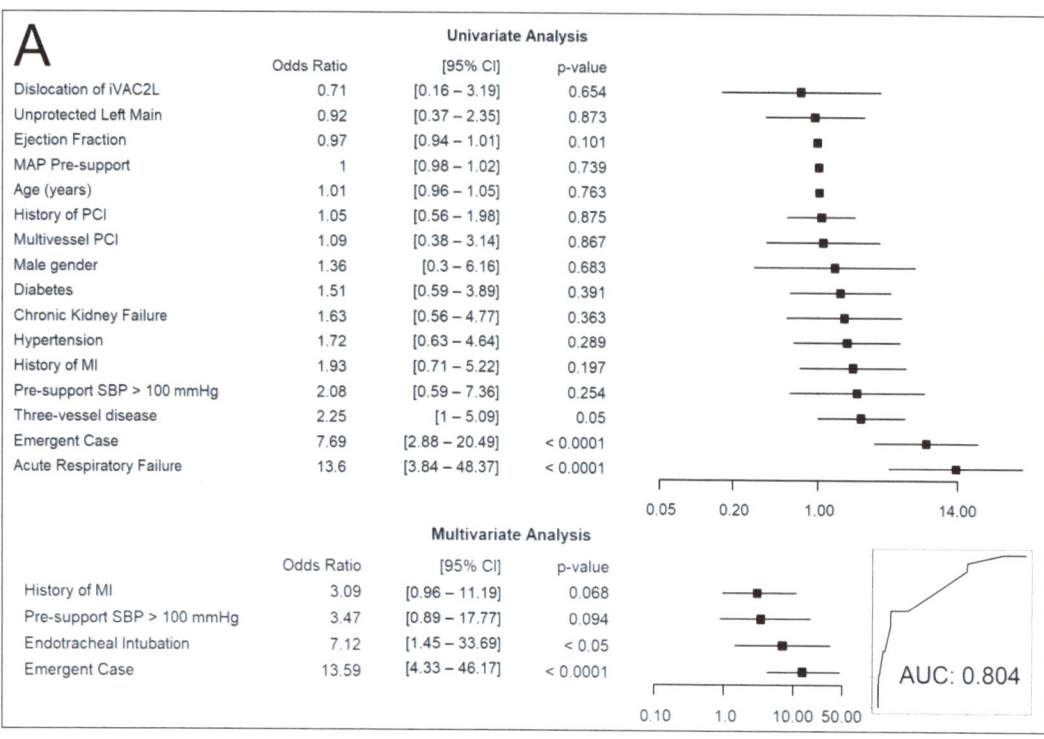
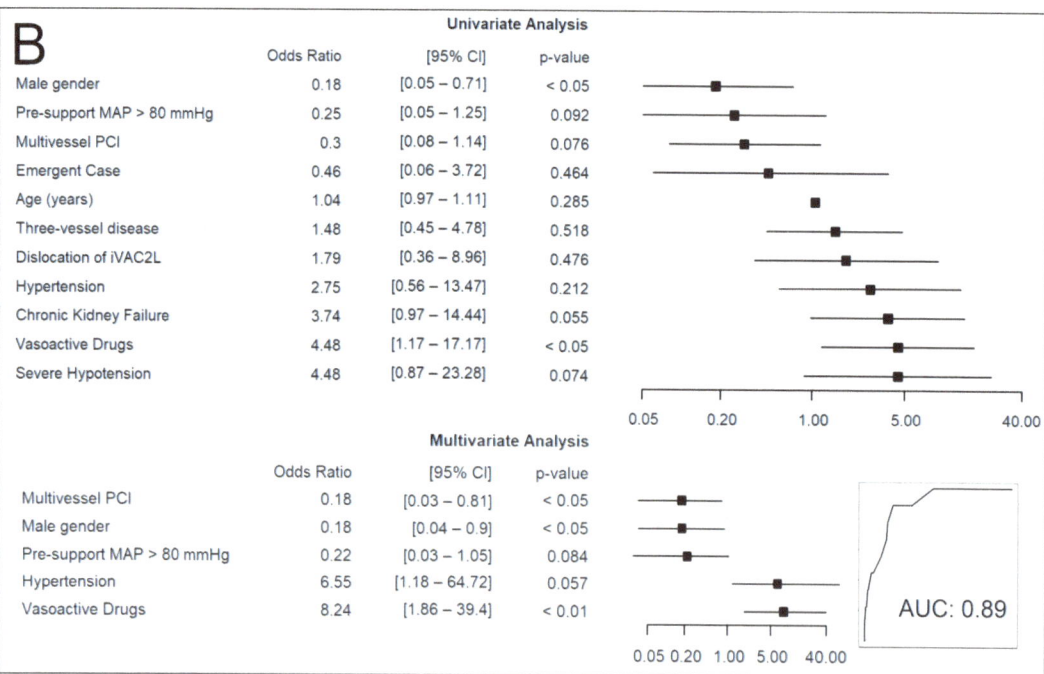

Figure 6. Uni- and multivariate logistic regression analysis: (**A**) predictors of intraprocedural severe hypotension; (**B**) predictors of in-hospital MACE; MACE: Major Adverse Cardiovascular Event. MAP: Mean Arterial Pressure; AUC: Area Under the Curve; PCI: Percutaneous Coronary Intervention.

4. Discussion

This study represents the most comprehensive compilation of clinical data on HR-PCI using PulseCath iVAC2L since the device received CE Mark approval in 2014. The in-hospital mortality rate was 1%, and the MACE rate was 3.1%. The findings also demonstrate beneficial effects on the systemic circulation, and the large sample size lends representativeness to real-world practice.

4.1. Previous Evidence on the iVAC2L

Since 2015, three prospective cohorts have been published, all in the context of elective HR-PCIs. Den Uil et al. reported hemodynamic improvements in elective HR-PCIs with no major adverse events. Samol et al. described that both iVAC2L and Impella 2.5 significantly increased the MAP, but Impella 2.5 precipitated hemolysis. The PULSE trial showed a 14% reduction in the metabolic demands, a 33% reduction in the native heart's cardiac output, and a 17% increase in the MAP [5]. The iVAC2L may be an alternative when there is a need for an LVAD that is less associated with hemolysis than a CFD or when there is great concern regarding the possibility of iatrogenic valvular damage that could precipitate circulatory collapse [8]. It may also be a more feasible alternative in hospitals where other percutaneous MCS devices are not yet reimbursed.

4.2. Study Findings

The output flow of the iVAC2L ranged between 1.0 and 2.5 L/min. This can be up to four times that of the IABP, approaching the output flow of Impella 2.5 (1.9 ± 0.27 L/min). It remains lower than that of the Impella CP (2.8 ± 0.4 L/min at P8), though [5,6,9].

The intraprocedural incidence of severe hypotension was 8.9%, which is lower than the rate observed in the Impella arm of the PROTECT II trial (10.2%) [3]. The PROTECT II evaluated the effects of Impella 2.5 versus IABP in elective HR-PCIs and remains the largest RCT in this population to date. As with the PROTECT II study, the iVAC2L Registry comprised a high-risk cohort with low EF, a high SYNTAX score, a history of frequent revascularization and/or AMI, and a high frequency of rotational atherectomy. It should be noted, however, that the registry also includes cases requiring emergent intervention. The odds of developing intraprocedural severe hypotension were 14 times higher in emergent cases compared to non-emergent cases. This parameter was identified as the strongest independent predictor of severe hypotension (Figure 6). In non-emergent cases, the incidence of severe hypotension was 3.5%, which is lower than that observed in elective and semi-elective studies using Impella, namely 7.1% (2015) and 4.6% (2018) [6,7]. While a 2.2% rate was recently reported in 2022 by O'Neill et al., it should be noted that patients in this study were healthier, with a SYNTAX score of 28 versus 31 in PROTECT II and 33 in the iVAC2L Registry. Our findings corroborate those of previous studies which have demonstrated that planned MCS is associated with less hemodynamic instability, which in turn is associated with lower odds of MACEs. Consonantly, previous data shows that non-emergent implantation leads to reduced rates of mortality, CPR, and lesser need for inotropes/vasopressors [10,11].

Activation of iVAC2L resulted in significant increases in MAP, SBP, DBP, CO, and CPO (Figure 5A). mPCWP decreased numerically with the activation of iVAC2L, but only in those receiving vasoactive medications during support. The aforementioned medications, which include vasoactive drugs such as inotropes and vasopressors, can be employed as surrogates for critical decompensated states in the majority of cases (Figure 5B). The observed changes are consistent with those reported in previous studies on the same device. Of particular clinical interest is the observed increase in CPO, as a CPO value below 0.6 Watts has been associated with worse clinical outcomes [12]. However, in the current study, CPO was only reported in 17% of cases, and thus it should be interpreted with caution.

The results demonstrate a reduction in the incidence of CPR episodes with iVAC2L (1.7%) in comparison to the Impella arm of PROTECT II (6.9%). This figure is also lower than the 3% reported by Alaswad et al. for the Impella device. However, it is comparable to the 1.6% reported in the PROTECT III report. Unlike Alaswad et al., PROTECT III predominantly used Impella CP rather than 2.5, suggesting equivalent performance between iVAC2L and Impella CP [3,7]. Although a reduction in mPCWP could only be detected in a critical state, only 3.7% of the total cohort required advanced airways compared to 5% with (mostly) CFDs in a previous study [5]. This may indicate that pulsatile flow (PF) facilitates improved unloading, although the observational design precludes the drawing of causal inferences.

The in-hospital mortality rate following mechanically assisted HR-PCI ranges from 3.2% to 11.5% [13]. The PROTECT II and the cVAD Registry reported in-hospital mortality rates of 4.6% and 3.3%, respectively [3,7]. In contrast, our findings indicate a 1% rate with iVAC2L, which is comparable to the 0.7% observed in the EUROPELLA registry [14]. The two studies exhibited similarities with regard to the frequency of left main stenting, history of CABG, and age distribution. However, the EUROPELLA excluded emergent cases (Supplementary Table S2). Recently, two studies have reported even higher rates of 7.4% with Impella CP and 14% with VA-ECMO, but they had small sample sizes and more complex interventions. While this compromises comparability with larger studies, the rate observed with ECMO is not unexpected, since this modality has been shown to increase mortality, vascular complications, and hemolysis [15–17].

The current analysis reveals a 3.1% incidence of in-hospital MACE which is less than the rates observed in the PROTECT II, PROTECT III, and the cVAD registry (10.2%, 5.4%, and 4.3%, respectively). This may be attributed to the utilization of PF, but also to the technical advancements since 2012. Although the PROTECT III was recently published, it employed rotational atherectomy more frequently, which might provide an explanation to the higher rate of MACE in comparison to iVAC2L [3,9]. Nevertheless, in the iVAC2L Registry, MACE was not determined by rotational atherectomy, but rather by the administration of vasoactive drugs, which are indicative of hemodynamic instability. As in clinical practice, the latter was primarily influenced by the urgency of the intervention. Another predictor of interest was multivessel PCI, a finding that has also been observed in large-scale studies where a more complete revascularization has been associated with superior outcomes. This finding suggests that the benefit observed in the FAME-2 and PROTECT II studies [3,18] at longer time frames may also be applicable in the short term. Moreover, this serves to reinforce the significance of the iVAC2L Registry as a reflection of contemporary clinical practice.

With the exception of CVE, all other clinical outcomes compared favorably with previous large studies (Supplementary Figure S2). Four patients had acute neurological deficits during or after the procedures. Notwithstanding, the observed incidence of stroke is lower than that expected for Impella, which is approximately 2.6% [13].

The use of PF instead of CF may be advantageous for several reasons. CF may reduce or eliminate aortic leaflet motion and coaptation, increasing the risk of acute thrombosis in the ascending aorta. It also decreases sensitivity to catecholamines in the peripheral vasculature and is reported to be less effective in maintaining end-organ perfusion while increasing aortic impedance and systemic vascular resistance [19]. The mechanisms involved include stiffening of the arterial system with obliteration of the Windkessel effect and increased backward propagation of reflected waves. This elevates the afterload and may jeopardize the unloading effect [4,12].

Counter-pulsation as applied by iVAC2L is probably less detrimental to LV afterload and more effective in unloading the LV chamber, resulting in more pronounced reductions in the myocardial metabolic demands. Previous reports have also documented significant reductions in intraventricular dyssynchrony [5,20]. In the peripheral circulation, PF can facilitate blood flow to end organs. It restores cyclic stress and delivers a greater amount of energy to the walls of peripheral vessels in comparison to CF. This has been linked to a reduction in postoperative mortality [4,19–21]. The evidence indicates that PF is more beneficial than CF for vital organ perfusion, as evidenced by studies on the stomach, liver, and kidney [22]. Consonantly, the levels of severe hypotension found in this analysis were remarkably low.

The aforementioned capabilities enhance the resilience of the cardiovascular system to ischemic injury, reducing hemodynamic instability, and consequently facilitating more extensive and meticulous interventions. The RESTORE-EF, PROTECT II, and Roma-Verona studies have demonstrated that patients who received a more complete revascularization exhibited greater improvements in LVEF after 90 days [3,23,24]. Concurrently, a meta-analysis including more than 17,000 individuals indicated that the utilization of intravascular imaging enhanced patient outcomes [25]. Furthermore, the augmented stability provided by MCS permits the broader deployment of hyperemic agents to evaluate lesion significance in patients with markedly impaired LV function, consequently reducing the incidence of repeat interventions [18].

5. Merits and Flaws

The present analysis includes a wide range of hospitals around the world and sheds light on the real-world use of iVAC2L in HR-PCI with focus on safety and efficacy. As in other relevant studies, the study population is characterized by a high-risk profile. The results also demonstrate a high prevalence of left main stenting and rotational atherectomy. Nevertheless, the observational design entails a risk of bias due to its potential for selective reporting, which precludes definitive conclusions on causality. Moreover, despite the lack of consistent follow-up beyond the immediate postoperative period, the initial hours were comprehensively documented. The majority of adverse events (approximately 70%) tend to occur within the first hours during and immediately after the PCI [26]. Therefore, while some limitations in follow-up may influenced the observed rates, this effect is most likely minor in magnitude.

It is not possible to discount the possibility that unmeasured confounders, such as the administration of intravenous fluids or the inherent effects of revascularization, may have influenced the results. Nevertheless, it can be argued that the observed hemodynamic response is consistent with that reported in previous studies [5]. Although arterial blood pressure data were widely available, pulmonary monitoring occurred in only 17% of cases, which limits the generalizability of the findings and reduces the study's power to draw definitive conclusions on the variations observed in CO and CPO. Additionally, the limited availability of angio-CT may have influenced the incidence of vascular complications. In light of these considerations, the present analysis should be regarded as hypothesis-generating only.

6. Future Research

Future research should incorporate more structured designs, such as matched cohorts, to address the limitations of the observational design. This should include the adoption of a prospective design, the incorporation of a clinical events committee, written informed consent, long-term follow-up for up to one year, and electronic centralized data collection. Hemodynamic evaluations should include details on timing relative to stenting, vasoactive drugs, intravenous fluids, and other confounders. In the coming years, the UNLOAD-CHIP trial will measure 30-day mortality or cardiogenic shock in 98 stable high-risk patients with low EF randomized to iVAC2L versus no MCS. The PULSE II trial will assess major adverse events (MAEs) at 90 days in 368 elective high-risk subjects randomized to iVAC2L (PF) or Impella CP (CF). In China, an RCT will investigate the incidence of MACEs at 30 days in 316 stable high-risk patients randomized to iVAC2L or IABP. By 2026, the PROTECT IV (NCT04763200) trial, which compares Impella CP with no MCS, will provide further evidence on CFDs. Additional gaps in knowledge include the impact of intermittent superior vena cava occlusion on the effects of iVAC2L and the impact of iVAC2L on the need for vasoactive drugs.

7. Conclusions

The PulseCath iVAC2L registry demonstrates low rates of in-hospital mortality and MACEs with the use of pulsatile MCS in a real-world setting. This demonstrates its potential to be a safe and effective tool to improve clinical outcomes after complex coronary interventions.

Supplementary Materials: The following supporting information can be downloaded at: https://www.mdpi.com/article/10.3390/jcm13185357/s1, Figure S1: The iVAC2L concept; Figure S2: Rates of in-hospital clinical outcomes; Table S1: Rates of Adverse Events; Table S2: Baseline data; Table S3: Hemodynamic measurements.

Author Contributions: J.B.: Writing—Review and Editing, Investigation. M.B.B.: Conceptualization, Methodology, Software, Validation, Formal Analysis, Investigation, Data curation, Writing original draft, Writing—Review and Editing, Visualization, Project administration, Reporting. O.H.: Writing—Review and Editing, Investigation, Reporting. O.M.: Funding acquisition, Conceptualization, Project administration. T.P.: Writing—Review and Editing, Investigation. M.D.: Writing—Review and Editing, Investigation. R.G.: Writing—Review and Editing, Investigation. All authors have read and agreed to the published version of the manuscript.

Funding: This research was funded by PulseCath BV.

Institutional Review Board Statement: Not applicable (the study is retrospective).

Informed Consent Statement: In order to guarantee strict adherence to the Declaration of Helsinki, it is recommended that operators seek verbal consent from patients regarding their willingness to have their data utilized for research purposes and to provide data only upon confirmation.

Data Availability Statement: Restrictions apply to the availability of these data. Data were obtained from PulseCath BV and are available from the authors with the permission of PulseCath BV.

Conflicts of Interest: Bulum received personal fees from PulseCath BV. Bastos received personal fees from PulseCath BV. Hlinomaz has no relationships relevant to the contents of this paper to disclose. Malkin is an employee of PulseCath BV. Pawlowski received personal fees from PulseCath BV. Dragula has no relationships relevant to the contents of this paper to disclose. Gil has no relationships relevant to the contents of this paper to disclose.

Abbreviations

AKI	Acute kidney injury
AMI	Acute myocardial infarction
CABG	Cardio-pulmonary bypass graft
CAD	Coronary artery disease
CO	Cardiac output
CF	Continuous flow
CFD	Continuous flow device
CPO	Cardiac power output
CVE	Cerebrovascular event
DBP	Diastolic blood pressure
EF	Ejection fraction
HR-PCI	High-risk percutaneous coronary intervention
IABP	Intra-aortic balloon pump
IQR	Interquartile range
LM	Left main
LV	Left ventricle
LVAD	LV assist device
MACE	Major adverse cardiovascular events
MAP	Mean arterial pressure
MCS	Mechanical circulatory support
mPCWP	Mean pulmonary artery wedge pressure
PCI	Percutaneous coronary intervention
PF	Pulsatile flow

RCT	Randomized controlled trial
SBP	Systolic blood pressure
VA-ECMO	Veno-arterial extra-corporeal membrane oxygenation

References

1. Chieffo, A.; Dudek, D.; Hassager, C.; Combes, A.; Gramegna, M.; Halvorsen, S.; Huber, K.; Kunadian, V.; Maly, J.; Møller, J.E.; et al. Joint EAPCI/ACVC expert consensus document on percutaneous ventricular assist devices. *Eur. Heart J. Acute Cardiovasc. Care* 2021, *10*, 570–583. [CrossRef] [PubMed]
2. Maini, B.; Naidu, S.S.; Mulukutla, S.; Kleiman, N.; Schreiber, T.; Wohns, D.; Dixon, S.; Rihal, C.; Dave, R.; O'Neill, W. Real-world use of the Impella 2.5 circulatory support system in complex high-risk percutaneous coronary intervention: The USpella Registry. *Catheter. Cardiovasc. Interv.* 2012, *80*, 717–725. [CrossRef] [PubMed]
3. O'Neill, W.W.; Anderson, M.; Burkhoff, D.; Grines, C.L.; Kapur, N.K.; Lansky, A.J.; Mannino, S.; McCabe, J.M.; Alaswad, K.; Daggubati, R.; et al. Improved outcomes in patients with severely depressed LVEF undergoing percutaneous coronary intervention with contemporary practices. *Am. Heart J.* 2022, *248*, 139–149. [CrossRef]
4. Thohan, V.; Stetson, S.J.; Nagueh, S.F.; Rivas-Gotz, C.; Koerner, M.M.; Lafuente, J.A.; Loebe, M.; Noon, G.P.; Torre-Amione, G. Cellular and hemodynamics responses of failing myocardium to CF mechanical circulatory support using the DeBakey–Noon LV assist device: A comparative analysis with pulsatile-type devices. *J. Heart Lung Transplant.* 2005, *24*, 566–575. [CrossRef]
5. Bastos, M.B.; van Wiechen, M.P.; Van Mieghem, N.M. PulseCath iVAC2L: Next-generation pulsatile mechanical circulatory support. *Future Cardiol.* 2020, *16*, 103–112. [CrossRef]
6. Cohen, M.G.; Matthews, R.; Maini, B.; Dixon, S.; Vetrovec, G.; Wohns, D.; Palacios, I.; Popma, J.; Ohman, E.M.; Schreiber, T.; et al. Percutaneous left ventricular assist device for high-risk percutaneous coronary interventions: Real-world versus clinical trial experience. *Am. Heart J.* 2015, *170*, 872–879. [CrossRef] [PubMed]
7. Alaswad, K.; Basir, M.B.; Khandelwal, A.; Schreiber, T.; Lombardi, W.; O'Neill, W. The Role of Mechanical Circulatory Support During Percutaneous Coronary Intervention in Patients Without Severely Depressed LV Function. *Am. J. Cardiol.* 2018, *121*, 703–708. [CrossRef]
8. Sef, D.; Kabir, T.; Lees, N.J.; Stock, U. Valvular complications following the Impella device implantation. *J. Card. Surg.* 2021, *36*, 1062–1066. [CrossRef]
9. Kapur, N.K.; Alkhouli, M.A.; DeMartini, T.J.; Faraz, H.; George, Z.H.; Goodwin, M.J.; Hernandez-Montfort, J.A.; Iyer, V.S.; Josephy, N.; Kalra, S.; et al. Unloading the Left Ventricle Before Reperfusion in Patients With Anterior ST-Segment-Elevation Myocardial Infarction. *Circulation* 2019, *139*, 337–346. [CrossRef]
10. O'Neill, B.P.; Grines, C.; Moses, J.W.; Ohman, E.M.; Lansky, A.; Popma, J.; Kapur, N.K.; Schreiber, T.; Mann'no, S.; O'Neill, W.W.; et al. Outcomes of bailout percutaneous ventricular assist device versus prophylactic strategy in patients undergoing nonemergent percutaneous coronary intervention. *Catheter. Cardiovasc. Interv.* 2021, *98*, E501–E512. [CrossRef]
11. Chieffo, A.; Ancona, M.B.; Burzotta, F.; Pazzanese, V.; Briguori, C.; Trani, C.; Piva, T.; De Marco, F.; Di Biasi, M.; Pagnotta, P.; et al. Observational multicentre registry of patients treated with IMPella mechanical circulatory support device in ITaly: The IMP-IT registry. *EuroIntervention* 2020, *15*, e1343–e1350. [CrossRef] [PubMed]
12. Burkhoff, D.; Naidu, S.S. The science behind percutaneous hemodynamic support: A review and comparison of support strategies. *Catheter. Cardiovasc. Interv.* 2012, *80*, 816–829. [CrossRef] [PubMed]
13. Elia, E.; Iannaccone, M.; D'Ascenzo, F.; Gallone, G.; Colombo, F.; Albani, S.; Attisani, M.; Rinaldi, M.; Boccuzzi, G.; Conrotto, F.; et al. Short term outcomes of Impella circulatory support for high-risk percutaneous coronary intervention a systematic review and meta-analysis. *Catheter. Cardiovasc. Interv.* 2022, *99*, 27–36. [CrossRef] [PubMed]
14. Sjauw, K.D.; Konorza, T.; Erbel, R.; Danna, P.L.; Viecca, M.; Minden, H.H.; Butter, C.; Engstrøm, T.; Hassager, C.; Machado, F.P.; et al. Supported high-risk percutaneous coronary intervention with the Impella 2.5 device the Europella registry. *J. Am. Coll. Cardiol.* 2009, *54*, 2430–2434. [CrossRef]
15. Van den Buijs, D.M.F.; Wilgenhof, A.; Knaapen, P.; Zivelonghi, C.; Meijers, T.; Vermeersch, P.; Arslan, F.; Verouden, N.; Nap, A.; Sjauw, K.; et al. Prophylactic Impella CP versus VA-ECMO in Patients Undergoing Complex High-Risk Indicated PCI. *J. Interv. Cardiol.* 2022, *2022*, 8167011. [CrossRef]
16. Griffioen, A.M.; Van Den Oord, S.C.H.; Van Wely, M.H.; Swart, G.C.; Van Wetten, H.B.; Danse, P.W.; Damman, P.; Van Royen, N.; Van Geuns, R.J.M. Short-Term Outcomes of Elective High-Risk PCI with Extracorporeal Membrane Oxygenation Support: A Single-Center Registry. *J. Interv. Cardiol.* 2022, *2022*, 7245384. [CrossRef]
17. Eckman, P.M.; Katz, J.N.; El Banayosy, A.; Bohula, E.A.; Sun, B.; van Diepen, S. Veno-Arterial Extracorporeal Membrane Oxygenation for Cardiogenic Shock: An Introduction for the Busy Clinician. *Circulation* 2019, *140*, 2019–2037. [CrossRef]
18. Fearon, W.F.; Nishi, T.; De Bruyne, B.; Boothroyd, D.B.; Barbato, E.; Tonino, P.; Jüni, P.; Pijls, N.H.J.; Hlatky, M.A.; FAME 2 Trial Investigators. Clinical outcomes and cost-effectiveness of fractional flow reserve-guided percutaneous coronary intervention in patients with stable coronary artery disease. *Circulation* 2018, *137*, 480–487. [CrossRef]
19. Travis, A.R.; Giridharan, G.A.; Pantalos, G.M.; Dowling, R.D.; Prabhu, S.D.; Slaughter, M.S.; Sobieski, M.; Undar, A.; Farrar, D.J.; Koenig, S.C. Vascular pulsatility in patients with a pulsatile- or continuous-flow ventricular assist device. *J. Thorac. Cardiovasc. Surg.* 2007, *133*, 517–524. [CrossRef]

20. Undar, A. Energy equivalent pressure formula is for precise quantification of different perfusion modes. *Ann. Thorac. Surg.* **2003**, *76*, 1777–1778. [CrossRef]
21. Ji, B.; Undar, A. An evaluation of the benefits of pulsatile versus nonpulsatile perfusion during cardiopulmonary bypass procedures in pediatric and adult cardiac patients. *ASAIO J.* **2006**, *52*, 357–361. [CrossRef] [PubMed]
22. Orime, Y.; Shiono, M.; Nakata, K.I.; Hata, M.; Sezai, A.; Yamada, H.; Iida, M.; Kashiwazaki, S.; Nemoto, M.; Kinoshita, J.I.; et al. The role of pulsatility in end-organ microcirculation after cardiogenic shock. *ASAIO J.* **1996**, *42*, M724–M729. [CrossRef] [PubMed]
23. Wollmuth, J.; Patel, M.P.; Dahle, T.; Bharadwaj, A.; Waggoner, T.E.; Chambers, J.W.; Ruiz-Rodriguez, E.; Mahmud, E.; Thompson, C.; Morris, D.L.; et al. Ejection fraction improvement following contemporary high-risk percutaneous coronary intervention: RESTORE EF study results. *J. Soc. Cardiovasc. Angiogr. Interv.* **2022**, *1*, 100350. [CrossRef] [PubMed]
24. Burzotta, F.; Russo, G.; Ribichini, F.; Piccoli, A.; D'Amario, D.; Paraggio, L.; Previ, L.; Pesarini, G.; Porto, I.; Leone, A.M.; et al. Long-term outcomes of extent of revascularization in complex high risk and indicated patients undergoing Impella-protected percutaneous coronary intervention: Report from the Roma-Verona registry. *J. Interv. Cardiol.* **2019**, *2019*, 5243913. [CrossRef] [PubMed]
25. Buccheri, S.; Franchina, G.; Romano, S.; Puglisi, S.; Venuti Ge D'Arrigo, P.; Francaviglia, B.; Scalia, M.; Condorelli, A.; Barbanti, M.; Capranzano, P.; et al. Clinical outcomes following intravascular imaging-guided versus coronary angiography-guided percutaneous coronary intervention with stent implantation: A systematic review and Bayesian network meta-analysis of 31 studies and 17,882 patients. *JACC Cardiovasc. Interv.* **2017**, *10*, 2488–2498. [CrossRef]
26. Thel, M.C.; Califf, R.M.; Tardiff, B.E.; Gardner, L.H.; Sigmon, K.N.; Lincoff, A.M.; Topol, E.J.; Kitt, M.M.; Blankenship, J.C.; Tcheng, J.E. Timing of and risk factors for myocardial ischemic events after percutaneous coronary intervention (IMPACT-II). Integrilin to Minimize Platelet Aggregation and Coronary Thrombosis. *Am. J. Cardiol.* **2000**, *85*, 427–434. [CrossRef]

Disclaimer/Publisher's Note: The statements, opinions and data contained in all publications are solely those of the individual author(s) and contributor(s) and not of MDPI and/or the editor(s). MDPI and/or the editor(s) disclaim responsibility for any injury to people or property resulting from any ideas, methods, instructions or products referred to in the content.

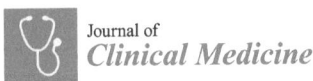

Article

Clinical Outcomes of Cardiac Transplantation in Heart Failure Patients with Previous Mechanical Cardiocirculatory Support

Michele D'Alonzo [1,*], Amedeo Terzi [2], Massimo Baudo [3], Mauro Ronzoni [1], Nicola Uricchio [2], Claudio Muneretto [1] and Lorenzo Di Bacco [1]

1. Cardiac Surgery Unit, Spedali Civili, University of Brescia, 25124 Brescia, Italy; m.ronzoni001@unibs.it (M.R.); cmuneretto@unibs.it (C.M.); lorenzo.dibacco@hotmail.it (L.D.B.)
2. Cardiac Surgery Unit, ASST Papa Giovanni XXIII, 24127 Bergamo, Italy; aterzi@asst-pg23.it (A.T.); nuricchio@asst-pg23.it (N.U.)
3. Department of Cardiac Surgery Research, Lankenau Institute for Medical Research, Main Line Health, Wynnewood, PA 19096, USA; massimo.baudo@icloud.com
* Correspondence: dalonzomi@gmail.com; Tel.: +39-3466316530

Abstract: Objectives: Heart failure (HF) remains a significant public health issue, with heart transplantation (HT) being the gold standard treatment for end-stage HF. The increasing use of mechanical circulatory support, particularly left ventricular assist devices (LVADs), as a bridge to transplant (BTT), presents new perspectives for increasingly complex clinical scenarios. This study aimed to compare long-term clinical outcomes in patients in heart failure with reduced ejection fraction (HFrEF) receiving an LVAD as BTT to those undergoing direct-to-transplant (DTT) without mechanical support, focusing on survival and post-transplant complications. **Methods:** A retrospective, single-center study included 105 patients who underwent HT from 2010. Patients were divided into two groups: BTT (n = 28) and DTT (n = 77). Primary endpoints included overall survival at 1 and 7 years post-HT. Secondary outcomes involved late complications, including organ rejection, renal failure, cardiac allograft vasculopathy (CAV), and cerebrovascular events. **Results:** At HT, the use of LVADs results in longer cardiopulmonary bypass and cross-clamping times in the BTT group; nevertheless, surgical complexity does not affect 30-day mortality. Survival at 1 year was 89.3% for BTT and 85.7% for DTT ($p = 0.745$), while at 7 years, it was 80.8% and 77.1%, respectively ($p = 0.840$). No significant differences were observed in the incidence of major complications, including permanent dialysis, organ rejection, and CAV. However, a higher incidence of cerebrovascular events was noted in the BTT group (10.7% vs. 2.6%). **Conclusions:** LVAD use as BTT does not negatively impact early post-transplant survival compared to DTT. At long-term follow-up, clinical outcomes remained similar across groups, supporting LVADs as a viable option for bridging patients to transplant.

Keywords: ventricular assist device; bridge to transplant; heart failure; heart transplantation

1. Introduction

The prevalence of heart failure (HF) is steadily rising in both genders, with a particular increase observed in the elderly cohorts of populations, a trend in part attributable to advancements in medical treatment and improved survival rates [1]. For patients with end-stage HF, refractory to medical treatment, heart transplantation (HT) remains to date the gold standard of care. Nevertheless, the limited availability of donor organs has resulted in a significant increase in the utilization and development of mechanical circulatory support

(MCS), such as left ventricular assist devices (LVADs), as a bridge to transplant (BTT) or bridge to candidacy (BTC) [2]. The widespread use of LVADs as a bridge to heart transplantation has improved survival rates for patients awaiting donor organs and has also enabled many candidates to endure extended waiting periods [3,4].

Although the therapeutic benefits of LVAD implantation are well documented [5], they are also associated with several complications, including gastrointestinal bleeding, neurological events, infection, pump thrombosis, and right ventricular failure [6,7]. Recent studies have also highlighted some negative effects of long-term LVADs on organ function, in particular, regarding liver [8] and renal dysfunction [9]. This has brought back into focus a highly controversial topic. It is therefore pivotal to better understand the long-term impact of patients who receive an LVAD as a bridge to HT. Early reports, particularly those that examined the earlier generations of LVADs, suggested that the use of LVADs could adversely affect survival following transplantation [10,11].

However, in the present day, survival outcomes of heart transplantation from durable mechanical circulatory support (MCS) using the latest devices (HeartMate III) are promising [5,12]. A literature review examined 428 papers on this subject, concluding that decreased survival was more likely in patients suffering from dilated cardiomyopathy, patients transplanted within two weeks of LVAD implantation, or patients who underwent BTT prior to 2003 [13]. Indeed, post-transplant outcomes in patients bridged to transplant with temporary mechanical circulatory support devices, like extracorporeal membrane oxygenation, were associated with a higher risk of mortality [14,15]. While the mechanisms underlying these outcomes remain complex, one established finding is that the duration of the LVAD does not have a direct effect on post-transplant survival [16].

More than a decade later, it has become essential to reassess these findings with a broader perspective: advances in technology, including smaller devices, longer battery life, and an improved understanding of the pathophysiology of circulation in patients with LVADs, reinforce the importance of these devices in the management of advanced heart failure without compromising long-term post-transplant outcomes.

This study aims to provide an overview of the long-term outcomes in patients in heart failure with reduced ejection fraction (HFrEF) receiving an LVAD as a bridge to heart transplantation compared to those receiving heart transplantation with medical therapy alone, and to offer insights into the various complications associated with pre-transplant mechanical support.

2. Materials and Methods

2.1. Ethical Statement

A retrospective, observational, single-center study was conducted analyzing clinical outcomes of 105 patients who underwent cardiac transplantation between January 2010 and June 2020 at Hospital "Papa Giovanni XIII" in Bergamo (Italy). Patients gave consent for surgical intervention and for data publication. Ethical review and approval were waived for this study due to the observational and retrospective nature of the study.

2.2. Patient Population

Adult patients (aged $\geq$ 18 years) with ischemic or dilated cardiomyopathy who underwent isolated heart transplantation were included in this study.

Patients with a left ventricular ejection fraction (LVEF) greater than 40% were excluded from the study, limiting the analysis to patients with heart failure with reduced ejection fraction (HFrEF). Patients with heart failure with mid-range ejection fraction (HFmrEF) or preserved ejection fraction (HFpEF) were not considered.

Exclusion criteria were congenital disease, other types of cardiomyopathy, and patients who died before heart transplantation. We analyzed patients who received an LVAD, either as a bridge to transplant (BTT) or bridge to candidacy (BTC), collectively categorized under the BTT group. The analysis included the following devices: HeartMate II (Thoratec Corporation; Pleasanton, CA, USA), HeartWare (Medtronic; Minneapolis, MN, USA), and HeartMate III (Abbott Laboratories; Chicago, IL, USA). Patients in this latter group were compared to those undergoing de novo heart transplantation (direct-to-transplant, DTT). Patients supported with extracorporeal LVADs, right ventricular assist devices, biventricular assist devices, and total artificial hearts were excluded.

2.3. Endpoints and Definitions

Follow-up was conducted up to January 2022 (mean follow-up was: 5.76 ± 3.8 years). The primary outcome of interest was overall survival at 1 and at 7 years. The secondary outcomes included the occurrence of adverse events during follow-up. Adverse events were defined as significant arrhythmias, cerebrovascular events (excluding those occurring before or during heart transplantation), renal failure (eGFR < 30 mL/min) or the need for permanent dialysis, organ rejection, and cardiac allograft vasculopathy (CAV), according to relative International Society for Heart and Lung Transplantation (ISHLT) classifications [17,18].

2.4. Data Collection and Follow-Up Protocols

Patients' clinical data and parameters were evaluated at four specific time-points:

- Baseline before HT: physical characteristics, assessment of clinical, history, heart failure etiology, echocardiographic, hemodynamic, and biochemical data of patients at the time of heart transplantation.
- LVAD-related complications between device implantation and heart transplantation (only for BTT group).
- Surgical data, early mortality (at 30-day), and morbidity during hospitalization, for heart transplantation.
- Evaluation of transplant-related complications by phone interview or direct clinical examination, at the last FU.

All patients underwent HT with bicaval anastomosis. All patients received antirejection therapy with calcineurin inhibitors, cyclosporine or tacrolimus, mycophenolate mofetil, and prednisone according to the hospital protocols. Endo-myocardial biopsies (EMBs) were performed at 1 year, to determine the occurrence of rejection, according to hospital protocols (one biopsy every week in the first month, one biopsy every two weeks until the third month, one biopsy every month until the sixth month, and one biopsy every two months until the twelfth month; after one year, no routine EMBs were performed if no clinical suspicion of rejection was present): biopsy classification followed the revised International Society for Heart and Lung Transplantation (ISHLT) staging classification [17].

To assess the presence of CAV, coronarography was scheduled at 3 and 5 years after transplantation, then every 5 years or following clinical suspicion. The grade of CAV was assessed using the ISHLT classification [18].

2.5. Statistical Analysis

The distribution of variables was evaluated using the Kolmogorov–Smirnov 1-sample test. Continuous variables were presented as mean ± standard deviation (SD) for variables with a normal distribution or as median (1st and 3rd interquartile) for data without Gaussian distribution. Categorical variables were expressed as absolute number of frequency (percentages). Independent t-tests were used to compare normally distributed data. For data without normal distribution, the Mann–Whitney test for unpaired continuous variables was used. The chi-square test was used to compare categorical data, and Fisher's exact test was used when the minimum cell size requirements for the chi-square test were not met. Kaplan–Meier estimates were used to assess long-term post-transplantation survival. Microsoft Office Excel (Microsoft, Redmond, WA, USA) was used for data extraction, and all analyses were performed in R, version 4.3.1 (R Software for Statistical Computing, Vienna, Austria) within RStudio. The R packages used were "survival", "survminer", "dplyr", and "ggplot2".

3. Results

Seventy-seven (n = 77) patients were in the DTT group, while twenty-eight patients were in the BTT group. Table 1 shows the baseline differences between the two groups. The BTT group had a higher BMI (26.4 ± 5.0 kg/m^2 vs. 23.1 ± 3.9, $p < 0.05$) with a lower percentage of patients with atrial fibrillation (n = 1, 3.6% vs. 20, 26.0%, $p = 0.004$). General comorbidities, such as liver and kidney function status, were comparable between the groups. The etiology of heart failure was balanced, with 50% of each group affected by ischemic heart disease and the other 50% by dilated cardiomyopathy ($p = 0.953$).

Table 1. Baseline characteristics before heart transplantation.

	BTT (n = 28)	DTT (n = 77)	p Value
Age, years	54 (43–58)	53 (42–49)	0.954
Gender, male	25 (89.3)	65 (84.4)	0.528
BMI, Kg/m^2	26.4 ± 5.0	23.1 ± 3.9	0.001
Etiology			0.953
ICM	14 (50.0)	39 (50.6)	
DCM	14 (50.0)	38 (49.4)	
Atrial fibrillation	1 (3.6)	20 (26.0)	0.004
Chronic dialysis	1 (3.6)	2 (2.6)	0.999
Hemodynamic status			
LVEF, %	24 (20–26)	20 (18–25)	0.137
sPAP, mmHg	41.8 ± 18.4	40.2 ± 15.4	0.686
Wedge, mmHg	18.5 ± 8.8	19.8 ± 9.3	0.561
CO, L	4.1 ± 1.0	3.5 ± 1.1	0.031
CI, L/m^2	2.0 (1.8–2.6)	1.9 (1.6–2.1)	0.128
PVR, WU	2.2 (1.4–2.9)	2.4 (1.5–3.3)	0.291
Laboratory			
Creatinine, mg/dL	1.1 ± 0.3	1.2 ± 0.4	0.392
Total bilirubin, mg/dL	1.1 ± 0.8	1.4 ± 1.8	0.349

BTT: bridge to transplant; CI: cardiac index; DCM: dilatative cardiomyopathy; ICM: ischemic cardiomyopathy; CO: cardiac output; DTT: direct-to-transplant; LVEF: left ventricular ejection fraction; PVR: pulmonary vascular resistance; sPAP: systolic pulmonary artery pression.

3.1. LVAD Population

The BTT population included 28 patients (mean age: 48.5 ± 11.4 years). Considering the broad recruitment period of the study (January 2010 to June 2020) and the availability of devices, 21 patients (75%) received a HeartWare implant, which was the most used LVAD, 3 patients (10.7%) received a HeartMate II, and 4 patients (14.3%) received a HeartMate III. The bridge-to-transplant duration was 554 ± 346 days, during which the complications outlined in Table 2 were recorded. It was not possible to trace patients who had LVAD implantation but were not transplanted for various reasons (death, refusal to transplant, transplantation to another hospital center, off transplant list).

Table 2. BTT details.

	BTT (n = 28)
Age at LVAD implant, years	48.5 ± 11.4
Implantable device	
HeartMate II	3 (10.7)
HeartMate III	4 (14.3)
HeartWare	21 (75.0)
Period of bridge, days (mean ± SD)	554 ± 346
Period of bridge, days (range)	(26–1559)
Complications	
Readmission for HF, n (%)	5 (17.9)
GI bleeding, n (%)	8 (28.6)
Cerebrovascular events, n (%)	11 (39.3)
Arrhythmias, n (%)	6 (21.4)
LVAD-related infection, n (%)	17 (60.7)

BTT: bridge to transplant; GI: gastrointestinal; LVAD: left ventricular assist device.

3.2. Heart Transplantation Hospitalization

Data at the time of hospitalization for heart transplantation are depicted in Table 3. Aortic cross-clamp and cardiopulmonary bypass times were longer in the BTT group, without impact on in-hospital mortality between the two groups, BTT: one patient (3.6%) vs. DTT: four patients (5.2%) ($p = 0.999$).

Table 3. Operative data and early outcomes after heart transplantation.

	BTT (n = 28)	DTT (n = 77)	p Value
CPB time, minutes	217.7 ± 58.3	146.2 ± 53.3	0.001
CC time, minutes	113.9 ± 29.4	79.3 ± 15.6	0.001
Bleeding requiring SR	4 (14.3)	7 (9.1)	0.442
Cerebrovascular events, n (%)	3 (10.7)	1 (1.3)	0.057
Hemodialysis, n (%)	13 (46.4)	39 (50.6)	0.702
Acute rejection, n (%)	2 (7.1)	9 (11.7)	0.723
ECMO, n (%)	7 (25.0)	22 (28.6)	0.717
Length of hospital stay, days	23 (20–28)	22 (20–27)	0.875
Hospital mortality, n (%)	1 (3.6)	4 (5.2)	0.999

BTT: bridge to transplant; CC: cross-clamping; CPB: cardiopulmonary bypass; DTT: direct-to-transplant; ECMO: Extra Corporeal Membrane Oxygenation.

A higher percentage of perioperative cerebrovascular events was observed in the BTT group: three patients, 10.7% vs. DTT: one patient, 1.3% ($p = 0.057$). No significant differences were observed in the incidence of various complications: acute organ rejection ($p = 0.723$), bleeding requiring surgery ($p = 0.442$), dialysis ($p = 0.702$), or ECMO ($p = 0.717$).

3.3. Primary Endpoint

Survival at 1 and at 7 years is shown in Figure 1. Of the 105 patients undergoing HT, 101 (96.2%) patients completed at 1-year FU. When stratified by surgical strategy for HT, there was no significant difference in terms of 1-year survival (BTT 89.3 ± 11.4% vs. DTT 85.7 ± 7.8%; $p = 0.745$). At 7-year follow-up, the survival rate was 80.8 ± 15.3% for the BTT group and 77.1 ± 9.6% for the DTT group ($p = 0.840$).

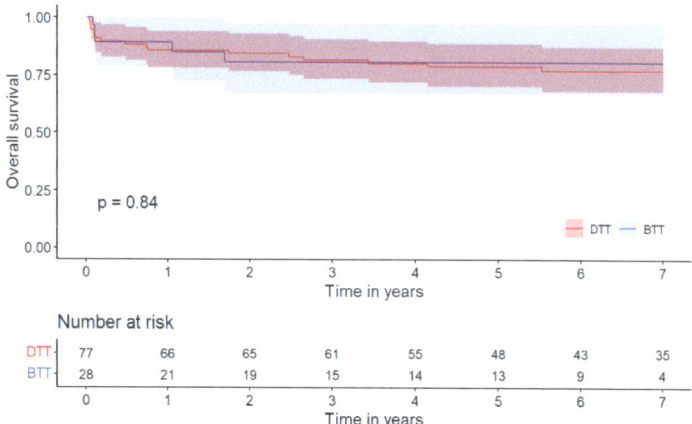

Figure 1. Kaplan–Meier curves for all-cause mortality in patients who underwent heart transplantation. DTT: direct-to-transplantation; BTT: bridge to transplantation.

3.4. Secondary Endpoints

The secondary outcomes during follow-up are depicted in Table 4. When considering cumulative arrhythmias (permanent atrial fibrillation, permanent pacemaker, or defibrillator), no significant differences were observed between the two groups ($p = 0.999$). Similarly, the incidence of cardiac allograft vasculopathy was comparable, with 14.2% in the BTT group and 18.2% in the DTT group ($p = 0.775$). A trend toward a higher incidence of postoperative cerebrovascular events was observed in the BTT group (10.7% vs. 2.6%, $p = 0.117$), while there was a greater need for dialysis in the DTT group (14.3% vs. 3.6%, $p = 0.175$). Regarding overall cardiac organ rejection, approximately one-quarter of patients in each group experienced this adverse event, with no statistically significant difference ($p = 0.644$); even when considering the more severe grades (grade IIIA and grade IIIB), no statistically significant difference was found.

Table 4. Secondary outcomes at last follow-up.

	BTT (n = 28)	DTT (n = 77)	p Value
Permanent AF/PM/ICD	3 (10.7)	8 (10.4)	0.999
Cerebrovascular events *	3 (10.7)	2 (2.6)	0.117
CAV	4 (14.2)	14 (18.2)	0.775
Grade I	2	10	
Grade II	0	3	
Grade III	2	1	
eGFR < 30 mL/min	4 (14.2)	18 (23.4)	0.420
Permanent dialysis	1 (3.6)	11 (14.3)	0.175
Organ rejection	21 (75.0)	61 (79.2)	0.644
Grade 1R	16	57	
Grade 2R	4	3	
Grade 3R	1	1	

AF: atrial fibrillation; BTT: bridge to transplant; CC: cross-clamping; CAV: cardiac allograft vasculopathy; DTT: direct-to-transplant; eGFR: estimated Glomerular Filtration Rate; ICD: Implantable Cardioverter-Defibrillator; PM: pacemaker; * previous cerebrovascular events were excluded.

4. Discussion

This study presents an updated analysis of long-term outcomes in patients in heart failure with reduced ejection fraction (HFrEF) undergoing heart transplantation after receiving mechanical circulatory support with a left ventricular assist device (LVAD). The main findings can be summarized as follows:

(I) At the time of heart transplantation, the use of an LVAD introduces technical challenges that result in longer cardiopulmonary bypass and cross-clamping times in the BTT (bridge to transplant) group; nevertheless, the increase in surgical complexity does not affect 30-day mortality.

(II) The overall survival at 1 year was comparable between the two groups, with no significant difference between the BTT and DTT (direct-to-transplant) patients.

(III) At 7 years, survival rates and comorbidities, including post-transplant complications such as cardiac allograft vasculopathy (CAV) and organ rejection, were similar between both groups.

(IV) Adverse neurological events (composite of TIA/stroke) occurred in 39.6% of patients during the BTT phase, indicating a concern on neurological risk mechanical support.

Heart transplantation is considered the gold standard treatment for patients with advanced heart failure [2]. However, nowadays, there is a trend toward the increasing use of LVADs as a bridge-to-transplant (BTT) or bridge-to-candidacy (BTC) solution. This phenomenon is mostly attributable to the increased number of patients with non-persistent contraindications to HT and the scarcity of heart organ donors [19,20]. Mechanical circulatory support gives patients a chance to reach the state of candidacy or transplant, but the surgical implications related to LVAD implantation should not be overlooked. Heart transplant surgical time tends to be longer for those patients, because of adhesions of previous cardiac surgery and LVAD removal, making surgery more technically demanding. The present study showed that the average aortic cross-clamp (ACC) and cardiopulmonary bypass (CPB) time were, respectively, 34.6 and 71.5 min shorter in the DTT group compared to the BTT group. Although the ACC and CPB duration are depicted from the literature as predictors of adverse outcomes, particularly in elective and low-risk procedures, we found no significant difference in early mortality between the two groups despite the significant difference in CPB and ACC times (hospital mortality: 3.6% BTT vs. 5.2% DTT, p: ns). The reported results in the BTT patients are consistent with the results of Fukuhara and colleagues in a cohort of patients with a similar bridge duration [21] with early mortality found to be slightly lower compared to the mortality rates in similar patient subsets reported in other studies, which range from 5% to 10% [15,22]. This finding could be explained by the hemodynamic support provided by LVADs prior to transplantation conferring a higher degree of clinical stability that can mitigate the potential negative impact of longer procedural times. Moreover, we found a 30-day mortality in the BTT group slightly lower than the previous literature in a similar subset of patients ranging from 5 to 10% [15,22]. In this series, the wide use of post-transplant support with ECMO (25% in BTT group and 28.6% in DTT group) might also have contributed to enhancing patients' survival in both groups. Post-transplant ECMO is typically used when the newly transplanted heart struggles to maintain adequate cardiac output due to primary graft dysfunction, rejection, or other complications such as severe pulmonary hypertension. The use of ECMO to unload the heart allowed the transplanted organ and lung to recover [23]. In addition, in this study, 89.3% of patients in the BTT group received a third-generation LVAD, namely HeartWare and HeartMate III, that can provide more benefits and less harm to patients who are waiting for HT [24].

Moreover, 1- and 7-year survival rates were also found to be comparable between the two groups (1-year: BTT 89.3 ± 11.4% vs. DTT 85.7 ± 7.8%; 7-year: BTT 80.8 ± 15.3% vs. DTT 77.1 ± 9.6% (p = 0.840), supporting the conclusion that the use of LVADs as a bridge-to-transplant strategy does not adversely affect early post-transplant survival.

These findings are consistent with the results reported in a French institution by Petroni et al. [25]. Conversely, the same differ from those of Truby et al's. [26] on an American population, where patients who had an LVAD as a bridge to HT experienced higher mortality within the first five years post-transplant. Although the primary outcome of the aforementioned papers is the same, it is crucial to consider the significant differences between the populations considered: Truby's and Petroni's studies included different ethnic groups, while our analysis exclusively involved Caucasian patients; racial differences in the population enrolled may represent an important risk factor for patients' survival. Furthermore, the etiology of heart failure varied considerably across these studies. In our cohort, there was a balance between ischemic and dilated cardiomyopathy, whereas in Petroni's study, ischemic cardiomyopathy accounted for only 32% of cases while Truby's analysis also included congenital heart diseases among the etiologies considered.

A further notable finding in the present study is that no significant differences were observed between the two groups in terms of major complications such as stroke, organ rejection, CAV, and chronic kidney failure. It is noteworthy, as previous authors have highlighted the risk of humoral sensitization in patients with LVAD implantation [12,27], suggesting that they may be more susceptible to graft rejection. In this regard, Arnaoutakis et al. identified a correlation between LVAD use and an increased rate of primary graft dysfunction, yet found no adverse effects on survival [28]. In our study, there was no significant difference in the incidence of any grade of CAV, nor in organ rejection. Petroni's analysis also reported a low morbidity rate among patients who underwent bridge to HT, compared to those who received only medical therapy [25]. This protective effect was attributed to improved systemic perfusion, which helped restore hemodynamic- and reverse kidney-related metabolic and cellular damage prior to HT, thereby also lowering the risk of post-transplant morbidity. The presented data support these findings, as demonstrated by the lower incidence of permanent dialysis (BTT 3.6% vs. DTT 14.3%) and higher eGFR values (Table 4) observed in patients who underwent LVAD implantation.

Despite several studies that attempted to investigate the short- and long-term clinical outcomes of patients treated with LVADs and those who undergo transplantation without bridging, the superiority of BTT over DTT is to date uncertain. The main reason lies in the absence of randomized trials due to the significant complexity of the patients and the limited availability of organs. Moreover, in retrospective registries and analysis, the populations compared are often highly heterogeneous as previously described.

Finally, the drawbacks related to the use of LVADs must be considered. The LVAD-related complications reported in the present study are comparable with the previous literature [29–31], while a higher incidence of neurological events during the BTT phase was reported when compared to previous experiences (39.6% in this analysis versus 8–25% [32,33]). This difference may be related to two factors. Firstly, most studies consider only major strokes (both ischemic and hemorrhagic) while in the present research, TIAs were also included. An additional consideration is that most of the latest studies primarily examine the outcomes of HeartMate devices within the first year, whereas our population had a higher prevalence of HeartWare devices. Notably, the HeartWare device was withdrawn from the market in 2021 due to an increased risk of neurological events and mortality compared to other devices. Moreover, as suggested by Fukuhara, the advantage of mechanical support with an LVAD gives the best results when the bridge period is shorter than 2 years; after this limit, BTT is associated with worse results in terms of survival after HT when compared to DTT and a shorter BTT period [21].

Strengths and Study Limitations

Only patients treated after 2010 were enrolled in this study. In our center, a post-transplant ECMO support protocol was routinely available if necessary as well as the newest anti-rejection protocol and third-generation LVAD devices, and the results of this study align with the results of larger studies on this topic. Furthermore, follow-up was completed in 96.2% of patients at one year, with very few patients lost at longer FU. Nevertheless, the current study has several limitations. It is a retrospective and single-center study; the small sample size was not eligible for multivariate analysis to identify primary endpoint predictive factors. Since this study was not randomized, assessing the superiority of one management over the other was not possible. Therefore, the adjustment of baseline characteristics, which is essential for accurate comparison among groups, was not possible, and consequently, we did not perform advanced statistical analyses such as multivariate analysis. Furthermore, despite the use of different types of LVADs, the results were mainly related to HeartWare implantation (75% of BTT patients). Lastly, we acknowledge as a limitation of this study the exclusion of etiologies other than ischemic and dilated cardiomyopathy.

5. Conclusions

Despite the progress in MCS support, heart transplantation remains the gold standard therapy for patients in heart failure with reduced ejection fraction (HFrEF). The one-year mortality post-transplantation was 13% (10.7% in BTT and 14.3% in DTT), in line with other European studies. Therefore, LVAD implantation as BTT does not increase the risk of mortality following heart transplant, as compared with patients bridged with medical therapy.

Author Contributions: Conceptualization, C.M.; data curation, M.R.; formal analysis, M.D. and M.B.; investigation, M.D. and M.R.; methodology, L.D.B.; supervision, C.M.; validation, A.T. and N.U.; visualization, M.D.; writing—original draft, M.D. and L.D.B.; writing—review and editing, M.B. and N.U. All authors have read and agreed to the published version of the manuscript.

Funding: This research received no external funding.

Institutional Review Board Statement: Ethical review and approval were waived for this study due to the observational and retrospective nature of the study.

Informed Consent Statement: Informed consent was obtained from all subjects involved in the study to publish this paper.

Data Availability Statement: The raw data supporting the conclusions of this article will be made available by the authors on request.

Conflicts of Interest: The authors declare no conflicts of interest.

References

1. Dunlay, S.M.; Roger, V.L.; Killian, J.M.; Weston, S.A.; Schulte, P.J.; Subramaniam, A.V.; Blecker, S.B.; Redfield, M.M. Advanced Heart Failure Epidemiology and Outcomes. *JACC Heart Fail.* **2021**, *9*, 722–732. [CrossRef] [PubMed]
2. McDonagh, T.A.; Metra, M.; Adamo, M.; Gardner, R.S.; Baumbach, A.; Böhm, M.; Burri, H.; Butler, J.; Čelutkienė, J.; Chioncel, O.; et al. 2021 ESC Guidelines for the diagnosis and treatment of acute and chronic heart failure: Developed by the Task Force for the diagnosis and treatment of acute and chronic heart failure of the European Society of Cardiology (ESC). With the special contribution of the Heart Failure Association (HFA) of the ESC. *Eur. J. Heart Fail.* **2022**, *24*, 4–131. [PubMed]
3. Han, J.J.; Elzayn, H.; Duda, M.M.; Iyengar, A.; Acker, A.M.; Patrick, W.L.; Helmers, M.; Birati, E.Y.; Atluri, P. Heart transplant waiting list implications of increased ventricular assist device use as a bridge strategy: A national analysis. *Artif. Organs* **2021**, *45*, 346–353. [CrossRef] [PubMed]
4. Miller, L.W.; Pagani, F.D.; Russell, S.D.; John, R.; Boyle, A.J.; Aaronson, K.D.; Conte, J.V.; Naka, Y.; Mancini, D.; Delgado, R.M.; et al. Use of a Continuous-Flow Device in Patients Awaiting Heart Transplantation. *N. Engl. J. Med.* **2007**, *357*, 885–896. [CrossRef]

5. Tedford, R.J.; Leacche, M.; Lorts, A.; Drakos, S.G.; Pagani, F.D.; Cowger, J. Durable Mechanical Circulatory Support. *J. Am. Coll. Cardiol.* **2023**, *82*, 1464–1481. [CrossRef]
6. Immohr, M.B.; Boeken, U.; Mueller, F.; Prashovikj, E.; Morshuis, M.; Böttger, C.; Aubin, H.; Gummert, J.; Akhyari, P.; Lichtenberg, A.; et al. Complications of left ventricular assist devices causing high urgency status on waiting list: Impact on outcome after heart transplantation. *ESC Heart Fail.* **2021**, *8*, 1253–1262. [CrossRef]
7. Rose, E.A.; Gelijns, A.C.; Moskowitz, A.J.; Heitjan, D.F.; Stevenson, L.W.; Dembitsky, W.; Long, J.W.; Ascheim, D.D.; Tierney, A.R.; Levitan, R.G.; et al. Long-Term Use of a Left Ventricular Assist Device for End-Stage Heart Failure. *N. Engl. J. Med.* **2001**, *345*, 1435–1443. [CrossRef]
8. Majumder, K.; Spratt, J.R.; Holley, C.T.; Roy, S.S.; Cogswell, R.J.; Liao, K.; John, R. Impact of Postoperative Liver Dysfunction on Survival After Left Ventricular Assist Device Implantation. *Ann. Thorac. Surg.* **2017**, *104*, 1556–1562. [CrossRef]
9. El Nihum, L.I.; Manian, N.; Arunachalam, P.; Al Abri, Q.; Guha, A. Renal Dysfunction in Patients with Left Ventricular Assist Device. *Methodist DeBakey Cardiovasc. J.* **2022**, *18*, 19–26. [CrossRef]
10. Patlolla, V.; Patten, R.D.; DeNofrio, D.; Konstam, M.A.; Krishnamani, R. The Effect of Ventricular Assist Devices on Post-Transplant Mortality. *J. Am. Coll. Cardiol.* **2009**, *53*, 264–271. [CrossRef]
11. Bull, D.A.; Reid, B.B.; Selzman, C.H.; Mesley, R.; Drakos, S.; Clayson, S.; Stoddard, G.; Gilbert, E.; Stehlik, J.; Bader, F.; et al. The impact of bridge-to-transplant ventricular assist device support on survival after cardiac transplantation. *J. Thorac. Cardiovasc. Surg.* **2010**, *140*, 169–173. [CrossRef] [PubMed]
12. Bartfay, S.; Bobbio, E.; Esmaily, S.; Bergh, N.; Holgersson, J.; Dellgren, G.; Bollano, E.; Karason, K. Heart transplantation in patients bridged with mechanical circulatory support: Outcome comparison with matched controls. *ESC Heart Fail.* **2023**, *10*, 2621–2629. [CrossRef]
13. Urban, M.; Pirk, J.; Dorazilova, Z.; Netuka, I. How does successful bridging with ventricular assist device affect cardiac transplantation outcome? *Interact. CardioVascular Thorac. Surg.* **2011**, *13*, 405–409. [CrossRef] [PubMed]
14. Zhou, A.L.; Etchill, E.W.; Shou, B.L.; Whitbread, J.J.; Barbur, I.; Giuliano, K.A.; Kilic, A. Outcomes after heart transplantation in patients who have undergone a bridge-to-bridge strategy. *JTCVS Open* **2022**, *12*, 255–268. [CrossRef] [PubMed]
15. Yin, M.Y.; Wever-Pinzon, O.; Mehra, M.R.; Selzman, C.H.; Toll, A.E.; Cherikh, W.S.; Nativi-Nicolau, J.; Fang, J.C.; Kfoury, A.G.; Gilbert, E.M.; et al. Post-transplant outcome in patients bridged to transplant with temporary mechanical circulatory support devices. *J. Heart Lung Transplant.* **2019**, *38*, 858–869. [CrossRef]
16. Grimm, J.C.; Magruder, J.T.; Crawford, T.C.; Fraser, C.D.; Plum, W.G.; Sciortino, C.M.; Higgins, R.S.; Whitman, G.J.R.; Shah, A.S. Duration of Left Ventricular Assist Device Support Does Not Impact Survival After US Heart Transplantation. *Ann. Thorac. Surg.* **2016**, *102*, 1206–1212. [CrossRef]
17. Stewart, S.; Winters, G.L.; Fishbein, M.C.; Tazelaar, H.D.; Kobashigawa, J.; Abrams, J.; Andersen, C.B.; Angelini, A.; Berry, G.J.; Burke, M.M.; et al. Revision of the 1990 Working Formulation for the Standardization of Nomenclature in the Diagnosis of Heart Rejection. *J. Heart Lung Transplant.* **2005**, *24*, 1710–1720. [CrossRef]
18. Mehra, M.R.; Crespo-Leiro, M.G.; Dipchand, A.; Ensminger, S.M.; Hiemann, N.E.; Kobashigawa, J.A.; Madsen, J.; Parameshwar, J.; Starling, R.C.; Uber, P.A. International Society for Heart and Lung Transplantation working formulation of a standardized nomenclature for cardiac allograft vasculopathy—2010. *J. Heart Lung Transplant.* **2010**, *29*, 717–727. [CrossRef]
19. Kirklin, J.K.; Naftel, D.C.; Pagani, F.D.; Kormos, R.L.; Stevenson, L.W.; Blume, E.D.; Myers, S.L.; Miller, M.A.; Baldwin, J.T.; Young, J.B. Seventh INTERMACS annual report: 15,000 patients and counting. *J. Heart Lung Transplant.* **2015**, *34*, 1495–1504. [CrossRef]
20. Moeller, C.M.; Valledor, A.F.; Oren, D.; Rubinstein, G.; Sayer, G.T.; Uriel, N. Evolution of Mechanical Circulatory Support for advanced heart failure. *Prog. Cardiovasc. Dis.* **2024**, *82*, 135–146. [CrossRef]
21. Fukuhara, S.; Takeda, K.; Polanco, A.R.; Takayama, H.; Naka, Y. Prolonged continuous-flow left ventricular assist device support and posttransplantation outcomes: A new challenge. *J. Thorac. Cardiovasc. Surg.* **2016**, *151*, 872–880.e5. [CrossRef] [PubMed]
22. Magruder, J.T.; Grimm, J.C.; Crawford, T.C.; Tedford, R.J.; Russell, S.D.; Sciortino, C.M.; Whitman, G.J.R.; Shah, A.S. Survival After Orthotopic Heart Transplantation in Patients Undergoing Bridge to Transplantation With the HeartWare HVAD Versus the Heartmate II. *Ann. Thorac. Surg.* **2017**, *103*, 1505–1511. [CrossRef] [PubMed]
23. Noly, P.-E.; Hébert, M.; Lamarche, Y.; Cortes, J.R.; Mauduit, M.; Verhoye, J.-P.; Voisine, P.; Flécher, E.; Carrier, M. Use of extracorporeal membrane oxygenation for heart graft dysfunction in adults: Incidence, risk factors and outcomes in a multicentric study. *Can. J. Surg.* **2021**, *64*, E567–E577. [CrossRef] [PubMed]
24. Sohn, S.H.; Kang, Y.; Hwang, H.Y.; Chee, H.K. Optimal timing of heart transplantation in patients with an implantable left ventricular assist device. *Korean J. Transpl.* **2023**, *37*, 79–84. [CrossRef]
25. Petroni, T.; D'Alessandro, C.; Combes, A.; Golmard, J.-L.; Brechot, N.; Barreda, E.; Laali, M.; Farahmand, P.; Varnous, S.; Weber, P.; et al. Long-term outcome of heart transplantation performed after ventricular assist device compared with standard heart transplantation. *Arch. Cardiovasc. Dis.* **2019**, *112*, 485–493. [CrossRef]

26. Truby, L.K.; Farr, M.A.; Garan, A.R.; Givens, R.; Restaino, S.W.; Latif, F.; Takayama, H.; Naka, Y.; Takeda, K.; Topkara, V.K. Impact of Bridge to Transplantation with Continuous-Flow Left Ventricular Assist Devices on Posttransplantation Mortality: A Propensity-Matched Analysis of the United Network of Organ Sharing Database. *Circulation* **2019**, *140*, 459–469. [CrossRef]
27. Chiu, P.; Schaffer, J.M.; Oyer, P.E.; Pham, M.; Banerjee, D.; Joseph Woo, Y.; Ha, R. Influence of durable mechanical circulatory support and allosensitization on mortality after heart transplantation. *J. Heart Lung Transplant.* **2016**, *35*, 731–742. [CrossRef]
28. Arnaoutakis, G.J.; George, T.J.; Kilic, A.; Weiss, E.S.; Russell, S.D.; Conte, J.V.; Shah, A.S. Effect of sensitization in US heart transplant recipients bridged with a ventricular assist device: Update in a modern cohort. *J. Thorac. Cardiovasc. Surg.* **2011**, *142*, 1236–1245.e1. [CrossRef]
29. Long, B.; Robertson, J.; Koyfman, A.; Brady, W. Left ventricular assist devices and their complications: A review for emergency clinicians. *Am. J. Emerg. Med.* **2019**, *37*, 1562–1570. [CrossRef]
30. Yuzefpolskaya, M.; Schroeder, S.E.; Houston, B.A.; Robinson, M.R.; Gosev, I.; Reyentovich, A.; Koehl, D.; Cantor, R.; Jorde, U.P.; Kirklin, J.K.; et al. The Society of Thoracic Surgeons Intermacs 2022 Annual Report: Focus on the 2018 Heart Transplant Allocation System. *Ann. Thorac. Surg.* **2023**, *115*, 311–327. [CrossRef]
31. Goldstein, D.J.; Meyns, B.; Xie, R.; Cowger, J.; Pettit, S.; Nakatani, T.; Netuka, I.; Shaw, S.; Yanase, M.; Kirklin, J.K. Third Annual Report From the ISHLT Mechanically Assisted Circulatory Support Registry: A comparison of centrifugal and axial continuous-flow left ventricular assist devices. *J. Heart Lung Transplant.* **2019**, *38*, 352–363. [CrossRef] [PubMed]
32. Tsukui, H.; Abla, A.; Teuteberg, J.J.; McNamara, D.M.; Mathier, M.A.; Cadaret, L.M.; Kormos, R.L. Cerebrovascular accidents in patients with a ventricular assist device. *J. Thorac. Cardiovasc. Surg.* **2007**, *134*, 114–123. [CrossRef] [PubMed]
33. Kadakkal, A.; Najjar, S.S. Neurologic Events in Continuous-Flow Left Ventricular Assist Devices. *Cardiol. Clin.* **2018**, *36*, 531–539. [CrossRef] [PubMed]

Disclaimer/Publisher's Note: The statements, opinions and data contained in all publications are solely those of the individual author(s) and contributor(s) and not of MDPI and/or the editor(s). MDPI and/or the editor(s) disclaim responsibility for any injury to people or property resulting from any ideas, methods, instructions or products referred to in the content.

Article

Evaluating a New Short Self-Management Tool in Heart Failure Against the Traditional Flinders Program

Pupalan Iyngkaran [1,2], David Smith [3], Craig McLachlan [2], Malcolm Battersby [4], Maximilian de Courten [5] and Fahad Hanna [2,*]

1. Melbourne Clinical School, University of Notre Dame, Melbourne, VIC 3000, Australia; pupalan.iyngkaran@students.torrens.edu.au
2. Centre for Healthy Futures, Torrens University Australia, Surry Hills, NSW 2000, Australia; craig.mclachlan@torrens.edu.au
3. College of Medicine & Public Health, Flinders University, Adelaide, SA 5042, Australia; david.smith@flinders.edu.au
4. College of Medicine and Public Health, Flinders University, Norwood, SA 5067, Australia; malcolm.battersby@flinders.edu.au
5. Australian Health Policy Collaboration, Institute for Health and Sport (IHES), Victoria University, Melbourne, VIC 8001, Australia; maximilian.decourten@vu.edu.au
* Correspondence: fahad.hanna@torrens.edu.au

Abstract: Background/Objective: Heart failure (HF) is a complex syndrome, with multiple causes. Numerous pathophysiological pathways are activated. Comprehensive and guideline-derived care is complex. A multidisciplinary approach is required. The current guidelines report little evidence for chronic disease self-management (CDSM) programs for reducing readmission and major adverse cardiovascular events (MACE). CDSM programs can be complex and are not user-friendly in clinical settings, particularly for vulnerable patients. The aim of this study was to investigate whether a simplified one-page CDSM tool, the *SCReening in Heart Failure (SCRinHF)*, is comparable to a comprehensive Flinders Program of Chronic Disease Management, specifically in triaging self-management capabilities and in predicting readmission and MACE. **Methods:** SELFMAN-HF is a prospective, observational study based on community cardiology. Eligible patients, consecutively recruited, had HF with left ventricular ejection fraction <40% and were placed on sodium–glucose co-transporter-2 inhibitors (SGLT2-i) within 3 months of recruitment. SGLT2-i is the newest of the four HF treatment pillars; self-management skills are assessed at this juncture. CDSM was assessed and scored independently via the long-form (*LF*) and short-form (*SF*) tools, and concordance between forms was estimated. The primary endpoint is the 80% concordance across the two CDSM scales for predicting hospital readmission and MACE. **Results:** Of the 117 patients, aged 66.8 years (±SD 13.5), 88 (75%) were male. The direct comparisons for *SF* versus *LF* patient scores are as follows: "good self-managers", 13 vs. 30 patients (11.1% vs. 25.6%); "average", 46 vs. 21 patients (39.3% vs. 17.9%), "borderline", 20 vs. 31 patients (17.1% vs. 26.5%), and "poor self-managers" (vulnerable), 38 vs. 35 patients (32.5% vs. 29.9%). These findings underscore the possibility of *SF* tools in picking up patients whose scores infer poor self-management capabilities. This concordance of the *SF* with the *LF* scores for patients who have poor self-management capabilities (38 vs. 35 patients $p = 0.01$), alongside readmission (31/38 vs. 31/35 $p = 0.01$) or readmission risk for poor self-managers versus good self-managers (31/38 vs. 5/13 $p = 0.01$), validates the simplification of the CDSM tools for the vulnerable population with HF. Similarly, when concurrent and predictive validity was tested on 52 patients, the results were 39 (75%) for poor self-managers and 14 (27%) for good self-managers in both groups, who demonstrated significant correlations between *SF* and *LF* scores. **Conclusions:** Simplifying self-management scoring with an *SF* tool to improve clinical translation is justifiable, particularly for vulnerable populations. Poor self-management capabilities and readmission risk for poor self-managers can be significantly predicted, and trends for good self-managers are observed. However, correlations of *SF* to *LF* scores across an HF cohort for self-management abilities and MACE are more complex. Translation to patients of all skill levels requires further research.

Citation: Iyngkaran, P.; Smith, D.; McLachlan, C.; Battersby, M.; de Courten, M.; Hanna, F. Evaluating a New Short Self-Management Tool in Heart Failure Against the Traditional Flinders Program. *J. Clin. Med.* **2024**, *13*, 6994. https://doi.org/10.3390/jcm13226994

Academic Editors: Cristina Tudoran and Larisa Anghel

Received: 23 October 2024
Revised: 9 November 2024
Accepted: 12 November 2024
Published: 20 November 2024

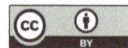

Copyright: © 2024 by the authors. Licensee MDPI, Basel, Switzerland. This article is an open access article distributed under the terms and conditions of the Creative Commons Attribution (CC BY) license (https://creativecommons.org/licenses/by/4.0/).

Keywords: clinical treatment; heart failure; Flinders Program; risk assessment; self-management; readmission

1. Introduction

Heart failure (HF) is a complex cardiovascular condition, arising from various contributing factors and typically accompanied by multiple comorbidities [1,2]. This multifaceted nature makes its management challenging for both healthcare providers and patients. Delivering comprehensive and optimal HF management requires several factors to be considered: first, the complex pathophysiology, with an attempt to improve function with medical treatments; second, a systems approach utilizing a multidisciplinary team to administer an integrative guideline-based management program (GDMT). The goal is maintaining quality of life, limiting preventable deteriorations (morbidity and mortality), and managing health resources [3,4]. There remain population-level gaps in preventing major adverse cardiovascular events (MACE), including hospital readmissions [5–9].

Chronic disease self-management (CDSM) is a health services approach and a domain within HF programs. In theory, CDSM can be a cost-effective approach to bridging gaps in HF care. While CDSM studies for most chronic diseases have reported positive outcomes [10,11], studies in HF have been relatively disappointing. In fact, recent guidelines have demoted this therapy in terms of both performance and quality measures, citing a lack of evidence [9]. CDSM tools can be complex. Their clinical roles can be difficult to navigate in clinical settings. There are structural issues with CDSM with respect to HF management. These include a lack of randomized trial evidence demonstrating efficacy [9] and a lack of clinical understanding on the value of CDSM [9,12] and how it fits within disease management domains [13], raising the question: could an important gap in CDSM programs for HF be within the tools themselves? The Flinders Program of Chronic Condition Management [*Flinders Program (*FP*®*)] is a gold-standard generic tool [14]. This generic unmodified tool, in its long form (*LF*), is the foundation from which this study is based. Short forms (*SF*) are uncommon and have not been tested in an HF population. Our team has demonstrated via a press publication the psychometrics of *FP* in *CHF* syndromes.

The **SELF**-**MAN**agement in Heart Failure *(SELFMAN-HF)* study [14] was derived to address one critical issue: can a novel *SF* CDSM tool (**SCRinHF*) be validated against the established and best-available *LF* in determining readmissions and MACE? To date, there are no proven CDSM tools that have been adapted from its generic form to a shorter version, and this includes HF. Numerous studies have concluded that the theoretical basis for CDSM is itself well established; the methods of delivery have been well studied, and these tools are the best means of delivering CDSM programs [10,15]. With a changing healthcare landscape, and with evidence for HF lacking, a novel simplified approach could be explored. There was also impetus from existing examples of simplifying other chronic disease tools—e.g., SF-36 to SF-12 [16] and PACIC to PACIC-plus [17]—for initiatives in HF [18–20].

Aims

Our aim was to validate the *SF* [14] against the established *LF* with respect to self-management capabilities, a primary endpoint of hospital readmission and a secondary outcome of MACE.

2. Materials and Methods

Detailed references for this study protocol, design, and methodology have been published [14]. The *SELFMAN-HF* is a prospective, observational case–cohort study that examined the feasibility and validity of the *SF* tool, comparing the novel one-page tool to the *LF* [14]. In brief, study patients were consecutively enrolled as they presented as community outpatients. Validity was explored with comparisons to the *LF* in a range of measures including self-management, clinical progress, and predicting 12 months MACE, including hospital readmissions. Feasibility was not a planned aim in this study.

2.1. Participants

The community service has 6 clinical sites treating HF. Participants were recruited and enrolled in one clinical site in Western Melbourne. A minimum of 80 patients with HF who met the inclusion criteria were offered the opportunity to participate. Eligible patients aged over 18 commenced sodium glucose cotransporter-2 inhibitor (SGLT-2I) within 3 months for systolic HF [echocardiographic ejection fraction (EF) < 40%]; they received care within the predefined health jurisdiction. Patients were excluded if concerns were raised by any medical staff; if they had a life expectancy of ≤6 months; or if they were receiving palliative or nursing home care. Patients of variant cognitive statuses and patients with dementia were not excluded if consent from a caring relative or legal guardian who would assist in the completion of the study was given. This study also excluded individuals with significant neurological or cognitive impairments, those unable to provide written informed consent for any reason, clients who did not typically reside in the region (preventing follow-up data collection), and patients for whom the dates of SGLT-2I prescriptions were unknown.

> * **SCR**eening **in H**eart **F**ailure (*SCRinHF*) *is designed as a* simplified triage tool *to risk-stratify CDSM capabilities and complement gold-standard tools. It is compared against* the Flinders Program of Chronic Condition Management [*Flinders Program (**FP**®)], *a gold-standard generic tool.* **SF** (short-form tools) and **LF** (long-form tools) will be the acronyms used to describe the tools and programs in this paper.

2.2. Sample Size Calculation

See Section 2.6.

2.3. Trial Instruments, Procedures and Treatment

Short-Form (SF) and Long-Form (LF) Tools (Flinders Program or FP®) Questionnaire

The **Flinders Program** (*FP*®) is a generic and comprehensive CDSM program that utilizes 4 tools to obtain a patient-centred and codesigned comprehensive and flexible program of care for patients [21]. The *FP*® is a gold-standard generic chronic disease management program and is on par with other CDSM programs in achieving outcomes; i.e., it assess self-management understanding and goals, and from this, an education and care plan can be tailored to achieve self-efficacy in managing chronic disease [21,22]. The tools used by the *FP* extract patient-reported outcomes (PRO) and health service data along 4 domains. A 2-day course certifies health workers to use the *LF* to conduct interviews with clients, which can take up to 90 min. The *LF* tools include the Partners in Health Scale (PIH), a self-rated questionnaire for the patient to assess 4 domains, namely, self-management knowledge, attitudes, behaviors, and the impacts of their chronic condition (Table 1); and the Cue and Response Interview (C&R), a health-worker-administered tool that explores the same PIH questions via open-ended questions and responses, rated from the health provider's perspective. The final 2 domains are not relevant for this study [21]. The programs questionnaire estimate a baseline and utilize other planning tools to attain the desired CDSM goal.

The *SF* tool is based on the principles of CDSM programs [14,21–24] and aims to simplify its use and broaden the usability of the application across the health continuum. The *SF* tool aims to assist with triaging patients at any health encounter along several domains, and self-management capabilities are one key domain (Table 1). This is unique and important as CDSM discussions that are often relegated to an exclusive aspect of a patient's health journey can now begin during any health encounter. Studies have shown that the *LF* can assess and deliver one client's capacity to self-manage, while the program then provides a generic set of tools in a structured process that enables health workers and patients to develop health goals collaboratively [14,21]. The *SF* tool is scored by the enrolling trial nurse based on information already recorded on the patient, with clarifications as needed. It does not require a lengthy patient interview [14].

Table 1. The CPFI, Partners in Health scale, and SCRinHF details and scoring.

A. PIH Domain	PIH Scale	SCRinHF Domain	SCRinHF Question
a. Knowledge	1. Overall, what I know about my health condition(s). 2. Overall, what I know about my treatment, including medications for my health condition(s).	1. Self-care maintenance/monitoring	a. Do you know "how to (skill)...to achieve (goal)"... 1. Problem Solve—e.g., (i) monitoring; 2. Decision making question 3. About Physical function—e.g., (i) exercise
b. Partnership in treatment	3. I take medications or carry out the treatments asked by my doctor or health worker. 4. I share in decisions made about my health condition(s) with my doctor or health worker. 5. I am able to deal with health professionals to get the services I need that fit with my culture, values and beliefs. 6. I attend appointments as asked by my doctor or health worker.	2. Self-management	b. Do you know "what to do if (skill) to achieve (goal)"... 4. Resource utilization e.g., (i) monitoring with action 5. Form patient provider partnership e.g., (i) engage health system 6. Action planning when self-tailoring
c. Recognizing and managing symptom	7. I keep track of my symptoms and early warning signs (e.g., blood sugar levels, peak flow, weight, shortness of breath, pain, sleep problems and mood). 8. I take action when my early warning signs and symptoms get worse.	3. Self-care efficacy/confidence	c. Do you know "how confident you are (skill)...when faced with (goal)" 7. Has client previously received Rehab/education? State level of Self-Care Confidence (SR, SE, TI, TE)—e.g., (i) adherence to diet ii) compliance
d. Coping	9. I manage the effect of my health condition(s) on my physical activity (e.g., walking and household tasks). 10. I manage the effect of my health condition(s) on how I feel (i.e., my emotions and spiritual well-being). 11. I manage the effect of my health condition(s) on my social life (i.e., how I mix with other people). 12. Overall, I manage to live a healthy life (e.g., no smoking, moderate alcohol, healthy food, regular physical activity and manage stress).	Operator assessment of care	Covered in another section of tool.

Table 1. *Cont.*

B. Correlation of PIH and SCRinHF—the column below highlights our approach to matching the domains and scores.
@At this point no correlation exists or has been tested between CFPI and SCRinHF. This process will also require validation.

		SCRinHF domain	PIH correlation
Scoring	Likert 0–8 Total 96	1	a, d (6 questions)
		2	b, c (6 questions)
		3	a, b, c, d (12 questions)
Interpretation	• SCRinHF is a risk score. Scores 0 indicated low risk, i.e., at least average ability to perform self-management task. Self-efficacy is more rigorous and compares to the entire PIH score. • The SCRinHF is compared to health-staff-administered PIH scale or C&R.	**@SCrinHF Score** 0 Good 1 Average 2 Borderline 3 Poor	**@PIH Pass Score** >8/16 (domain a or c—2 questions/domain) >16/32 (domain b or d 4 questions/domain) >48/96 (combined CFPIscore)
Validation	• Construct and factor validity. • Face and content validity. • Criterion related validity (concurrent, predictive).	Ref [25] Delphi process	• Research design and conduct. • Expert, patient consultation with study data. • Association to gold standard, predict outcomes.

(A) The Partners in Health scale (PIH) is a patient-reported outcome tool and the first part of The Flinders Program. Four domains are assessed. In contrast, the SCRinHF extracts three components; the coping domain is rested here and extracted in another tool domain. (B) The PIH is scored 0 to 8 in each care dimension and, overall, achieves a score of 96. With respect to scoring, the SCRinHF domain 1 and 2 correlate with the respective PIH domains. The third domain of self-effectiveness correlates with all PIH domains. Each SCRinHF domain has a score of 0 (competent) or 1 poor. In interpretation, SCRinHF patients can have a combined score of 0, 1, 2, or 3. A score of 3 equates to a PIH total score of <48. Individually, a score of 1 in each SCRinHF domain will equate to <16 for the PIH domains. Pass scores in PIH are >4/8 per question, >8/16 or 16/32 for specific domains, or >48/96 overall are not being assessed.

2.4. Data Collection

2.4.1. Comparing the Scores of Self-Management Domains

SF has 4 steps [14] and works on the basis of the following (Table 1): first (domain 1), understanding a client's generic baseline readmission risk; second (domain 2), determining the buffers to counter this risk; this includes three parts, patients' living-at-home skills and goals determined via 3 questions on self-management maintenance, 3 on self-management, and 1 on self-management confidence or efficacy; third (domain 3), support for living at home; fourth, (domain 4) the chronology is employed as an introspective element when understanding where a client is and where they should aspire to be in the context of their journeys. The scoring system (domains 5 and 6) has not been tested clinically. The rationale for scores are matched to *LF* scales and are described in [14].

2.4.2. Scoring of Outcomes

MACE was measured at 6 and 12 months as the number of planned and unplanned hospitalizations, cardiovascular events, and mortality. Side effects are listed as those in the manufacturers' brochure and documented as reducing the dose, ceasing medications, and worsening renal function [WRF: 25% reduction in eGFR or increase in serum Creatinine (SCr)]. Attendance was calculated, in years, from the day of starting the SGLT-2 inhibitor and documented as visits for test and clinical review as per the number of clinical bookings and non-attendance.

2.4.3. Scoring of Established Tools (Appendix)

Baseline scores were completed and presented as per published tool guidelines. Multiple tools measuring well-being were used. The references for its clinical justification are provided as follows: PIH [14,21–24,26–31], Charlson Comorbidity Index (CCI https://www.mdcalc.com/calc/3917/charlson-comorbidity-index-cci, accessed on 17 May 2024) [27], SF-12 (https://orthotoolkit.com/sf-12, accessed on 17 May 2024) [28], and PHQ-9 [29]. The scoring is described in the results section (Table 1).

2.4.4. Scoring of the *SF* and the *LF*

The *SF* tool extracts 3 CDSM domains from the PIH scale and allows for health staff to score in a binary fashion. Specifics are provided in Table 1, published methods [14]. Client (or dyad) contribution in PRO tools makes up a component of the non-controlled information extracted from carers and health systems. Thus, with any scoring, a degree of judgement is required, and the removal of the 8-point Likert scores challenges health staff to commit to clinical decision making

2.5. Ethical Considerations

This study has been approved by the St Vincent's ethics committees committee (approval no. LRR 177/21). All participants completed a written informed consent form prior to enrolment in the study. The study results will be disseminated widely via local and international health conferences and peer-reviewed publications.

2.6. Statistical Aspects and Data Analysis

The study cohort assesses validity, which will allow for the appropriate parameters to determine sample size power calculations for future studies that will utilize a controlled design. Initial data analysis will investigate the distribution characteristics of each primary and secondary outcome measure and determine either a parametric or semi-parametric statistical approach to the main data analysis. Descriptive statistics for baseline demographics and clinical characteristics will be presented as means (standard deviation) for continuous data and count (%) for categorical data. As an example, the previous publication provides estimates for pilot sample size calculations for categorical data [32–36]. Latest-edition IBM SPSS (2024) Statistics 29 has been utilized for this analysis.

3. Results

From May 2022 to January 2024, 210 patients were screened for SGLT-2I, with 120 patients heart failure with reduced ejection fraction (HFrEF) consenting to participate in this study (Figure 1). All patients completed baseline criteria and were enrolled. At the time of final follow-up and study closure, no patient withdrew consent; however, nine patients were lost to follow-up. Their reasons for being lost to follow-up were confirmed by a relative or their general practitioner, including travel overseas ($n = 2$), relocating ($n = 2$), mental health ($n = 1$), and no contact being made ($n = 4$).

3.1. Baseline Characteristics

The study population comprises 117 patients. Baseline study characteristics are summarized in Tables 2 and 3. The population was 66.8 years old (SD: 13.5); 88 (75%) were male and 29 were female. The majority of patients ethnicity were Caucasian [90 (77%)], followed by South Asian, Asian, African, or Indigenous. Most patients were married [75 (64%)]. At least 71 (65%) described their spouses as family support. A majority of 90 (76.9%) patients had received an education up to high school level. As many as 30 (25.6%) of patients did not record any associated comorbidity at baseline, 26 (22.3%) had one, and the remainder had three or more. Hypertension and hypercholesterolemia were the most common comorbidity, being present in 79 (68%) and 73 (62.4%) patients, respectively. Renal impairment, defined as eGFR < 60 mL/min, was recorded in 48 (39%) patients. Coronary artery disease (CAD) and diabetes were recorded in 51 (44%) and 42 (36%) patients, respectively. Obstructive sleep apnea was also common, recorded in 31 (26.5%) patients in the cohort. Smoking history was recorded in 53 patients (45%). CHF was not a new diagnosis, i.e., a chronic condition, having been diagnosed prior to 12 months in 34 (29%) of the cohort. Further details are described in Appendix A.

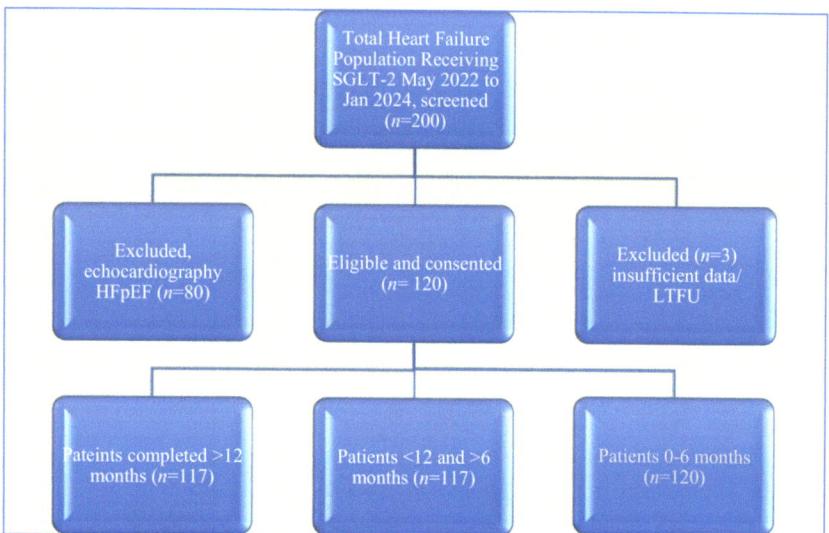

Figure 1. Study flowchart. Abbreviations: f; HFpEF—heart failure with preserved ejection fraction; LTFU—lost to follow-up; n—number of patients.

Table 2. Baseline descriptive statistics of cohort sociodemographic and clinical variables.

Variable	Cohort (n = 117)	%
Age (yo)	66.8 mean	SD 13.5
Sex, (men)	88	75
Ethnicity		
Caucasian	90	77
South Asian	7	6
Asian	3	3
African	10	8
Aboriginal/Pacific Is	7	6
Marital Status		
Married	75	64
Divorced/Separated	23	19
Widowed	15	13
Never married/Single	4	3
Lives/Support		
Alone	46	39
With spouse/Family	71	61
Education Level		
Less than high school graduate	43	36.7
High school graduate	47	40.2
Community college education	18	15.4
Baccalaureate graduate	9	7.7
Graduate school	0	0

Table 2. *Cont.*

Variable	Cohort (n = 117)	%
Body Mass Index (BMI) (kg/m^2)		
BMI < 20	6	5
BMI < 25 (Normal)	21	17.9
25 ≤ BMI < 30 (Overweight)	32	27.4
30 ≤ BMI < 35 (Obese 1)	27	23.1
BMI ≥35–40 (Obese II)	14	12
BMI > 40 (Obese III)	17	14.6
Smoking History		
No	53	45
Ex/Yes	64	55
Comorbidities		
CRI		
1 > 60	69	59
30–60	39	33.3
15–30	7	6
<15	2	1.7
CAD	51	44
DM	42	36
HT	79	68
Chol	73	62.4
OSA	31	26.5
Years with HF Diagnosis		
Less than 1 year	83	71
1–4 years	21	18
5–10 years	13	11
LVEF (%)		
Grade 2 (40–49)	1	0.8
Grade 3 (30–39)	84	71.2
Grade 4 (20–29)	29	25
Grade 5 < 20	4	3
Number of Comorbidities		
Causative/nil	30	25.6
>1	26	22.3
>3	59	50.4
>6	2	1.7
* Comorbidity		
IHD	37	31.6
Viral Idio	21	18
AF/Rhythm	31	26.5
Others (VHD/Met Obese, OSA/Chemo-Ca-amyloid)	2/4/4	8.5
A/D	9/9	15.4
BP (mmHg)		
<100/60	42	36
>100/60	75	64
Medications		
Aspirin	69	59
NOAC	47	41
ACEI/ATRA	34	29.1
ARNI	77	66
BB	112	96
SGLT-2	109	93
Statin	74	63
MRA	46	39
Diuretic	67	57
COVID-19 vaccine	98	84

Table 2. *Cont.*

Variable	Cohort (n = 117)	%
Number of prescribed medications		
≤5	37	32
>5 ≤ 10	57	47
>10	24	21
CR		
Within 6 months of diagnosis	16	14
nil	102	86

* Some have two causes; the first documented aetiology is stated. Abbreviations: ACEI—novel oral anticoagulant; A/D—alcohol and illicit drugs; AF—atrial fibrillation; ATRA—angiotensin receptor antagonist; ARNI—angiotensin receptor neprilysin inhibitor; BB—beta-blocker; BMI—body mass index; BP—blood pressure; Ca—cancer; CAD—coronary artery disease; Chemo—chemotherapy; Chol—hypercholesterolemia; CR—cardiac rehabilitation; CRI—chronic renal impairment; DM—diabetes mellitus; Ex—ex-smoker; HF—heart failure; HT—hypertension; Idio—idiopathic; Is—island; kg/m^2—weight and height in kilograms and meters; LVEF—left ventricular ejection fraction; Met—metabolic; MRA—mineralocorticoid receptor antagonist; NOAC—novel oral anticoagulant; OSA—obstructive sleep apnea; SGLT-2—sodium–glucose co-transporter inhibitor; yo—years old; VHD—valvular heart disease.

Table 3. Summary of health scores at baseline.

Variable	Cohort (n = 117)	Cohort %
NYHA classification at discharge		
I	0	0
II	73	62.4
III	41	35
IV	3	2.6
PHQ-9		
1–4	36	31.5
5–9	27	23.1
>9	52	44.4
SF-12 score, mean (SD)		
Physical Component Summary > 50	4	3.5
Mental Component Summary > 42	69	59
Charlson comorbidity index		
0	0	0
Mild (<2)	27	23.1
Moderate (>2 < 4)	25	21.4
Severe (>5)	65	55.5

See Appendixes A–C for guide to interpreting scores. Abbreviations: n—number of patients; NYHA—New York Heart Association; PHQ—Patient Health Questionnaire; SD—standard deviation; SF-12—Short-Form Survey.

3.2. Self-Management Scores in the Cohort

The *LF* scores are highlighted in Table 4. For the 117 patients, the number and scores for knowledge (K), coping (C), partnership in treatment (P), and management and recognition of symptoms (M) are scored as 16, 32, 32, and 16 points, respectively, for a maximum of 96 points. With the *SF* domain 1, for self-maintenance (*Ma*) 76 patients (65%) scored as good, and 41 patients (35%) scored as average to poor. In comparison, the *LF* scores combining K and C at similar levels are 15 (12.8%) for good and 27 (23.1%), 48 (41.9%), and 27 (22.2%) average to poor. For *SF* dimension 2, or self-tailoring (*Mx*), 61 (52.1%) showed good capabilities, while 56 (48.9%) of patients were average to poor. In comparison, the *LF* scores combining P and M at similar levels are 35 (29.9%) for good and 43 (36.8%), 26 (22.2%), and 13 (11.1%) for average to poor. When both tools are looked at in combination, the *SF* has the capacity for a wider scoring range. The direct comparisons for *SF* versus *LF* are as follows: good, 13 vs. 30 (11.1% vs. 25.6%); and average, 46 vs. 21 (39.3% vs. 17.9%), 20 vs. 31 (17.1% vs. 26.5%), and 38 vs. 35 (32.5% vs. 29.9% [$p < 0.01$]*).

Table 4. Comparison of actual and predicted readmission using combined SF scores.

Self-Management Variable *	Self-Management SCORE #	n = 117	%	Mean	SD	Range
	CFPI					
#K, M (16/96)	K					
0 Good ≥ 12	0	6	5.1	6.12	2.41	0–12
1 Ave ≥ 9–11	1	10	8.5			
2 BL = 6–8	2	49	41.9			
3 Poor ≤ 6	3	53	45.3			
#P, C (32/96)	P					
0 Good ≥ 20	0	33	28.2	17.67	5.27	5–35
1 Ave ≥ 17–20	1	33	28.2			
2 BL = 12–16	2	38	32.5			
3 Poor ≤ 12	3	13	11.1			
#P,C,K,M (96/96)	M					
0 Good ≥ 56	0	19	16.2	8	2.62	2–14
1 Ave ≥ 49–56	1	19	16.2			
2 BL = 41–48	2	64	54.7			
3 Poor ≤ 40	3	15	12.8			
#KC & PM (48/96)	C					
0 Good ≥ 30	0	17	14.5	15.75	4.01	5–24
1 Ave = 24–30	1	24	20.5			
2 BL = 18–23	2	62	53			
3 Poor ≤ 18	3	14	12			
	KC			21.9	5.67	9–36
	0	15	12.8			
	1	27	23.1			
	2	48	41.9			
	3	27	22.2			
	PM					
	0	35	29.9	25.67	7.58	7–45
	1	43	36.8			
	2	26	22.2			
	3	13	11.1			
	Total					
	0	*30*	*25.6*	47.55	12.7	16–79
	1	21	17.9			
	2	31	26.5			
	3	*35*	*29.9*			
* SF						
0 Good **	*0*	*13*	*11.1*			
1 Ave	1	46	39.3	1.71	1.04	0–3
2 BL	2	20	17.1			
3 Poor	*3*	*38*	*32.5*			
1. Ma (K+C)	*0*	76	65	na	na	na
2. Mx (P+M)	*0*	61	52.1	na	na	na
3. Mse (K+C+P+M) **	*0*	*13*	*11.1*	na	na	na

This table highlights the combined *SF* scores for patients compared to the combined *LF* scores for the matching self-management domains, as well as the total *LF* score. ** All patients who had good self-tailoring were good in terms of the *SF* score. No patient who scored poorly in *LF* scored well in *SF*, although the *SF* under-identified good patients, with 13 (11.1%) identified in *SF* and 30 (25.6%) identified in *LF*. Poor self-managers aligned closer with 38 (32.5%) versus 35 (29.9%). * Self-management variables: (a) *LF* has four domains: C—coping; K—knowledge; M—recognition and management of symptoms; P—partnership in treatment; (b) *SF* has three domains: Ma—self-maintenance/monitoring; Mx—self-management/tailoring; Mse—self-efficacy or good chronic disease self-management; (c) Combining scores: domains are combined to match and compare the *SF* and *LF*. Domains that overlap are (1) Ma = K + C; (2) Mx = P + M; (3) Mse = K + C + P + M. # Self-management scores (first row): (a) *LF* questions are scored from 0 to 8. Two domains (K,M) have two questions and combined scores range from 0 to 16; two domains have four questions and combined scores range from 0 to 32; the total score is 96. Different combinations for *LF* scores are compared to the *SF* score to match self-management capabilities. (b) The *SF* domain is scored 0 or 1, and the total score varies from 0 to 3. Abbreviations: Ave—average and above; BL—borderline; *LF*—Flinders Program of chronic condition management (Flinders Program or FP); na—not applicable; SF—Screen in Heart Failure Tool (SCRinHF).

3.3. Readmission and MACE

Among 117 patients, 6 patients died within the 12-month follow-up. One patient had cardiac amyloid and renal failure, two from complications of CHF or cardiac procedure (who were 86 and 92 years old, respectively), and three had CHF secondary to illicit drug use. The total number with five or more hospital admissions came to 14 (12.0%) over the 12-month period. Among these, 2 patients had terminal cancer, several were elderly with dementia and other requiring cardiac and non-cardiac care; 31 (26.5%) had between one and three admissions; 17 (14.5%) had one admission; and 55 (47%) did not have an unplanned cardiac or non-cardiac admission. In terms of attendance to the clinic, 34% failed to attend >25% of pre-booked appointments. These patients had the highest readmission rates. Reasons documented for cardiovascular readmissions include HF (17), cardiovascular reasons (21), AF (9) (AF ablation and cardioversions), and 13 had angiography, device insertion, and bypass surgery. Adverse events, including reduced, ceased, and worsening renal function, as well as other medication side effects, occurred in 53 (45.2%) of the patients. Among the 38 patients who scored 0 ($n = 13$) or 3 ($n = 38$) in *SF*, 4 vs. 0 died, and 4 vs. 1 were lost to follow-up; unplanned cardiovascular admissions, including HF and death, amounted to 5 vs. 31 ($p < 0.01$). Repeat admissions of >5 were seen in 5 vs. 1 patients, and between 1 and 3 readmissions were seen in 13 and 2 patients, respectively. The breakdown for admissions for poor and good self-management scores is highlighted in Table 5 and Figure 2.

Table 5. SF and LF correlation with readmission and MACE.

Self-Management Score			Events			
SF Score/(n)	LF (n) Mean Range	Clinic Appointments/ FTA (>25%)	CV Adm HF Adm	NCV/Multiple	S/E	Deceased ($n = 6$)
0 (13)	30 59.8 24–76	21.3 (10–34) 3	5 * 4	5/13	2	Nil
3 (38)	35 36.13 16–53	22.7 (4–48) 17	31 * 25	29	24	4 32.4 (16–47)

Poor self-managers identified by **SF** and **LF** had significantly more cardiovascular admissions than good self-managers. * Statistically significant association with the χ^2 (chi squared = 8.69) test at 1 degree of freedom between the observed **SF** score of 0 (mean **LF** 59.8) and heart failure admissions compared to the **SF** score of 3 (mean **LF** 36.13) $p < 0.01$. Abbreviations: Adm—admission; **LF**—Flinders Program of chronic condition management; CV—cardiovascular; FTA—failure to attend clinical review (>25% of appointments); n—patient numbers NCV—non cardiovascular; **SF**—Screen in Heart Failure tool (SCRinHF); S/E—side effect. NB// Figure 2 is graphical representation of Table 5 results.

3.4. Validity

Concurrent and predictive validity was tested on 52 patients' data (Appendix A). These patients comprised 39 poor and 14 good self-managers, both of which demonstrated significant correlations between *LF* (PIH scale) and *SF* scores. For concurrent validity, an association was noted between *LF* and *SF* when adjusting for age, sex, and the number of co-morbidities. Multivariate analysis shows that the *LF* (PIH scale) score correlates with *SF* [with coefficient −14.692, SE 4.268217; t = −3.44; $p > 0.001$ (95% CI −23.27855 to −6.105458)]. For predictive validity from 48 observations, similar associations were not demonstrated [coefficient −1.327082, SE 1.039514; t = −1.28; $p > 0.209$ (95% CE −3.423462 to 0.7692982).

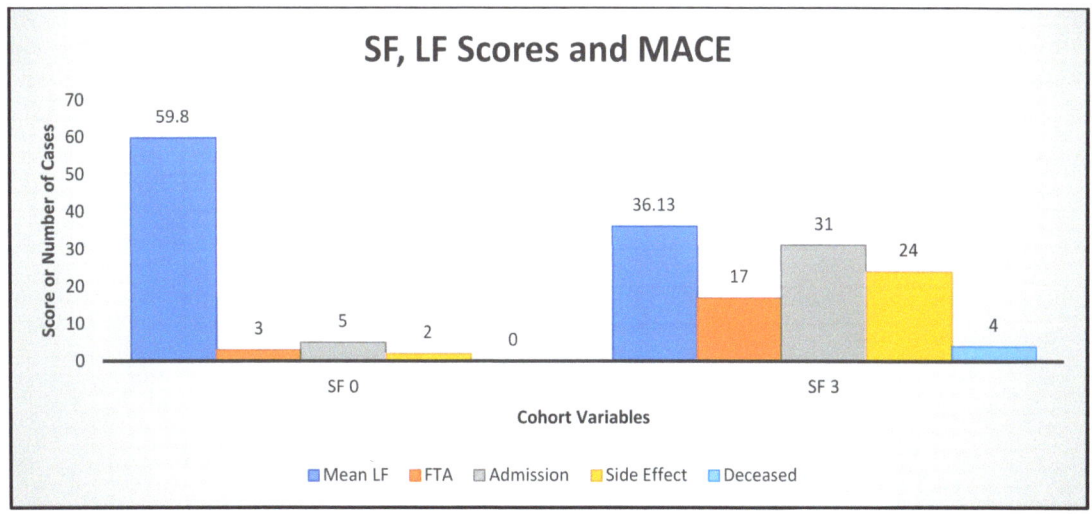

Figure 2. SF and LF correlation with readmission and MACE.

4. Discussion

This study has shown that it is feasible to simplify established CDSM principles as a triage tool, and they can predict readmission and probably MACE. The **SF** tool, a binary questionnaire with a pooled score ranging from 0 to 3, correlates significantly with the **LF** in identifying poor self-managers (a vulnerable patient cohort), who are characteristically at a significant risk of readmissions. This tool displayed some trends with respect to good self-managers in predicting lower readmission and MACE, albeit with gaps as assessed with the **LF**. Patients who were borderline or average self-managers did not show similar correlations.

Concerning the study's stated aim of predicting self-management capabilities based on **SF** and **LF** scores, our study found that patients who score poorly (poor self-managers) in most domains of the **LF** correlate with a matched "poor" score in the **SF**. What appears more ambiguous are the borderline and average cases, where patients have a range of abilities. The **SF** tool missed 3/5 good self-managers, which raises the issue of the sensitivity of binary scoring in extrapolating broader nuances in CDSM capabilities. This raises the possibility of a role for confounders here, which could include patient factors, supports, previous CDSM education, and a range of other factors. An area that is receiving greater attention is the role of dyads [37]. If we look at a previously published experience on short forms, interestingly, in an older publication of SF-36 scores (noted despite the loss to patients' response opportunities), the authors found that SF-36 binary recoding provided the possibility of a newer, easier, smarter method to administer, compile, and score tests and process data [38]. In 1248 HF patients who completed a PRO tool [Kansas City Cardiomyopathy Questionnaire-12 (KCCQ-12)], Sandhu et al. found that with respect to the correlation with the four-scoring item NYHA class and KCCQ-12, patients' perceptions were greatest when clinicians accessed patients' KCCQ-12 scale [25]. Another study in support of multi-response PRO tools was the FAIR-HF trial of 3459 HF patients with iron deficiency who were randomly assigned to receive intravenous iron (ferric carboxymaltose) or saline (placebo). For the secondary endpoint of HRQoL, using the KCCQ score, scores started at 53 points in both groups. The ferric carboxymaltose group had an improvement of 14 points, and the placebo group of 6 points. This effect was significant in favor of ferric carboxymaltose ($p < 0.001$) [39]. This area will thus require further attention in the ongoing analysis of how and where long- and short-form tools can best be utilized in research and clinical settings. Larger sample sizes and randomization may be required.

In reference to our other endpoint, readmissions, this study's findings also showed significant concordance between poor self-managers and higher readmission, and trends correlating good self-managers with lower readmissions. Poor self-managers are a vulnerable group and are naturally associated with a higher risk of readmissions. There are a range of factors, and these includes sociodemographic factors. These can be identified with both the *LF* and *SF* tools. This finding has significance in today's HF healthcare resourcing, where readmission is the largest contributor to cost (around 2% of health budgets) [1,3,4]. Furthermore, identifying poor self-managers leads to the identification of behaviors relevant for self-management capabilities, making this an identifiable and modifiable risk factor. The opportunity to optimize GDMT then presents itself, i.e., through triaging these patients at various healthcare encounters and providing these high-risk patients with early, patient-focused direction and longer-term readmission planning. Patient- and resource-centric care seem a feasible objective. Nonetheless, the true value of the clinical tools can only be gauged after they have undergone rigorous validation. The construct validity of the *PIH* in HF is established in [40,41]. The next phase is to establish face and content validity via a Delphi process.

With regards to predictive validity, this study suggests that there are significant observations to support patients who have low scores in self-management skills; and in risk prediction, these are also the patients who are at higher risk of readmission and adverse outcomes. This trend (Appendix A) needs to be tested in a larger sample, and at the next or subsequent stage removal of bias must be undertaken through blinding and randomization. Good and poor self-managers make up 51/117 patients in the cohort. To advance this concept for future consideration, the scoring process is explored. To help interpret the complex scoring process, the range of scores from the *LF* in this study ranged from 16 to 79 points. There were differences in domain scores, with the partnership (P) domain being the highest mean score for good (17.67). The knowledge (K) domain appears to be the hardest to score well. Thus, to understand the nuances of *SF* scores fully, greater understanding of CDSM domains is needed, as well as of their potential weighted impacts on self-efficacy (i.e., overall self-management abilities). This may well then present an opportunity to understand better the role of simplifying scores and to achieve concordance with *LF* across all self-management capabilities. This study, however, was not intended to compare the individual components of each domains score.

4.1. Limitations

This study has several limitations. First, on the issue of the generalizability of the findings, while there are positive signs with respect to observations of the *SF* tool's effectiveness, this study lacks randomization and a control. Any follow-up study will require this design. Second, the types of readmissions include planned and unplanned cardiac or medical procedures, complications, or delays from the planned procedures, as well as other forms of care. This study was not designed to accurately interrogate these confounders in detail. Third, this was an observational longitudinal study; MACE data were presented for the lowest (0, good self-manager) and the highest (3, poor self-manager) groups; i.e., no significant data were observed for the intermediate groups. In future, a larger cohort, multi-site, controlled, and randomized trial would help to factor in the various confounders. Finally, on scoring nurse-aided vs. PRO tools, this tool is only tested on nurse-aided.

4.2. Current Findings and Future Research

There are numerous recognized simplifications of established tools. This is the first (that we know of) for the generic CDSM tool. As the concepts and self-management domains are established, it was encouraging to see signals for poor and good self-managers. There are gaps in triaging the intermediate group and also with respect to broader generalizability. Thus, future studies will need to consider the following: First, on self-management capabilities, our observation suggests that the self-management domains, when utilized in the *S*, may require weighting; a simple start would be to understand how each of the individual four domains (K, P, M, C) correlates to MACE. Second, in interpreting the association between readmission and MACE, readmission is a complex issue. Uptake of GDMT [3,4] and the hospital care programs processes [5,7] are established, and when implemented, they improve outcome [42–44] Heterogeneity (e.g., disease phenotype, comorbidities, certain demographics, and risk factors that play important roles), HF disease chronology and phases, specific identifiable vulnerable phases (including non-HF), and status following HF hospitalizations are established factors [45–49]. In this study, patients were recruited at the point where the diagnosis of HF was already made; however, in 11% of patients, the diagnosis of HF was made more than 5 years before the SGLT-2 was started. At recruitment, many HF pillars (i.e., beta-blockers, RAAS inhibitors, and aldosterone antagonists) were already commenced. However. low cardiac rehabilitation, with only 14% at baseline, could also influence and skew MACE rates. These factors point to the need to tighten controls in study design and to introduce multi-site recruitment to confirm if the current observations have generalizability beyond this study population. A final point to consider with respect to how tools are used; future designs will need to factor in trialing this tool as a PRO tool in addition to health staff use.

What is new and important

1. The SF tool can identify poor self-managers.
2. The SF tool can be used in many health encounters for triaging risk based on self-management capabilities.
3. A binary scoring system can be used in short-form tools.
4. Important gaps exist in identifying higher levels of self-management.

---

5. Conclusions

The **SELFMAN-HF**, for the first time, tested an *SF* tool against validated *LF* tools in the Flinders Program in HF. This study, importantly, has highlighted the potential to simplify CDSM tools for the targeted purpose of risk stratification and triage in patients with HF. Poor self-mangers, a vulnerable cohort, can be identified with the risk correlating to both readmissions and MACE. Trends for good self-managers are noted. More than half of the cohort who were of borderline and average capabilities could not be risk-stratified against the gold standard. This early finding requires more robust interrogation to assess the short-form tool as a PRO tool, along with its validity, reliability, sensitivity, and specificity in HF, as well as in a spectrum of chronic diseases. CDSM remains a challenging area.

Author Contributions: P.I., F.H., C.M. and M.d.C. participated in research design, data analysis, and writing of the paper; P.I., F.H. and D.S. participated in performance of the research and data collection; P.I., F.H., M.B. and M.d.C. provided advice and support; P.I. assisted D.S. in statistical analysis. All authors have read and agreed to the published version of the manuscript.

Funding: Dr Iyngkaran is supported by the RACP Fellows contribution scholarship. This research received no external funding.

Institutional Review Board Statement: This study was conducted in accordance with the Declaration of Helsinki. St Vincent's ethics committees committee (approval no. LRR 177/21) 17 May 20202.

Informed Consent Statement: Informed consent was obtained from all subjects involved in the study.

Data Availability Statement: We abide by the data sharing policy. Details of CFPI and SCRinHF can be obtained from https://www.frontiersin.org/articles/10.3389/fmed.2023.1059735/full.

Acknowledgments: Support from relevant University and clinic administration.

Conflicts of Interest: Professor Malcolm Battersby is co-inventor of the "Flinders Model of Chronic Condition Self-Management" and has received competitive and Federal Government funding for research in chronic condition self-management. All other authors have received government and non-governmental funding. None pose a conflict of interest for this publication.

Appendix A. Association Between PIH and SCRinHF When Adjusting for Age, Sex, and Number of Co-Morbidities

Concurrent validity

```
reg pih i.Self sex age no of comorbidities if time == 1

      Source |       SS           df       MS      Number of obs   =        52
-------------+----------------------------------   F(4, 47)        =      5.04
       Model |  3180.65322         4  795.163306   Prob > F        =    0.0018
    Residual |   7417.4237        47  157.817526   R-squared       =    0.3001
-------------+----------------------------------   Adj R-squared   =    0.2406
       Total |  10598.0769        51   207.80543   Root MSE        =    12.563

---------------------------------------------------------------------------------
      pihscore | Coefficient  Std. err.      t    P>|t|     [95% conf. interval]
---------------+-----------------------------------------------------------------
        1.self |    -14.692   4.268217    -3.44   0.001    -23.27855    -6.105458
           sex |  -6.613667   3.953303    -1.67   0.101    -14.56669     1.339352
           age |   .2282114   .1276815     1.79   0.080    -.0286506     .4850735
noofcomorbidities| -.9578241  1.1221      -0.85   0.398    -3.215198     1.29955
         _cons |   77.40082   11.38127     6.80   0.000     54.50466      100.297
---------------------------------------------------------------------------------
```

Predictive margins of self with 95% CIs

Predictive validity

Does Baseline Selfman predict Na⁺ levels at Time 2 when adjusting for covariates?

```
replace na = " " if na == "na"
replace na = " " if na == "0"
replace na = " " if na == "4.7"

reg sodium i.self age sex no of comorbidities if time == 2

      Source |       SS           df       MS      Number of obs   =        48
-------------+----------------------------------   F(4, 43)        =      0.67
       Model |  23.9000786        4  5.97501965    Prob > F        =    0.6186
    Residual |  385.349921       43  8.96162608    R-squared       =    0.0584
-------------+----------------------------------   Adj R-squared   =   -0.0292
       Total |     409.25        47  8.70744681    Root MSE        =    2.9936

---------------------------------------------------------------------------------
        sodium | Coefficient  Std. err.      t    P>|t|     [95% conf. interval]
---------------+-----------------------------------------------------------------
        1.self |  -1.327082   1.039514    -1.28   0.209    -3.423462     .7692982
           age |  -.0045624   .0318131    -0.14   0.887    -.0687196     .0595949
           sex |  -.1285864    .990904    -0.13   0.897    -2.126935     1.869762
noofcomorbidities| .3442489   .2785337     1.24   0.223    -.2174678     .9059656
         _cons |    140.424    2.91873    48.11   0.000     134.5378      146.3102
---------------------------------------------------------------------------------
```

Appendix B. Heart Failure and Illness Burden of Cohort (Tables 1 and 2)

To interpret the table, the description of the cohort is provided. At baseline, all patients had commenced SGLT-2i within 6 months of identification for study enrolment. At this point, at least three of the four HF pillars were already started in patients diagnosed prior to 12 months. Most patients with a diagnosis of HF within the 12-month period were also optimized on CHF pillar therapy [beta-blocker, renin–angiotensin aldosterone, and/or neprilysin inhibitor (RAAS/ARNI) or mineralocorticoid receptor antagonist (MRA)]. As was the requirement for eligibility of SGLT-2i, all patients were NYHA class II or more, with left ventricular ejection fraction (LVEF) class III (<40%) and greater. HF therapy was good; all patients were on antiplatelet or anticoagulant at baseline. HF pillars were 112 (96%) for beta blockers, 111 (95.1%) for RAAS/ARNI, and 46 (39%) for MRA. Polypharmacy was common: 101 (68%) had at least five prescribed medications classes. Cardiac rehabilitation was only recorded among 16 (14%) patients. At baseline, patient symptoms were NYHA class II in 73 (62.4%) and 41 (35%) NYHA class III. Only three patients were NYHA IV from the urgent referrals, as is expected for community outpatients. On imaging, 1 patient (0.8%) had grade 2 LVEF, while 84 (71.2%), 29 (25%), and 4 (3%) had grades 3, 4, and 5, respectively. The etiology of HF was most commonly ischemic heart disease (IHD) (37, 31.6%), followed by atrial fibrillation (AF) (31, 26.5%) and viral or idiopathic diseases (21, 18%). Patients with drug (amphetamine) (9) and alcohol abuse (9) accounted for 18 cases (15.4%); miscellaneous combination of metabolic syndrome, valvular heart disease, amyloid, and chemotherapy accounted for several cases individually, totaling 10 patients (8.55%). Blood pressure was lower than 100/60 mmHg in 42 (36%) patients, although this study was not equipped to report on the impact of drug dosing and delivering guideline-based medical therapies (GDMT). A limited number (16m 14%)—predominately IHD—who received treatment underwent cardiac rehabilitation within 6 months of their recorded diagnosis. Health scores for depression with PHQ-9 were negligible for 36 patients (31.5%), intermediate for 27 (23.1), and high risk for 52 (44.4%). In comparison, the SF-12 highlighted 48 patients (41%) at high risk. The SF-12 physical score highlighted high physical disability in the cohort for 113 (96.5) patients, with moderate or greater limitations. The Charlson Comorbidity Index (CCI) highlighted an elevated comorbidity risk, with mild, moderate, and severe scores for 27 (23.1%), 25 (21.4%), and 65 (55.5%) patients, respectively, with the older cohort having higher scores.

Appendix C. PHQ-9 Scores

How to Score the PHQ-9

Major depressive disorder (MDD) is suggested if:
- Of the 9 items, 5 or more are checked as at least 'more than half the days'
- Either item 1 or 2 is checked as at least 'more than half the days'

Other depressive syndrome is suggested if:
- Of the 9 items, between 2 to 4 are checked as at least 'more than half the days'
- Either item 1 or 2 is checked as at least 'more than half the days'

PHQ-9 scores can be used to plan and monitor treatment. To score the instrument, tally the numbers of all the checked responses under each heading (not at all = 0, several days = 1, more than half the days = 2, and nearly every day = 3). Add the numbers together to total the score on the bottom of the questionnaire. Interpret the score by using the guide listed below.

Guide for Interpreting PHQ-9 Scores

Score	Depression Severity	Action
0–4	None-minimal	Patient may not need depression treatment
5–9	Mild	Use clinical judgment about treatment, based on patient's duration of symptoms and functional impairment
10–14	Moderate	Use clinical judgment about treatment, based on patient's duration of symptoms and functional impairment
15–19	Moderately severe	Treat using antidepressants, psychotherapy or a combination of treatment
20–27	Severe	Treat using antidepressants with or without psychotherapy

Functional Health Assessment
The instrument also includes a functional health assessment. This asks the patient how emotional difficulties or problems impact work, life at home, or relationships with other people. Patient response of 'very difficult' or 'extremely difficult' suggest that the patient's functionality is impaired. After treatment begins, functional status and number score can be measured to assess patient improvement.

Note: Depression should not be diagnosed or excluded solely on the basis of a PHQ-9 score. A PHQ-9 score ≥ 10 has a sensitivity of 88% and a specificity of 88% for major depression. Since the questionnaire relies on patient self-report, the practitioner should verify all responses. A definitive diagnosis is made taking into account how well the patient understood the questionnaire, as well as other relevant information from the patient.

PHQ-9 is adapted from PRIME-MD TODAY, developed by Drs Spitzer, Williams, Kroenke and colleagues, with an educational grant from Pfizer Inc. Use of the PHQ-9 may only be made in accordance with the Terms of Use available at www.pfizer.com Copyright © 1999 Pfizer Inc. All rights reserved. PRIME-MD TODAY is a trademark of Pfizer Inc.

Reference: Kroenke K, Spitzer RL, Williams JB. The PHQ-9: Validity of a brief depression severity measure. J Gen Intern Med. 2001;16(9):606-613.

Reference: Kroenke et al., 2001 [29].

Appendix D. SF-12 Scoring

Scores range from 0 to 100, with higher scores indicating better physical and mental health functioning [28]. A score of 50 or less on the PCS-12 has been recommended as a cut-off to determine a physical condition, while a score of 42 or less on the MCS-12 may be indicative of "clinical depression"

Reference: Soh et al., 2021 [30].

Appendix E. Charlson Comorbidity Score

A cut-off of 50 or less can be used to identify a physical condition, while a score of 42 or less may signify clinical depression.

Reference: Charlson et al., 1987 [31].

References

1. Roger, V.L. Epidemiology of heart failure: A contemporary perspective. *Circ. Res.* **2021**, *128*, 1421–1434. [CrossRef] [PubMed]
2. Mann, D.L.; Felker, G.M. Mechanisms and models in heart failure: A translational approach. *Circ. Res.* **2021**, *128*, 1435–1450. [CrossRef] [PubMed]
3. Heidenreich, P.A.; Bozkurt, B.; Aguilar, D.; Allen, L.A.; Byun, J.J.; Colvin, M.M.; Deswal, A.; Drazner, M.H.; Dunlay, S.M.; Evers, L.R.; et al. 2022 AHA/ACC/HFSA Guideline for the Management of Heart Failure: A Report of the American College of Cardiology/American Heart Association Joint Committee on Clinical Practice Guidelines. *J. Am. Coll. Cardiol.* **2022**, *79*, e263–e421. [PubMed]
4. McDonagh, T.A.; Metra, M.; Adamo, M.; Gardner, R.S.; Baumbach, A.; Böhm, M.; Burri, H.; Butler, J.; Čelutkienė, J.; Chioncel, O.; et al. ESC Scientific Document Group, 2021 ESC Guidelines for the diagnosis and treatment of acute and chronic heart failure: Developed by the Task Force for the diagnosis and treatment of acute and chronic heart failure of the European Society of Cardiology (ESC) With the special contribution of the Heart Failure Association (HFA) of the ESC. *Eur. Heart J.* **2021**, *42*, 3599–3726.
5. Fonarow, G.C.; Abraham, W.T.; Albert, N.M.; Stough, W.G.; Gheorghiade, M.; Greenberg, B.H.; O'Connor, C.M.; Pieper, K.; Sun, J.L.; Yancy, C.W.; et al. Influence of a performance-improvement initiative on quality of care for hospitalized patients with heart failure: Results of the organized program to initiate lifesaving treatment in hospitalized patients heart failure (OPTIMIZE-HF). *Arch. Intern. Med.* **2007**, *167*, 1493–1502. [CrossRef]
6. Reza, N.; Nayak, A.; Lewsey, S.C.; De Filippis, E.M. Representation matters: A call for inclusivity and equity in heart failure clinical trials. *Eur. Heart J. Suppl.* **2022**, *24* (Suppl. L), L45–L48. [CrossRef]
7. Fonarow, G.C.; Albert, N.M.; Curtis, A.B.; Stough, W.G.; Gheorghiade, M.; Heywood, J.T.; McBride, M.L.; Inge, P.J.; Mehra, M.R.; O'Connor, C.M.; et al. Improving evidence-based care for heart failure in outpatient cardiology practices: Primary results of the Registry to Improve the Use of Evidence-Based Heart Failure Therapies in the Outpatient Setting (IMPROVE HF). *Circulation* **2010**, *122*, 585–596. [CrossRef]
8. DeVore, A.D.; Granger, B.B.; Fonarow, G.C.; Al-Khalidi, H.R.; Albert, N.M.; Lewis, E.F.; Butler, J.; Piña, I.L.; Allen, L.A.; Yancy, C.W.; et al. Effect of a Hospital and Postdischarge Quality Improvement Intervention on Clinical Outcomes and Quality of Care for Patients with Heart Failure With Reduced Ejection Fraction: The CONNECT-HF Randomized Clinical Trial. *JAMA* **2021**, *326*, 314–323. [CrossRef]
9. Heidenreich, P.A.; Fonarow, G.C.; Breathett, K.; Jurgens, C.Y.; Pisani, B.A.; Pozehl, B.J.; Spertus, J.A.; Taylor, K.G.; Thibodeau, J.T.; Yancy, C.W.; et al. 2020 ACC/AHA Clinical Performance and Quality Measures for Adults with Heart Failure: A Report of the American College of Cardiology/American Heart Association Task Force on Performance Measures. *J. Am. Coll. Cardiol.* **2020**, *76*, 2527–2564. [CrossRef]
10. Iyngkaran, P.; Toukhsati, R.S.; Harris, M.; Connors, C.; Kangaharan, N.; Ilton, M.; Nagel, T.; KMoser, D.; Battersby, M. Self-Managing Heart Failure in Remote Australia—Translating Concepts into Clinical Practice. *Curr. Cardiol. Rev.* **2016**, *12*, 270–284. [CrossRef]
11. Reynolds, R.; Dennis, S.; Hasan, I.; Slewa, J.; Chen, W.; Tian, D.; Bobba, S.; Zwar, N. A systematic review of chronic disease management interventions in primary care. *BMC Fam. Pract.* **2018**, *19*, 11. [CrossRef] [PubMed]
12. Toukhsati, S.R.; Jaarsma, T.; Babu, A.S.; Driscoll, A.; Hare, D.L. Self-Care Interventions That Reduce Hospital Readmissions in Patients With Heart Failure; Towards the Identification of Change Agents. *Clin. Med. Insights Cardiol.* **2019**, *13*, 1179546819856855. [CrossRef] [PubMed]
13. Krumholz, H.M.; Currie, P.M.; Riegel, B.; Phillips, C.O.; Peterson, E.D.; Smith, R.; Yancy, C.W.; Faxon, D.P. American Heart Association Disease Management Taxonomy Writing Group. A taxonomy for disease management: A scientific statement from the American Heart Association Disease Management Taxonomy Writing Group. *Circulation* **2006**, *114*, 1432–1445. [CrossRef] [PubMed]
14. Iyngkaran, P.; Hanna, F.; Andrew, S.; Horowitz, J.D.; Battersby, M.; De Courten, M.P. Comparison of short and long forms of the Flinders program of chronic disease SELF-management for participants starting SGLT-2 inhibitors for congestive heart failure (SELFMAN-HF): Protocol for a prospective, observational study. *Front. Med.* **2023**, *10*, 1059735. [CrossRef]

15. Grady, P.A.; Gough, L.L. Self-management: A comprehensive approach to management of chronic conditions. *Am. J. Public Health* **2014**, *104*, e25–e31. [CrossRef]
16. Lin, Y.; Yu, Y.; Zeng, J.; Zhao, X.; Wan, C. Comparing the reliability and validity of the SF-36 and SF-12 in measuring quality of life among adolescents in China: A large sample cross-sectional study. *Health Qual. Life Outcomes.* **2020**, *18*, 360. [CrossRef]
17. Schmittdiel, J.; Mosen, D.M.; Glasgow, R.E.; Hibbard, J.; Remmers, C.; Bellows, J. Patient Assessment of Chronic Illness Care (PACIC) and improved patient-centered outcomes for chronic conditions. *J. Gen. Intern. Med.* **2008**, *23*, 77–80. [CrossRef]
18. Dineen-Griffin, S.; Garcia-Cardenas, V.; Williams, K.; Benrimoj, S.I. Helping patients help themselves: A systematic review of self-management support strategies in primary health care practice. *PLoS ONE* **2019**, *14*, e0220116. [CrossRef]
19. Smith, S.M.; Wallace, E.; O'Dowd, T.; Fortin, M. Interventions for improving outcomes in patients with multimorbidity in primary care and community settings. *Cochrane Database Syst. Rev.* **2021**, CD006560. [CrossRef]
20. Coulter, A.; Entwistle, V.A.; Eccles, A.; Ryan, S.; Shepperd, S.; Perera, R. Personalised care planning for adults with chronic or long-term health conditions. *Cochrane Database Syst. Rev.* **2015**, *3*, CD010523. [CrossRef]
21. The Flinders Program Evidence Summary. Available online: https://www.flindersprogram.com.au/wp-content/uploads/Flinders-Program-Evidence-Summary.pdf (accessed on 1 October 2022).
22. Iyngkaran, P.; Majoni, V.; Nadarajan, K.; Haste, M.; Battersby, M.; Ilton, M.; Harris, M. AUStralian Indigenous Chronic Disease Optimisation Study (AUSI-CDS) prospective observational cohort study to determine if an established chronic disease health care model can be used to deliver better heart failure care among remote Indigenous Australians: Proof of concept-study rationale and protocol. *Heart Lung Circ.* **2013**, *22*, 930–939. [PubMed]
23. O'Connell, S.; Mc Carthy, V.J.C.; Savage, E. Frameworks for self-management support for chronic disease: A cross-country comparative document analysis. *BMC Health Serv. Res.* **2018**, *18*, 583. [CrossRef] [PubMed]
24. Rolstad, S.; Adler, J.; Ryden, A. Response Burden and Questionnaire Length: Is Shorter Better? A Review and Meta-analysis. *Value Health* **2011**, *14*, 1101–1108. [CrossRef] [PubMed]
25. Sandhu, A.T.; Zheng, J.; Kalwani, N.M.; Gupta, A.; Calma, J.; Skye, M.; Lan, R.; Yu, B.; Spertus, J.A.; Heidenreich, P.A. Impact of Patient-Reported Outcome Measurement in Heart Failure Clinic on Clinician Health Status Assessment and Patient Experience: A Substudy of the PRO-HF Trial. *Circ. Heart Fail.* **2023**, *16*, e010280. [CrossRef] [PubMed] [PubMed Central]
26. Higgins, R.; Murphy, B.; Worcester, M.; Daffey, A. Supporting chronic disease self-management: Translating policies and principles into clinical practice. *Aust. J. Prim. Health.* **2012**, *18*, 80–87. [CrossRef]
27. Available online: https://www.mdcalc.com/calc/3917/charlson-comorbidity-index-cci# (accessed on 1 October 2022).
28. Available online: https://orthotoolkit.com/sf-12/ (accessed on 1 October 2022).
29. Kroenke, K.; Spitzer, R.L.; Williams, J.B. The PHQ-9: Validity of a brief depression severity measure. *J. Gen. Intern. Med.* **2001**, *16*, 606–613. [CrossRef]
30. Soh, S.E.; Morello, R.; Ayton, D.; Ahern, S.; Scarborough, R.; Zammit, C.; Brand, M.; Stirling, R.G.; Zalcberg, J. Measurement properties of the 12-item Short Form Health Survey version 2 in Australians with lung cancer: A Rasch analysis. *Health Qual Life Outcomes* **2021**, *19*, 157. [CrossRef]
31. Charlson, M.E.; Pompei, P.; Ales, K.L.; MacKenzie, C.R. A new methoRed of classifying prognostic comorbidity in longitudinal studies: Development and validation. *J. Chronic Dis.* **1987**, *40*, 373–383. [CrossRef]
32. Chen, Y.; Lu, M.; Jia, L. Psychometric properties of self-reported measures of self-management for chronic heart failure patients: A systematic review. *Eur. J. Cardiovasc. Nurs.* **2023**, *22*, 758–764. [CrossRef]
33. Cameron, J.; Worrall-Carter, L.; Driscoll, A.; Stewart, S. Measuring self-care in chronic heart failure: A review of the psychometric properties of clinical instruments. *J. Cardiovasc. Nurs.* **2009**, *24*, E10–E22. [CrossRef]
34. Vaughan Dickson, V.; Lee, C.S.; Yehle, K.S.; Mola, A.; Faulkner, K.M.; Riegel, B. Psychometric Testing of the Self-Care of Coronary Heart Disease Inventory (SC-CHDI). *Res. Nurs. Health* **2017**, *40*, 15–22. [CrossRef] [PubMed]
35. Wang, X.; Jiang, Y.; Kang, X.; Ji, S.; Zhang, J. Reliability and Validity of the Chinese Version of the Partners in Health Scale in Patients with Chronic Heart Failure Chinese General. *Practice* **2022**, *25*, 497–504.
36. Iyngkaran, P.; McLachlan, C.; Battersby, M.; De Courten, M.; Smith, D.; Hanna, F. Clinical Audit—Validation of Psychometric Properties of The Partners in Health Scale in Heart Failure. *J. Clin. Med.* **2024**. in review.
37. Yu, D.S.; Qiu, C.; Li, P.W.C.; Lau, J.; Riegel, B. Effects of dyadic care interventions for heart failure on patients' and caregivers' outcomes: A systematic review, meta-analysis and meta-regression. *Int. J. Nurs. Stud.* **2024**, *157*, 104829. [CrossRef] [PubMed]
38. Grassi, M.; Nucera, A.; Zanolin, E.; Omenaas, E.; Anto, J.M.; Leynaert, B. European Community Respiratory Health Study Quality of Life Working Group. Performance comparison of Likert and binary formats of SF-36 version 1.6 across ECRHS II adults populations. *Value Health.* **2007**, *10*, 478–488. [CrossRef] [PubMed]
39. Ferreira, J.P. Health-related quality of life scores: Ending the minimum 5-point difference as the clinically meaningful threshold. *Eur. J. Heart Fail.* **2020**, *22*, 1006–1008. [CrossRef] [PubMed]
40. Trevethan, R. Sensitivity, Specificity, and Predictive Values: Foundations, Pliabilities, and Pitfalls in Research and Practice. *Front. Public Health* **2017**, *5*, 307. [CrossRef]
41. Iyngkaran, P.; Usmani, W.; Hanna, F.; de Courten, M. Challenges of Health Data Use in Multidisciplinary Chronic Disease Care: Perspective from Heart Failure Care. *J. Cardiovasc. Dev. Dis.* **2023**, *10*, 486. [CrossRef]

42. Lawson, C.; Crothers, H.; Remsing, S.; Squire, I.; Zaccardi, F.; Davies, M.; Bernhardt, L.; Reeves, K.; Lilford, R.; Khunti, K. Trends in 30-day readmissions following hospitalisation for heart failure by sex, socioeconomic status and ethnicity. *eClinicalMedicine* **2021**, *38*, 101008. [CrossRef]
43. Khan, M.S.; Sreenivasan, J.; Lateef, N.; Abougergi, M.S.; Greene, S.J.; Ahmad, T.; Anker, S.D.; Fonarow, G.C.; Butler, J. Trends in 30- and 90-Day Readmission Rates for Heart Failure. *Circ. Heart Fail.* **2021**, *14*, e008335. [CrossRef]
44. Bergethon, K.E.; Ju, C.; DeVore, A.D.; Hardy, N.C.; Fonarow, G.C.; Yancy, C.W.; Heidenreich, P.A.; Bhatt, D.L.; Peterson, E.D.; Hernandez, A.F. Trends in 30-Day Readmission Rates for Patients Hospitalized with Heart Failure: Findings from the Get with The Guidelines-Heart Failure Registry. *Circ. Heart Fail.* **2016**, *9*, e002594. [CrossRef] [PubMed]
45. Chamberlain, R.S.; Sond, J.; Mahendraraj, K.; Lau, C.S.; Siracuse, B.L. Determining 30-day readmission risk for heart failure patients: The Readmission After Heart Failure scale. *Int. J. Gen. Med.* **2018**, *11*, 127–141. [CrossRef] [PubMed]
46. Gracia, E.; Singh, P.; Collins, S.; Chioncel, O.; Pang, P.; Butler, J. The vulnerable phase of heart failure. *Am. J. Ther.* **2018**, *25*, e456–e464. [CrossRef] [PubMed]
47. Greene, S.J.; Fonarow, G.C.; Vaduganathan, M.; Khan, S.S.; Butler, J.; Gheorghiade, M. The vulnerable phase after hospitalization for heart failure. *Nat. Rev. Cardiol.* **2015**, *12*, 220–229. [CrossRef]
48. Allan, L.A.; Stevenson, L.W.; Grady, K.L.; Goldstein, N.E.; Matlock, D.D.; Arnold, R.M.; Cook, N.R.; Felker, G.M.; Francis, G.S.; Hauptman, P.J.; et al. Decision Making in Advanced Heart Failure. A Scientific Statement from the American Heart Association. *Circulation* **2012**, *125*, 1928–1952. [CrossRef]
49. Liljeroos, M.; Kato, N.P.; van der Wal, M.H.; Brons, M.; Luttik, M.L.; van Veldhuisen, D.J.; Strömberg, A.; Jaarsma, T. Trajectory of self-care behaviour in patients with heart failure: The impact on clinical outcomes and influencing factors. *Eur. J. Cardiovasc. Nurs.* **2020**, *19*, 421–432. [CrossRef]

Disclaimer/Publisher's Note: The statements, opinions and data contained in all publications are solely those of the individual author(s) and contributor(s) and not of MDPI and/or the editor(s). MDPI and/or the editor(s) disclaim responsibility for any injury to people or property resulting from any ideas, methods, instructions or products referred to in the content.

MDPI AG
Grosspeteranlage 5
4052 Basel
Switzerland
Tel.: +41 61 683 77 34

Journal of Clinical Medicine Editorial Office
E-mail: jcm@mdpi.com
www.mdpi.com/journal/jcm

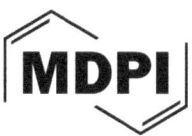

Disclaimer/Publisher's Note: The title and front matter of this reprint are at the discretion of the Guest Editors. The publisher is not responsible for their content or any associated concerns. The statements, opinions and data contained in all individual articles are solely those of the individual Editors and contributors and not of MDPI. MDPI disclaims responsibility for any injury to people or property resulting from any ideas, methods, instructions or products referred to in the content.

www.ingramcontent.com/pod-product-compliance
Lightning Source LLC
LaVergne TN
LVHW072327090526
838202LV00019B/2368